Planning, Implementing, and Evaluating Health Promotion Programs

A Primer

SIXTH EDITION

James F. McKenzie, Ph.D., M.P.H., M.C.H.E.S.
Ball State University
Penn State Hershey

Brad L. Neiger, Ph.D., M.C.H.E.S.
Brigham Young University

Rosemary Thackeray, Ph.D., M.P.H.
Brigham Young University

Boston   Columbus   Indianapolis   New York   San Francisco   Upper Saddle River
Amsterdam   Cape Town   Dubai   London   Madrid   Milan   Munich   Paris   Montréal   Toronto
Delhi   Mexico City   São Paulo   Sydney   Hong Kong   Seoul   Singapore   Taipei   Tokyo

Executive Editor: *Sandra Lindelof*
Project Editor: *Meghan Zolnay*
Editorial Assistant: *Briana Verdugo*
Managing Editor: *Deborah Cogan*
Production Project Manager and Manufacturing Buyer: *Dorothy Cox*
Production Management and Composition: *Jouve*
Interior Design: *Hespenheide Design*
Cover Designer: *Angelyn Navasca/Riezebos Holzbaur Design Group*
Marketing Manager: *Neena Bali*
Text Printer: *RR Donnelley*
Cover Printer: *RR Donnelley*
Cover Photo Credit: © *Color Symphony/Shutterstock*

Credits and acknowledgments borrowed from other sources and reproduced, with permission, in this textbook appear on the appropriate page within the text and on page 493.

Library of Congress Cataloging-in-Publication Data

McKenzie, James F.
   Planning, implementing, and evaluating health promotion programs : a primer / James F. McKenzie, Brad L. Neiger, Rosemary Thackeray. — 6th ed.
      p. ; cm.
   Includes bibliographical references.
   ISBN 978-0-321-78850-4 — ISBN 0-321-78850-8
I. Neiger, Brad L.   II. Thackeray, Rosemary.   III. Title.
   [DNLM: 1. Health Promotion—United States.   2. Health Education—United States.
3. Health Planning—United States.   4. Program Evaluation—United States. WA 590]

   613.0973—dc23

                                                                    2011053408

                                          ISBN-10: 0-321-78850-8
                                          ISBN-13: 978-0-321-78850-4

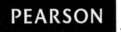

www.pearsonhighered.com   1 2 3 4 5 6 7 8 9 10—RRD—16 15 14 13 12

This book is dedicated to seven special people—
Bonnie, Anne, Greg, Mitchell, Julia, Sherry, and Callie Rose

and to our teachers and mentors—
Marshall H. Becker (deceased), Mary K. Beyer, Noreen Clark, Enrico A. Leopardi, Brad L. Neiger, Lynne Nilson, Terry W. Parsons, Glenn E. Richardson, Irwin M. Rosenstock (deceased), Yuzuru Takeshita, and Doug Vilnius

Contents

Preface

This book is written for students who are enrolled in their first professional course in health promotion program planning. It is designed to help them understand and develop the skills necessary to carry out program planning regardless of the setting. The book is unique among the health promotion planning textbooks on the market in that it provides readers with both theoretical and practical information. A straightforward, step-by-step format is used to make concepts clear and the full process of health promotion planning understandable. This book provides, under a single cover, material on all three areas of program development: planning, implementing, and evaluating.

Learning Aids

Each chapter includes chapter objectives, a list of key terms, presentation of content, chapter summary, review questions, activities, and Weblinks. In addition, many of the key concepts are further explained with information presented in boxes, applications, figures and tables. There is also an Appendix with the *Code of Ethics for the Health Education Profession*, an extensive list of references, and a Glossary.

Chapter Objectives

The chapter objectives identify the content and skills that should be mastered after reading the chapter, answering the review questions, completing the activities, and using the Weblinks. Most of the objectives are written using the cognitive and psychomotor (behavior) educational domains. For most effective use of the objectives, we suggest that they be reviewed before reading the chapter. This will help readers focus on the major points in each chapter and facilitate answering the questions and completing the activities at the end.

Key Terms

Key terms are introduced in each chapter and are important to the understanding of the chapter. The terms are presented in a list at the beginning of each chapter and then are printed in boldface at the appropriate points within the chapter. In addition, all the key terms are presented in the Glossary. Again, as with the chapter objectives, we suggest that readers skim the list before reading the chapter. Then as the chapter is read, particular attention should be paid to the definition of each term.

Presentation of Content

Although each chapter could be expanded—in some cases, entire books have been written on topics we have covered in a chapter or less—we believe that each chapter contains the necessary information to help students understand and develop many of the skills required to be a successful health promotion planner, implementer, and evaluator.

Responsibilities and Competencies Boxes

Within the first few pages of each chapter, readers will find a box that contains the responsibilities and competencies for health education specialists that are applicable to the content of the chapter. The responsibilities and competencies presented in each chapter are the result of the National Health Educator Job Analysis 2010 (HEJA2010) and are published in *A Competency-Based Framework for Health Education Specialists—2010* (NCHEC, SOPHE, & AAHE, 2010). These boxes will help readers understand how the chapter content applies to the various roles and responsibilities assumed by health education specialists. In addition, these boxes should help guide candidates as they prepare to take either the Certified Health Education Specialist (CHES) or Master Certified Health Education Specialist (MCHES) exam.

Chapter Summary

At the end of each chapter, readers will find a one- or two-paragraph review of the major concepts covered in the chapter.

Review Questions

The questions at the end of each chapter provide readers with some feedback regarding their mastery of the content. These questions also reinforce the objectives and key terms presented in each chapter.

Activities

Each chapter includes several activities that allow students to use their new knowledge and skills. The activities are presented in several different formats for the sake of variety and to appeal to the different learning styles of students. It should be noted that, depending on the ones selected for completion, the activities in one chapter can build on those in a previous chapter and lead to the final product of a completely developed health promotion program.

Weblinks

The final portion of each chapter consists of a list of updated links on the World Wide Web. These links encourage students to explore a number of different Websites that are available to support planning, implementing, and evaluating programs.

New to This Edition

In revising this textbook, we incorporated as many suggestions from reviewers, colleagues, and former students as possible. In addition to updating material throughout the text, the following points reflect the major changes in this new edition:

- Chapter 1 includes information about the revised areas of responsibility, competencies, and subcompetencies based on the National Health Educator Job Analysis (NCHEC, SOPHE, & AAHE, 2010). Along with this information is an explanation of the new Master Certified Health Education Specialist (MCHES) credential. In addition, the generalized model is introduced with information on the pre-planning.

- Chapter 2, which was Chapter 3 in the previous edition, has been expanded to include information on return on investment (ROI), social math, and increased coverage of evidence-based practice to help in creating program rationales. In addition, a section has been added on writing problem statements.

- Chapter 3, which was Chapter 2 in the previous edition, has been reorganized and updated. Greater emphasis and explanation has been added on the Generalized Model. Specifically, more information has been provided on pre-planning and how knowledge of this model serves as a foundation for understanding all others. Information is also presented on other key planning models, such as PRECEDE-PROCEED, Mobilizing for Action through Planning and Partnerships (MAPP), MAP-IT, and SMART. The chapter concludes with brief explanations of six planning models including SWOT, Healthy Communities, the Health Communication Model, Intervention Mapping, and Healthy Plan-It.

- Chapter 4 has been expanded with additional information on community capacity, electronic interviews, and photovoice. In addition, the chapter includes new information on the BPR model 2.0 for prioritizing the needs identified through the needs assessment process, and new information on health impact assessment.

- Chapter 5 has been updated and focuses on various aspects of measurement and sampling with enhanced descriptions of the measurement process within the context of planning and evaluation as well as more comprehensive explanations of the levels of measurement used in data collection and analysis.

- Chapter 6 includes new information on methods for setting targets for objectives, *Healthy People 2020* goals and objectives, and MAP-IT: the Action Model to Achieve *Healthy People* Goals.

- Chapter 7 has been expanded and several new theories and models have been added including the protection motivation theory, the information-motivation-behavioral skills model, social capital theory, and social network theory.

- Chapter 8 features new information on health communication strategies including the impact of health literacy and health numeracy, the use of social media, adult learning, health policy, incentives, and GINA. We've also added information on using best practices in the creation of health education interventions.

- Chapter 9 includes additional information on creating community coalitions.

- Chapter 10 has been expanded with more information on personnel-related issues such as technical assistance, volunteers, teamwork, and cultural factors. In addition, the section on preparing and monitoring budgets is presented in greater detail.

- Chapter 11 has been reworked and includes a more thorough description of the process for segmenting priority populations, tips for working with marketing or public relations agencies to develop promotional communications and materials, and a discussion of the six key areas that make the social marketing approach unique to program development. We've also added a new section on pretesting, including new boxes for what questions to ask when pretesting products, messages, and materials, and a new box that compares using focus groups and intercept interviews in pretesting.

- Chapter 12 content now includes information on logic models, more information on managing resources during implementation, and information on working with program participants who have disabilities.

- Chapter 13 has been reworked to help the reader better conceptualize and understand the purposes, sequence, and process of program evaluation. Specifically, we now employ the terminology of formative and summative evaluation as opposed to process and summative. The two basic purposes for evaluation—assessing quality and measuring effectiveness—are clearly labeled and defined, and the CDC framework for program evaluation provides a clear foundation for all evaluation efforts.

- Chapter 14 has been expanded with the elements of a comprehensive formative evaluation, and additional distinctions are drawn between formative and process evaluations.

- Chapter 15 clarifies and more appropriately sequences the elements of evaluation reporting, and guidelines for how to more effectively present data are provided.

- All chapters include more real-life planning examples, and where appropriate new application boxes have been added to chapters.

- A revised test bank has been created for this edition and is available in Microsoft Word and TestGen formats.

- A new *Instructor Manual* has been created for this edition and is available for download.

- Again, as with the previous edition, PowerPoint® presentations are available online.

- The Companion Website (http://www.aw-bc.com/mckenzie) has been updated and includes chapter objectives, practice quizzes, Responsibilities and Competencies boxes, Weblinks, some new example program plans created by former students, the

Glossary and flashcards, and instructor resources (i.e., instructor manual, test bank, and PowerPoint® presentations).

- All electronic instructor resources are available for download on the Pearson Instructor Resource Center. Go to http://www.pearsonhighered.com and search for the title to access and download the PowerPoint® presentations, electronic Instructor Manual and Test Bank, and TestGen Computerized Test Bank. Students will also be able to purchase the ebook version of this text from this page.

Students will find this book easy to understand and use. We are confident that if the chapters are carefully read and an honest effort is put into completing the activities and visiting the Weblinks, students will gain the essential knowledge and skills for program planning, implementation, and evaluation.

Acknowledgments

A project of this nature could not have been completed without the assistance and understanding of many individuals. First, we thank all our past and present students, who have had to put up with our working drafts of the manuscript.

Second, we are grateful to those professionals who took the time and effort to review and comment on various editions of this book. For the first edition, they included Vicki Keanz, Eastern Kentucky University; Susan Cross Lipnickey, Miami University; Fred Pearson, Ricks College; Kerry Redican, Virginia Tech; John Sciacca, Northern Arizona University; and William K. Spath, Montana Tech. For the second edition, reviewers included Gordon James, Weber State; John Sciacca, Northern Arizona University; and Mark Wilson, University of Georgia. For the third edition, reviewers included Joanna Hayden, William Paterson University; Raffy Luquis, Southern Connecticut State University; Teresa Shattuck, University of Maryland; Thomas Syre, James Madison University; and Esther Weekes, Texas Women's University. For the fourth edition, reviewers included Robert G. LaChausse, California State University, San Bernardino; Julie Shepard, Director of Health Promotion, Adams County Health Department; Sherm Sowby, California State University, Fresno; and William Kane, University of New Mexico. For the fifth edition, the reviewers included Sally Black, St. Joseph's University; Denise Colaianni, Western Connecticut State University; Sue Forster-Cox, New Mexico State University; Julie Gast, Utah State University; Ray Manes, York College CUNY; and Lois Ritter, California State University East Bay. For this edition, reviewers included Jacquie Rainey, University of Central Arkansas; Bridget Melton, Georgia Southern University; Marylen Rimando, University of Iowa; Beth Orsega-Smith, University of Delaware; Aimee Richardson, American University; Heather Diaz, California State University, Sacramento; Steve McKenzie, Purdue University; Aly Williams, Indiana Wesleyan University; Jennifer Banas, Northeastern Illinois University; and Heidi Fowler, Georgia College and State University.

Third, we thank our friends for providing valuable feedback on various editions of this book: Robert J. Yonker, Ph.D., Professor Emeritus in the Department of Educational Foundations and Inquiry, Bowling Green State University; Lawrence W. Green, Dr. P. H., Adjunct Professor, Department of Epidemiology and Biostatistics, University of California,

San Francisco (UCSF), and UCSF Comprehensive Cancer Center; Bruce Simons-Morton, Ed.D., M.P.H., Senior Investigator, Prevention Research Branch, National Institute of Child Health and Human Development, National Institutes of Health; and Jerome E. Kotecki, H.S.D., Professor, Department of Physiology and Health Science, Ball State University. We would also like to thank Jan L. Smeltzer, Ph.D., coauthor, for her contributions to the first four editions of the book.

Fourth, we appreciate the work of the Benjamin Cummings employees Sandra Lindelof, acquisitions editor for health and kinesiology, who has always been very supportive of our work, and Meghan Zolnay, developmental editor, whose hard work and encouragement ensured we created a quality product. We also appreciate the careful work of Jouve North America and Jouve India.

Finally, we express our deepest appreciation to our families for their support, encouragement, and understanding of the time that writing takes away from our family activities.

J. F. M.
B. L. N.
R. T.

Health Education, Health Promotion, Health Education Specialists, and Program Planning

CHAPTER OBJECTIVES

After reading this chapter and answering the questions at the end, you should be able to:

- Explain the relationship among good health behavior, health education, and health promotion.
- Explain the difference between health education and health promotion.
- Write your own definition of health education.
- Explain the role of the health educator as defined by the Role Delineation Project.
- Explain how a person becomes a Certified Health Education Specialist or a Master Certified Health Education Specialist.
- Explain how the Competency-Based Framework for Health Education Specialist is used by colleges and universities, the National Commission for Health Education Credentialing, Inc. (NCHEC), the National Council for the Accreditation of Teacher Education (NCATE), and the SOPHE/AAHE Baccalaureate Program Approval Committee (SABPAC).
- Identify the assumptions upon which health education is based.
- Define the term *pre-planning*.

KEY TERMS

advanced-level 1 health
   educator
advanced-level 2 health
   educator
decision makers
entry-level health educator
Framework

health behavior
health education
health education specialist
health educator
health promotion
Healthy People
pre-planning

primary prevention
priority population
Role Delineation Project
secondary prevention
stakeholders
tertiary prevention

History has shown that much progress was made in the health and life expectancy of Americans in the twentieth century. Since 1900, we have seen a sharp drop in infant mortality (Miniño, Xu, & Kochanek, 2010); the eradication of smallpox; the elimination of poliomyelitis in the Americas; the control of measles, rubella, tetanus, diphtheria, Haemophilus influenzae type b, and other infectious diseases; better family planning (CDC, 1999b); and an increase of 29.5 years in the average life span of a person in the United States (NCHS, 2011). Over this same time, we have witnessed disease prevention change "from focusing on reducing environmental exposures over which the individual had little control, such as providing potable water, to emphasizing behaviors such as avoiding use of tobacco, fatty foods, and a sedentary lifestyle" (Breslow, 1999, p. 1030). Yet, even with this change in focus most Americans have not changed their lifestyle enough to reduce their risk of illness, disability, and premature death. As a result, unhealthy lifestyle characteristics have lead to the United States ranking 89th (out of 225 countries) in crude death rate and 50th (out of 223 countries) in life expectancy (CIA, 2011).

Today in the United States, much of the death and disability of Americans is associated with chronic diseases. Seven out of every 10 deaths among Americans each year are from chronic diseases, while heart disease, cancer, and stroke account for more than 50% of deaths each year (CDC, 2009a). In addition, more than 75% of all health care spending in the United States is on people with chronic conditions (Anderson, 2004). Chronic diseases are not only the most common, deadly, and costly, they are also the most preventable of all health problems in the United States (NCCDPHP, 2009). They are the most preventable because "four modifiable risk behaviors—lack of physical activity, poor nutrition, tobacco use, and excessive alcohol consumption—are responsible for much of the illness, suffering, and early death related to chronic diseases" (NCCDPHP, 2009, p. 5) (see **Table 1.1**). In fact, one study estimates that all causes of mortality could be cut by 55% by never smoking, engaging in regular physical activity, eating a healthy diet, and avoiding being overweight (van Dam, Li, Spiegelman, Franco, & Hu, 2008).

Table 1.1   Comparison of Most Common Causes of Death and Actual Causes of Death

Most Common Causes of Death, United States, 2008*	Actual Causes of Death, United States, 2000**
1. Diseases of the heart	1. Tobacco
2. Malignant neoplasms (cancers)	2. Poor diet and physical inactivity
3. Chronic lower respiratory diseases	3. Alcohol consumption
4. Cerebrovascular diseases (stroke)	4. Microbial agents
5. Accidents (unintentional injuries)	5. Toxic agents
6. Alzheimer's disease	6. Motor vehicles
7. Diabetes mellitus	7. Firearms
8. Influenza and pneumonia	8. Sexual behavior
9. Nephritis, nephrotic syndrome, and nephrosis	9. Illicit drug use
10. Septicemia	

*Miniño, Xu, & Kochanek (2010).
**Mokdad, Marks, Stroup, & Greberding (2004, 2005).

But modifying risk behaviors does not come easy to Americans. One study (Reeves & Rafferty, 2005) has shown that only 3% of U.S. adults adhere to four healthy lifestyle characteristics (not smoking, engaging in regular physical activity, maintaining a healthy weight, and eating five fruits and vegetables a day). If moderate alcohol use were included in the healthy lifestyle characteristics the percentage would be even lower (King, Mainous, Carnemolla, & Everett, 2009). Now in the second decade of the twenty-first century, behavior patterns continue to "represent the single most prominent domain of influence over health prospects in the United States" (McGinnis, Williams-Russo, & Knickman, 2002, p. 82).

Though the focus on good health, wellness, and **health behavior** (those behaviors that impact a person's health) seem commonplace in our lives today, it was not until the last fourth of the twentieth century that health promotion was recognized for its potential to help control injury and disease and to promote health.

> Most scholars, policymakers, and practitioners in health promotion would pick 1974 as the turning point that marks the beginning of health promotion as a significant component of national health policy in the twentieth century. That year Canada published its landmark policy statement, *A New Perspective on the Health of Canadians* (Lalonde, 1974). In the United States, Congress passed PL 94-317, the Health Information and Health Promotion Act, which created the Office of Health Information and Health Promotion, later renamed the Office of Disease Prevention and Health Promotion (Green 1999, p. 69).

This paved the way for the U.S. government's *Healthy People: The Surgeon General's Report on Health Promotion and Disease Prevention* (USDHEW, 1979), which brought together much of what was known about the relationship of personal behavior and health status. The document also presented a "personal responsibility" model that provided Americans with a prescription for reducing their health risks and increasing their chances for good health.

It may not have been the content of *Healthy People* that made the publication so significant, because several publications written before it provided a similar message. Rather, *Healthy People* was important because it summarized the research available up to that point, presented it in a very readable format, and made the information available to the general public. *Healthy People* was followed by the release of the first set of health goals and objectives for the nation, titled *Promoting Health/Preventing Disease: Objectives for the Nation* (USDHHS, 1980). These goals and objectives, now in their fourth generation (USDHHS, 2010a), have defined the nation's health agenda and guided its health policy since their inception. And, in part, they have kept the importance of good health visible to all Americans.

This focus on good health has given many people in the United States a desire to do something about their health. This desire, in turn, has increased the need for good health information that can be easily understood by the average person. One need only look at the current best-seller list, read the daily newspaper, observe the health advertisements delivered via the electronic mass media, or consider the increase in the number of health-promoting facilities (not illness or sickness facilities) to verify the interest that American consumers have in health. Because of the increased interest in health and changing health behavior, health professionals are now faced with providing the public with the information. However, obtaining good information does not mean that those who receive it will make healthy decisions and then act on those decisions. Good health education and health promotion programs are needed to assist people in reducing their health risks in order to obtain and maintain good health.

Health Education and Health Promotion

There is more to health education than simply disseminating health information (Auld et al., 2011). Health education is a much more involved process. Two formal definitions of health education have been frequently cited in the literature. The first comes from the *Report of the 2011 Joint Committee on Health Education and Promotion Terminology* (Joint Committee on Terminology, 2012). The committee defined **health education** as "[a]ny combination of planned learning experiences using evidence-based practices and/ or sound theories that provide the opportunity to acquire knowledge, attitudes, and skills needed to adopt and maintain healthy behaviors" (Joint Committee on Terminology, 2012). The second definition was presented by Green and Kreuter (2005), who defined health education as "any planned combination of learning experiences designed to predispose, enable, and reinforce voluntary behavior conducive to health in individuals, groups, or communities" (p. G-4).

Another term that is closely related to health education, and sometimes incorrectly used in its place, is health promotion. *Health promotion* is a broader term than *health education*. The Joint Committee on Terminology (2012) defined **health promotion** as "[a]ny planned combination of educational, political, environmental, regulatory, or organizational mechanisms that support actions and conditions of living conducive to the health of individuals, groups, and communities." Green and Kreuter (2005) offered a slightly different definition of *health promotion*, calling it "any planned combination of educational, political, regulatory and organizational supports for actions and conditions of living conducive to the health of individuals, groups, and communities" (p. G-4).

To help us further understand and operationalize the term *health promotion*, Breslow (1999) has stated, "Each person has a certain degree of health that may be expressed as a place in a spectrum. From that perspective, promoting health must focus on enhancing people's capacities for living. That means moving them toward the health end of the spectrum, just as prevention is aimed at avoiding disease that can move people toward the opposite end of the spectrum" (p. 1031). According to these definitions of health promotion, health education is an important component of health promotion and firmly implanted in it (see **Figure 1.1**). "Health promotion takes into account that human behavior is not only governed by personal factors (e.g., knowledge, expectancies, competencies, and well-being), but also by structural aspects of the environment" (Vogele, 2005, p. 272). However, "without health education, health promotion would be a manipulative social engineering enterprise" (Green & Kreuter, 1999, p. 19).

The effectiveness of health promotion programs can vary greatly. However, the success of a program can usually be linked to the planning that takes place before implementation of the program. Programs that have undergone a thorough planning process are usually the most successful. As the old saying goes, "If you fail to plan, your plan will fail."

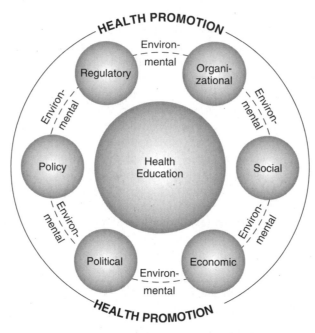

Figure 1.1 Relationship of Health Education and Health Promotion

Health Education Specialists

The individuals best qualified to plan health promotion programs are health educators. A **health educator** is a "professionally prepared individual who serves in a variety of roles and is specifically trained to use appropriate educational strategies and methods to facilitate the development of policies, procedures, interventions, and systems conducive to the health of individuals, groups, and communities" (Joint Committee on Terminology, 2001, p. 100). Based on the results of a marketing study conducted by Hezel Associates (2007) for five health education profession member organizations and the National Commission for Health Education Credentialing, Inc. (NCHEC) (Gambescia et al., 2009), it has been recommended that the profession de-emphasize the term *health educator* and use the term *health education specialist* in its place. A **health education specialist** has been defined as "[a]n individual who has met, at a minimum, baccalaureate-level required health education academic preparation qualifications, who serves in a variety of settings, and is able to use appropriate educational strategies and methods to facilitate the development of policies, procedures, interventions, and systems conducive to the health of individuals, groups, and communities" (Joint Committee on Terminology, 2012). Therefore, throughout the remainder of this book the term *health education specialist* will be used except when the term *health educator* is a part of a title or when the term carries historical relevance. Today, health education specialists can be found working in a variety of settings, including schools (K–12, colleges, and universities), community health agencies (governmental and nongovernmental), worksites (business, industry, and other work settings), and health care settings (e.g., clinics, hospitals, and managed care organizations).

The role of the health education specialist in the United States as we know it today is one that has evolved over time based on the need to provide people with educational interventions to enhance their health. The earliest signs of the role of the health education specialist appeared in the mid-1800s with school hygiene education, which was closely associated with physical activity. By the early 1900s, the need for health education spread to the public health arena, but it was the writers, journalists, social workers, and visiting nurses who were doing the educating—not health education specialists as we know them today (Deeds, 1992). As we gained more knowledge about the relationship between health, disease, and health behavior, it was obvious that the writers, journalists, social workers, visiting nurses, and primary caregivers—mainly physicians, dentists, other independent practitioners, and nurses—were unable to provide the needed health education. The combination of the heavy workload of the primary caregivers, the lack of formal training in the process of educating others, and the need for education at all levels of prevention—primary, secondary, and tertiary—(see **Figure 1.2**) created a need for health education specialists.

As the role of the health education specialist grew over the years, there was a movement by those in the discipline to clearly define their role so that people inside and

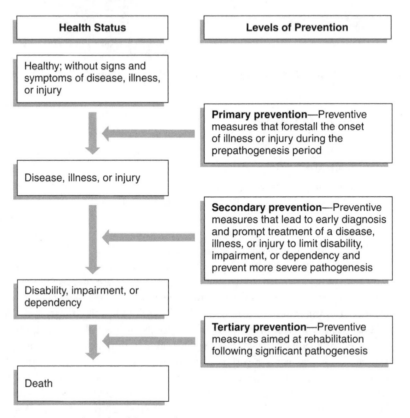

Figure 1.2 Levels of Prevention

Source: Public Health: Administration and Practice. George E. Pickett and John J. Hanlon. Copyright © 1990 by McGraw Hill Education. Adapted with permission.

outside the profession would have a better understanding of what the health education specialist did. In January 1979, the **Role Delineation Project** began (National Task Force on the Preparation and Practice of Health Educators, 1985). Through a comprehensive process, this project yielded a generic role for the **entry-level health educator**—that is, responsibilities for health education specialists taking their first job regardless of their work setting. Once the role of the entry-level health educator was delineated, the task became to translate the role into a structure that professional preparation programs in health education could use to design competency-based curricula. The resulting document, *A Framework for the Development of Competency-Based Curricula for Entry Level Health Educators* (NCHEC, 1985), and its revised version, *A Competency-Based Framework for the Professional Development of Certified Health Education Specialists* (NCHEC, 1996), provided such a structure. These documents, simply referred to as the *Framework* were comprised of the seven major areas of responsibility, which defined the scope of practice, and several different competencies and subcompetencies, which further delineated the responsibilities.

Even though the seven areas of responsibility defined the role of the entry-level health educator, they did not fully express the work of the health education specialist with an advanced degree. Thus, over a four-year period beginning in 1992, the profession worked to define the role of an advanced-level practitioner. By July 1997, the governing boards of the National Commission for Health Education Credentialing, Inc. (NCHEC), the American Association of Health Education (AAHE), and the Society for Public Health Education (SOPHE) had endorsed three additional responsibilities for the advanced-level health educator. Those responsibilities revolved around research, administration, and the advancement of the profession (AAHE, NCHEC, & SOPHE, 1999).

The seven entry-level and three additional advanced-level responsibilities served the profession well, but during the mid- to late-1990s it became obvious that there was a need to revisit the responsibilities and competencies and to make sure that they still defined the role of the health educator. Thus in 1998, the profession launched a six-year multiphase research study known as the *National Health Educator Competencies Update Project* (CUP) to reverify the entry-level health educator responsibilities, competencies, and subcompetencies and to verify the advanced-level competencies and subcompetencies (Airhihenbuwa et al., 2005).

What became obvious from the analysis of the CUP data was that the seven responsibilities and many of the competencies and subcompetencies identified in the earlier Role Delineation Project were still valid. However, the wording of the responsibilities was changed slightly, some competencies and subcompetencies were dropped, and a few new ones were added. Also, certain subcompetencies were reported as more important and performed more regularly by health education specialists who had both more work experience and academic degrees beyond the baccalaureate level. Thus, the CUP model that emerged included responsibilities, competencies, and subcompetencies and the development of a three-tiered (i.e., **Entry, Advanced-Level 1**, and **Advanced-Level 2**) hierarchical model reflecting the role of the health education specialist (see **Table 1.2** for levels of practice). The results of the CUP, which were published approximately 20 years after the initial role delineation project, lead to the creation of a revised framework titled *A Competency-Based Framework for Health Educators* (NCHEC, SOPHE, & AAHE, 2006).

Table 1.2   CUP Model Hierarchical Approach

Level of Practice	Competencies/Subcompetencies
Entry (less than 5 years of experience; baccalaureate or master's degree)	Entry
Advanced 1 (5 or more years of experience; baccalaureate or master's degree)	Entry + Advanced 1
Advanced 2 (doctorate and 5 or more years of experience)	Entry + Advanced 1 + Advanced 2

Source: "Overview of the National Health Educator Competencies Update Project, 1998–2004." Gary David Gilmore, Larry K. Olsen, Alyson Taub, David Connell from *Health Education & Behavior, 32*(6), pp. 725–737. Copyright © 2005 by SAGE Publications. Reprinted with Permission.

The most recent edition of the *framework* titled *A Competency-Based Framework for Health Education Specialist–2010* (NCHEC, SOPHE, AAHE, 2010) is the result of the National Health Educator Job Analysis (HEJA-2010). Like the CUP before it, HEJA-2010 was undertaken "to validate the contemporary practice of entry- and advanced-level health education specialists" (NCHEC, SOPHE, & AAHE, 2010, p. 10). However, unlike the CUP, HEJA-2010 was undertaken after a much shorter gap of time (i.e., 5 versus 20 years) than the previous validation study. This shorter gap in time was necessary, in part, to meet the best practice accreditation standards of the National Commission for Certifying Agencies (NCCA) (NCHEC, SOPHE, & AAHE, 2010). It is NCCA that accredits the entry-level credential (i.e., Certified Health Education Specialist [CHES]) of National Commission for Health Education Credentialing, Inc. (NCHEC).

Over the years, the Areas of Responsibility outlined in the *Framework* have remained fairly consistent (see **Table 1.3** for a comparison of the Responsibilities from 1995 to 2010). What has changed over the years is the number and wording of the competencies and subcompetencies found under the Areas of Responsibility. In the 2010 *Framework*, there are 34 competencies and 223 subcompetencies (162 Entry-level and 61 Advanced-level) (NCHEC, SOPHE, & AAHE, 2010).

In reviewing the current seven areas of responsibility, it is obvious that four of the seven are directly related to program planning, implementation, and evaluation and that the other three could be associated with these processes, depending on the type of program being planned. In effect, these responsibilities distinguish health education specialists from other professionals who try to provide health education experiences.

The importance of the defined role of the health education specialist is becoming greater as the profession of health promotion continues to mature. This is exhibited by its use in several major professional activities. First, the *Framework* has provided a guide for all colleges and universities to use when designing and revising their curricula in health education to prepare future health education specialists. Second, the *Framework* was used by the National Commission for Health Education Credentialing, Inc. (NCHEC) to develop the core criteria for certifying individuals as health education specialists (Certified Health Education Specialists, or CHES). The first group of individuals (N=1,558) to receive the CHES credential did so between October 1988 and December 1989, during the charter certification period. "Charter certification allows qualified individuals to be certified based

Table 1.3   Comparison of Areas of Responsibility (1985–2010)

Entry-Level Framework (1985)	Graduate-Level Framework (1999)	CUP Model (2006)	HEJA Model (2010)
I. Assessing individual and community needs for health education	I. Assessing individual and community needs for health education	I. Assess individual and community needs for health education	I. Assess needs, assets, and capacity for health education
II. Planning effective health education programs	II. Planning effective health education programs	II. Plan health education strategies, interventions, and programs	II. Plan health education
III. Implementing health education programs	III. Implementing health education programs	III. Implement health education strategies, interventions, and programs	III. Implement health education
IV. Evaluating effectiveness of health education programs	IV. Evaluating effectiveness of health education programs	IV. Conduct evaluation and research related to health education	IV. Conduct evaluation and research related to health education
V. Coordinating provision of health education services	V. Coordinating provision of health education services	V. Administer health education strategies, interventions, and programs	V. Administer and manage health education
VI. Acting as a resource person in health education	VI. Acting as a resource person in health education	VI. Serve as a health education resource person	VI. Serve as a health education resource person
VII. Communicating health and health education needs, concerns, and resources	VII. Communicating health and health education needs, concerns, and resources	VII. Communicate and advocate for health and health education	VII. Communicate and advocate for health and health education
	VIII. Applying appropriate research principles and techniques in health education		
	IX. Administering health education programs		
	X. Advancing the profession of health education		

Source: "Overview of the National Health Educator Competencies Update Project, 1998–2004" by Gary David Gilmore, Larry K. Olsen, Alyson Taub, David Connell from *Health Education & Behavior, 32*(6), pp. 725–737 as adapted in *A Competency-Based Framework for Health Education Specialists, 2010*, p. 61. Copyright © 2005 by SAGE Publications. Reprinted with Permission.

on their academic training, work experience, and references without taking the exam" (Cottrell, Girvan, & McKenzie, 2012, p. 178). In 1990, using a criterion-referenced examination based on the *Framework*, the nationwide testing program to certify health education specialists was begun by NCHEC, Inc.

In 2011, again using a criterion-referenced examination based on the *Framework*, NCHEC began offering an examination to certify advanced-level health education specialists. Those who passed the examination were awarded the Master Certified Health Education Specialist (MCHES) credential. Prior to the first MCHES examination, this new certification was made available to those who had held active CHES status since 2005 and who could demonstrate that they were practicing health education at an advanced-level. This process was known as the Experience Documentation Opportunity (EDO). All those who successfully completed the EDO were granted the MCHES credential in April 2011. Currently, both the CHES and MCHES examinations are given twice a year—once in April and once in October—at approximately 120 college-campus locations around the United States. Both examinations are composed of 165 questions (150 are scored and 15 are pilot questions) and are offered in a paper-and-pencil format (NCHEC, 2011). Information about eligibility for the examinations and the percentage of questions from each Area of Responsibility are available on the NCHEC Website (see the link for the Website in the Weblinks section at the end of the chapter).

Third, the *Framework* is used by program accrediting and approval bodies to review college and university academic programs in health education. The National Council for the Accreditation of Teacher Education (NCATE) uses the *Framework* to review and accredit teacher preparation programs in health education at institutions of higher education. Also, a joint committee of the Society for Public Health Education, Inc. (SOPHE) and the American Association for Health Education, known as the SOPHE/AAHE Baccalaureate Program Approval Committee (SABPAC), uses the *Framework* to review and approve undergraduate community health education programs via self-study and external reviewers.

The use of the *Framework* by the profession to guide academic curricula, provide the core criteria for the health education specialist examinations, and form the basis of program approval processes has done much to advance the health education profession. "In 1998 the U.S. Department of Commerce and Labor formally acknowledged 'health educator' as a distinct occupation. Such recognition was justified, based to a large extent, on the ability of the profession to specify its unique skills" (AAHE, NCHEC, & SOPHE, 1999, p. 9). In 2010, the U.S. Department of Labor Bureau of Labor Statistics (BLS) described the work of health educators (Standard Occupation Classification [SOC] 21-1091) using the following language:

> Provide and manage health education programs that help individuals, families, and their communities maximize and maintain healthy lifestyles. Collect and analyze data to identify community needs prior to planning, implementing, monitoring, and evaluating programs designed to encourage healthy lifestyles, policies, and environments. May serve as resource to assist individuals, other health professionals, or the community, and may administer fiscal resources for health education programs (USDL, BLS, 2010).

Assumptions of Health Promotion

So far, we have discussed the need for health, what health education and health promotion are, and the role health education specialists play in delivering successful health promotion programs. We have not yet discussed the assumptions that underlie health promotion—all the things that must be in place before the whole process of health promotion begins.

In the mid-1980s, Bates and Winder (1984) outlined what they saw as four critical assumptions of health education. Their list has been modified by adding several items, rewording others, and referring to them as "assumptions of health promotion." This expanded list of assumptions is critical to understanding what we can expect from health promotion programs. Health promotion is by no means the sole answer to the nation's health problems or, for that matter, the sole means of getting a smoker to stop smoking or a nonexerciser to exercise. Health promotion is an important part of the health system, but it does have limitations. Here are the assumptions:

1. Health status can be changed.

2. "Health and disease are determined by dynamic interactions among biological, psychological, behavioral, and social factors" (Pellmar, Brandt, & Baird, 2002, p. 217).

3. Disease occurrence theories and principles can be understood (Bates & Winder, 1984).

4. Appropriate prevention strategies can be developed to deal with the identified health problems (Bates & Winder, 1984).

5. "Behavior can be changed and those changes can influence health" (Pellmar et al., 2002, p. 213).

6. "Individual behavior, family interactions, community and workplace relationships and resources, and public policy all contribute to health and influence behavior change" (Pellmar et al., 2002, p. 217).

7. "Initiating and maintaining a behavior change is difficult" (Pellmar et al., 2002, p. 217).

8. Individual responsibility should not be viewed as victim blaming, yet the importance of health behavior to health status must be understood.

9. For health behavior change to be permanent, an individual must be motivated and ready to change.

The importance of these assumptions is made clearer if we refer to the definitions of health education and health promotion presented earlier in the chapter. Implicit in those definitions is the goal of having program participants voluntarily adopt actions conducive to health. To achieve such a goal, the assumptions must indeed be in place. We cannot expect people to adopt lifelong health-enhancing behavior if we force them into such change. Nor can we expect people to change their behavior just because they have been exposed to a health promotion program. Health behavior change is very complex, and health education specialists should not expect to change every person with whom they come in contact. However, the greatest chance for success will come to those who have the knowledge and skills to plan, implement, and evaluate appropriate programs.

Program Planning

Because many of health education specialists' responsibilities are involved in some way with program planning, implementation, and evaluation, health education specialists need to become well versed in these processes. "Planning an effective program is more difficult than implementing it. Planning, implementing, and evaluating programs are all interrelated, but good planning skills are prerequisite to programs worthy of evaluation" (Minelli & Breckon, 2009, p. 137). All three processes are very involved, and much time, effort, practice, and on-the-job training are required to do them well. Even the most experienced health education specialists find program planning challenging because of the constant changes in settings, resources, and priority populations.

Hunnicutt (2007a) offered four reasons why systematic planning is important. The first is that planning forces planners to think through details in advance. Detail plans can help to avoid future problems. Second, planning helps to make a program transparent. Good planning keeps the program **stakeholders** (any person or organization with a vested interest in a program; e.g., decision makers, partners, clients) informed. The planning process should not be mysterious or secretive. Third, planning is empowering. Once **decision makers** (those who have the authority to approve a plan; e.g., administrator of an organization, governing board, chief executive officer) give approval to the resulting comprehensive program plan, planners and facilitators are empowered to implement the program. Without an approved plan, planners will spend a great deal of time waiting for the "next step" to be approved and risk losing program momentum. And fourth, planning creates alignment. Once the decision makers have approved the program, all organization members have a better understanding of where it "fits" in the organization and the importance that the plan carries.

A general understanding of all that is involved in creating a health promotion program can be obtained by reviewing the Generalized Model (see **Figure 1.3**). (Also see a more in-depth explanation of this model in Chapter 3.) This model includes the five major steps involved in planning a program. However, prior to undertaking the first step in the Generalized Model, it is important to do some pre-planning. **Pre-planning** allows a core group of people (or steering committee) to gather answers to key questions (see **Table 1.4**) that are critical to the planning process before the actual planning process begins. It also helps to clarify and give direction to planning, and helps stakeholders avoid confusion as the planning progresses.

Also prior to starting the actual planning process, planners need to have a very good understanding of the community where the program will be implemented. Understanding the community means finding out as much as possible about the **priority population** (those for whom the program is intended to serve) and the environment in which it exists. Each setting and group is unique with its own nuances, resources, and culture. These are important to know at the beginning of the process. Planners should never assume they "know" a community. The more background information that planners secure, the better the resulting program can be. However, it is not enough to understand the community,

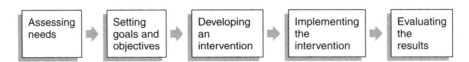

Figure 1.3 Generalized Model

Table 1.4   Example Key Questions to Be Answered in the Pre-Planning Process

Purpose of program
- How is the community defined?
- What are the desired health outcomes?
- Does the community have the capacity and infrastructure to address the problem?
- Is a policy change needed?

Scope of the planning process
- Is it intra- or inter-organizational?
- What is the time frame for completing the project?

Planning process outcomes (deliverables)
- Written plan?
- Program proposal?
- Program documentation or justification?

Leadership and structure
- What authority, if any, will the planners have?
- How will the planners be organized?
- What is expected of those who participate in the planning process?

Identifying and engaging partners
- How will the partners be selected?
- Will the planning process use a top-down or bottom-up approach?

Identifying and securing resources
- How will the budget be determined?
- Will a written agreement (i.e., MOA—memorandum of agreement) outlining responsibilities be needed?
- If MOA is needed, what will it include?
- Will external funding (i.e., grants or contracts) be needed?
- Are there community resources (e.g., volunteers, space, donations) to support the planned program?
- How will the resources be obtained?

planners also need to engage members of the priority population. Engaging the priority population means involving those in the priority population or a representative group from the priority population in the planning process.

Finally, before the actual planning begins thought must be given to "when the best time is to plan such a program, what data are needed, where the planning should occur, what resistance can be expected, and generally, what will enhance the success of the project" (Minelli & Breckon, 2009, p. 138).

The remaining chapters of this book present a process that health education specialists can use to plan, implement, and evaluate successful health promotion programs and will introduce you to the necessary knowledge and skills to carry out these tasks.

SUMMARY

The increased interest in personal health, behavior change, and the flood of new health information have expanded the need for quality health promotion programs. Individuals are seeking guidance to enable them to make sound decisions about behavior that is conducive to their health. Those best prepared to help these people are health education specialists who receive appropriate training. Properly trained health education specialists are aware of the limitations of the discipline and understand the assumptions on which health promotion is based.

REVIEW QUESTIONS

1. Explain the role *Healthy People* played in the relationship between the American people and health.
2. How is *health education* defined by the Joint Committee on Terminology (2012)?
3. What are the key phrases in the definition of health education presented by Green and Kreuter (2005)?
4. What is the relationship between health education and health promotion?
5. Why is there a need for health education specialists?
6. What is the Role Delineation Project?
7. How is the *Competency-Based Framework for Health Education Specialists* used by colleges and universities? By NCHEC? By NCATE? By SABPAC?
8. How does one become a Certified Health Education Specialist (CHES)?
9. How does one become a Master Certified Health Specialist (MCHES)?
10. What are the seven major responsibilities of health education specialists?
11. What is the National Health Educator Competencies Update Project (CUP)?
12. What is the Health Educator Job Analysis – 2010 (HEJA-2010)?
13. What assumptions are critical to health promotion?
14. What are the steps in the Generalized Model?
15. What is meant by the term *pre-planning*?

ACTIVITIES

1. Based on what you have read in this chapter and your knowledge of the profession of health education, write your own definitions for *health, health education, health promotion*, and *health promotion program*.

2. Write a response indicating what you see as the importance of each of the nine assumptions presented in the chapter. Write no more than one paragraph per assumption.

3. With your knowledge of health promotion, what other assumptions would you add to the list presented in this chapter? Provide a one-paragraph rationale for each.

4. If you have not already done so, go to the government documents section of the library on your campus and read *Healthy People: The Surgeon General's Report on Health Promotion and Disease Prevention* (USDHEW, 1979).

5. Say you are in your senior year and will graduate next June with a bachelor's degree in health education. What steps would you have to take in order to be able to take the CHES exam in April prior to your graduation? (Hint: Check the Website of the National Commission for Health Education Credentialing, Inc.).

6. In a one-page paper describe the differences and similarities in the two credentials— CHES and MCHES—available to health education specialists (Hint: Check the Website of the National Commission for Health Education Credentialing, Inc.).

7. Visit the Website of the Coalition of National Health Education Organizations (www.cnheo.org). At this site click on the "Publications" link and read the "Marketing the Profession: Executive Summary." After reading the executive summary be prepared to discuss its contents in class. Do you agree with all of the recommendations? Was there anything in this document that surprised you? To get further information and clarification on this report you may want to read the article written by Gambescia and his colleagues (2009).

WEBLINKS

1. http://www.healthypeople.gov

   Healthy People

   This is the Webpage for the U.S. government's Healthy People initiative including a complete presentation of *Healthy People 2020*.

2. http://www.nchec.org/

   National Commission for Health Education Credentialing, Inc. (NCHEC)

   The NCHEC, Inc. Website provides the most current information about the CHES and MCHES credentials.

3. http://www.cnheo.org

   Coalition of National Health Education Organizations (CNHEO)

   At CNHEO's Website you will find information about issues that are common to the health education profession.

PART I

PLANNING A HEALTH PROMOTION PROGRAM

The chapters in this section of the book provide the basic information needed to plan a health promotion program. Each chapter presents readers with the tools they will need to develop a successful program in a variety of settings. The chapters and topics presented in this section are:

2

Starting the Planning Process

After reading this chapter and answering the questions at the end, you should be able to:

- Develop a rationale for planning and implementing a health promotion program.
- Explain the importance of gaining the support of decision makers.
- Identify the individuals who could make up a planning committee.
- Explain what planning parameters are and the impact they have on program planning.

advisory board
cost-benefit analysis (CBA)
doers
epidemiology
evidence
evidence-based practice

*Guide to Community
    Preventive Services*
influencers
institutionalized
literature
organizational culture
planning committee

planning parameters
planning team
program ownership
return on investment (ROI)
social math
steering committee

As noted earlier (Chapter 1), planning a health promotion program is a multistep process that begins after doing pre-planning. "To plan is to engage in a process or a procedure to develop a method of achieving an end" (Minelli & Breckon, 2009, p. 137). However, because of the many different variables and circumstances of any one setting, the multistep process of planning does not always begin the same way. There are times when the need for a program is obvious and there is recognition that a new program should be put in place. For example, if a community's immunization rate for its children is less than half the national average, a program should be created. There are other times when a program has been successful in the past but needs to be changed or reworked slightly before being implemented again. And, there are situations where planners have been given the independence and authority to create the programs that are needed in a community in order to improve the health and quality of life. However, when the need is not so obvious, or when there has not been successful health promotion programming

---

Box 2.1 RESPONSIBILITIES AND COMPETENCIES FOR HEALTH
EDUCATION SPECIALISTS

The content of this chapter includes information on several tasks that occur early in
the program planning process. These tasks are not associated with a single area of
responsibility, but rather five areas of responsibility of the health education specialist:

Responsibility I: Assess Needs, Assets, and Capacity for Health Education

Competency 1.2: Access Existing Information and Data Related
to Health

Competency 1.6: Examine Factors that Enhance or Compromise
the Process of Health Education

Responsibility II: Plan Health Education

Competency 2.1: Involve Priority Populations and Other
Stakeholders in the Planning Process

Responsibility V: Administer and Manage Health Education

Competency 5.2: Obtain Acceptance and Support for Programs

Competency 5.3: Demonstrate Leadership

Competency 5.5: Facilitate Partnerships in Support of Health
Education

Responsibility VI: Serve as a Health Education Resource Person

Competency 6.1: Obtain and Disseminate Health-Related
Information

Responsibility VII: Communicate and Advocate for Health and Health Education

Competency 7.4: Engage in Health Education Advocacy

Source: NCHEC, SOPHE, & AAHE (2010).

---

in the past, the planning process often begins with the planners creating a rationale to
gain the support of key people in order to obtain the necessary resources to ensure that
the planning process and the eventual implementation proceed as smoothly as possible.

This chapter presents the steps of creating a program rationale to obtain the support
of decision makers, identifying those who may be interested in helping to plan the program, and establishing the parameters in which the planners must work. **Box 2.1** identifies
the responsibilities and competencies for health education specialists that pertain to the
material presented in this chapter.

The Need for Creating a Rationale to Gain the Support of Decision Makers

No matter what the setting of a health promotion program—whether a business, an
industry, the community, a clinic, a hospital, or a school—it is most important that the
program have support from the highest level (e.g., the administration, chief executive

officer, church elders, board of health, or board of directors) of the "community" for which the program is being planned (Allen & Hunnicutt, 2007; Chapman, 1997, 2006; Hunnicutt & Leffelman, 2006; Ryan, Chapman, & Rink, 2008). It is the individuals in these top-level decision-making positions who are able to provide the necessary resource support for the program.

> "Resources" usually means money, which can be turned into staff, facilities, materials, supplies, utilities, and all the myriad number of things that enable organized activity to take place over time. "Support" usually means a range of things: congruent organizational policies, program and concept visibility, expressions of priority value, personal involvement of key managers, a place at the table of organizational power, organizational credibility, and a role in integrated functioning (Chapman, 1997, p. 1).

There will be times when the idea for, or the motivating force behind, a program comes from the top-level people. When this happens, it is a real boon for the program planners because they do not have to sell the idea to these people to gain their support. However, this scenario does not occur frequently.

Often, the idea or the big push for a health promotion program comes from someone other than one who is part of the top-level of the "community." The idea could start with an employee, an interested parent, a health education specialist within the organization, a member of the parish or congregation, or a concerned individual or group from within the community. The idea might even be generated by an individual outside the "community," such as one who may have administrative or oversight responsibilities for activities in a community. An example of this arrangement is the employee of a state health department who provides consultative services to a local health department. Or it may be an individual from a regional agency who is partnering with a group within the community to carry out a collaborative project. When the scenario begins at a level below the decision makers, those who want to create a program must "sell" it to the decision makers. In other words, in order for resources and support to flow into health promotion programming, decision makers need to clearly perceive a set of values or benefits associated with the proposed program (Chapman, 2006). Without the support of decision makers, it becomes more difficult, if not impossible, to plan and implement a program. A number of years ago Behrens (1983) stated that health promotion programs in business and industry have a greater chance for success if all levels of management, including the top, are committed and supportive. This is still true today of health promotion programs in all settings, not just programs in business and industry (see **Box 2.2**).

If they need to gain the support of decision makers, program planners should develop a rationale for the program's existence. Why is it necessary to sell something that everyone knows is worthwhile? After all, does anyone doubt the value of trying to help people gain and maintain good health? The answer to these and similar questions is that few people are motivated by health concerns alone. Decisions by top-level management to develop new programs are based on a variety of factors, including finances, policies, public image, and politics, to name a few. Thus to sell the program to those at the top, planners need to develop a rationale that shows how the new program will help decision makers to meet the organization's goals and, in turn, to carry out its mission. In other words, planners need to position their program rationale politically, in line with the organization.

Box 2.2 MEASURING DECISION MAKERS' SUPPORT FOR HEALTH PROMOTION

Though the importance of decision makers' support to the success of health promotion programs has been known for a number of years, it is only recently that efforts have been put forth to actually measure decision makers' support for health promotion programs. Della, DeJoy, Goetzel, Ozminkowski, and Wilson (2008) created a valid instrument to assess leadership support for health promotion programs in work settings. The measurement tool, referred to as the Leading by Example (LBE) Instrument, is a four-factor scale. The four factors are (1) business assignment with health promotion objectives, (2) awareness of the economics of health and worker productivity, (3) worksite support for health promotion, and (4) leadership support for health promotion (Della et al., 2010). Della and colleagues feel that the LBE could be used in two ways. The first would be through a single administration "to assess specific areas in which the health promotion climate might support/hinder programmatic efforts" (p. 139). The second would be to administer the LBE two different times to monitor change in support for health promotion programs over time.

Steps in Creating a Program Rationale

Planners must understand that gaining the support of decision makers is one of the most important steps in the planning process and it should not be taken lightly. Many program ideas have died at this stage because the planners were not well prepared to sell the program to decision makers. Thus, before making an appeal to decision makers, planners need to have a sound rationale for creating a program that is supported by evidence that the proposed program will benefit those for whom it is planned.

There is no formula or recipe for writing a rationale, but through experience, the authors have found a logical format for putting ideas together to help guide planners (see **Figure 2.1**). Note that Figure 2.1 is presented as an inverted triangle. This inverted triangle is symbolic in design to reflect the flow of a program rationale beginning at the top by identifying a health problem in global terms and moving toward a more focused solution at the bottom of the triangle.

Step 1: Identify Appropriate Background Information

Before planners begin to write a program rationale, they need to identify appropriate sources of information and data that can be used to sell program development. The place to begin the process of identifying appropriate sources of information and data to support the development of a program rationale is to conduct a search of the existing literature. **Literature** includes the articles, books, government publications, and other documents that explain the past and current knowledge about a particular topic. By conducting a search, planners gain a better understanding of the health problem(s) of concern, approaches to reducing or eliminating the health problem, and an understanding of the people for whom the program is intended (remember these individuals

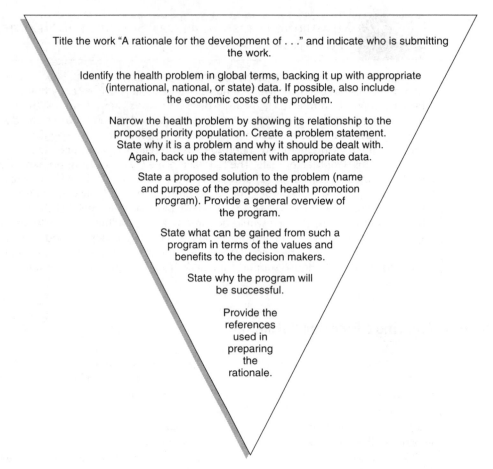

Title the work "A rationale for the development of . . ." and indicate who is submitting the work.

Identify the health problem in global terms, backing it up with appropriate (international, national, or state) data. If possible, also include the economic costs of the problem.

Narrow the health problem by showing its relationship to the proposed priority population. Create a problem statement. State why it is a problem and why it should be dealt with. Again, back up the statement with appropriate data.

State a proposed solution to the problem (name and purpose of the proposed health promotion program). Provide a general overview of the program.

State what can be gained from such a program in terms of the values and benefits to the decision makers.

State why the program will be successful.

Provide the references used in preparing the rationale.

Figure 2.1 Creating a Rationale

are referred to as the priority population). There are a number of different ways that planners can carry out a review of the literature (see Chapter 4 for an explanation of the literature search process).

In general, the types of information and data that are useful in writing a rationale include those that (1) express the needs and wants of the priority population, (2) describe the status of the health problem(s) within a given population, (3) show how the potential outcomes of the proposed program align with what the decision makers feel is important, (4) show compatibility with the health plan of a state or the nation, (5) provide evidence that the proposed program will make a difference, and (6) show how the proposed program will protect and preserve the single biggest asset of most organizations—the people. Though many of these types of information and data are generated through a review of the literature, the first one discussed below—needs and wants of the priority population—is not.

Information and data that express the needs and wants of the priority population can be generated through a needs assessment. A *needs assessment* is the process of identifying, analyzing, and prioritizing the needs of a priority population. Needs assessments are carried out through a multiple-step process in which data are collected and analyzed. The analysis generates a prioritized list of needs of the priority population (see Chapter 4 for a detailed explanation of the needs assessment process). Even though information and data that express the needs and wants of the priority population can be very useful in generating a rationale for a proposed program, more than likely at this point in the planning process, a formal needs assessment will not have been completed. Often, a complete needs assessment does not take place until decision makers give permission for the planning to begin. However, the review of literature may generate information about a needs assessment of another related or similar program. If so, it can provide valuable information and data that can help to develop the rationale.

Information and data that describe the status of a health problem within a population can be obtained by analyzing epidemiological data. Epidemiological data are those that result from the process of **epidemiology**, which has been defined as "the study of the distribution and determinants of health-related states or events in specific populations, and the application of this study to control health problems" (*Dictionary of Epidemiology* as cited in Last, 2007, p. 111). Epidemiological data are available from a number of different sources and include but are not limited to the *U.S. Census*, the *Statistical Abstract of the United States*, the *Monthly Vital Statistics Report*, *Morbidity and Mortality Weekly Report*, the *National Health Interview Survey*, the *National Health and Nutrition Examination Survey*, the *Behavioral Risk Factor Surveillance System (BRFSS)*, the *Youth Risk Behavior Surveillance System (YRBSS)*, the *National Hospital Discharge Survey*, and the *National Hospital Ambulatory Medical Care Survey*.

Epidemiological data gain additional significance when it can be shown that the described health problem(s) is/are the result of modifiable health behaviors and that spending money to promote healthy lifestyles and prevent health problems makes good economic sense. Here are a couple examples where modifiable health behaviors and health-related costs have been connected. The first deals with smoking. Approximately 20.6% of U.S. adults 18 years of age and older are cigarette smokers (CDC, 2010b). It has been estimated that the cost of ill effects from smoking in the United States totals approximately $193 billion per year. Almost equal amounts come from smoking-attributable health-care expenditures ($96 billion) and productivity losses (~ $97 billion) (CDC, 2008). The second example deals with diabetes. It has been estimated that annual costs associated with diabetes are approximately $174 billion; $116 billion from direct medical costs and $58 billion in direct costs related to disability, work loss, and premature death (CDC, 2010a). We know that not all cases of diabetes are related to health behavior, but it is known "for people with prediabetes, lifestyle changes, including a 5%–7% weight loss and at least 150 minutes of physical activity per week, can reduce the rate of onset of type 2 diabetes by 58%" (CDC, 2010a, para. 4). In addition, we know "people with diagnosed diabetes have medical expenditures that are about 2.3 times higher than medical expenditures for people without diabetes" (CDC, 2010a, para. 3).

When a rationale includes an economic component it is often reported based on a **cost-benefit analysis (CBA)**. A CBA of a health promotion program will yield the dollar benefit received from the dollars invested in the program. A common way of reporting a CBA is through a metric called **return on investment (ROI)**. ROI "measures the costs

---

Box 2.3 RETURN ON INVESTMENT

In general, ROI compares the dollars invested in something to the benefits produced by that investment:

$$\text{ROI} = \frac{(\text{benefits of investment} - \text{amount invested})}{\text{amount invested}}$$

In the case of an investment in a prevention program, ROI compares the savings produced by the intervention, net of the cost of the program, to how much the program cost:

$$\text{ROI} = \frac{\text{net savings}}{\text{cost of intervention}}$$

When ROI equals 0, the program pays for itself. When ROI is greater than 0, then the program is producing savings that exceed the cost of the program.

Source: Copyright © 2009 by Trust for America's Health. Reprinted with permission.

---

of a program (i.e., the investment) versus the financial return realized by that program" (Cavallo, 2006, p. 1) (see **Box 2.3** for formula to calculate ROI). An example of ROI is a study that examined the economic impact of an investment of $10 per person per year in a proven community-based program to increase physical activity, improve nutrition, and prevent smoking and other tobacco use. The results of the study showed that the nation could save billions of dollars annually and have an ROI in one year of 0.96 to 1, 5.6 to 1 in 5 years, and 6.2 to 1 in 10–20 years (TFAH, 2009).

However, it should be noted that "proving" the economic impact of many health promotion programs is not easy. There are a number of reasons for this including the multiple causes of many health problems, the complex interventions needed to deal with them, and the difficulty of carrying out rigorous research studies. Additionally, McGinnis and colleagues (2002) feel that part of the problem is that health promotion programs are held to a different standard than medical treatment programs when cost-effectiveness is being considered.

> In a vexing example of double standards, public investments in health promotion seem to require evidence that future savings in health and other social costs will offset the investments in prevention. Medical treatments do not need to measure up to the standard; all that is required here is evidence of safety and effectiveness. The cost-effectiveness challenge often is made tougher by a sense that the benefits need to accrue directly and in short term to the payer making investments. Neither of these two conditions applies in many interventions in health promotion. (p. 84)

For those planners interested in using economic impact and cost-effectiveness of health promotion programs as part of a program rationale, we recommend that the work of the following authors be reviewed: Aldana (2001, 2009), Chapman (2003a, 2005b, 2006), Cohen, Neumann, & Milton (2008), Edington (2001), Goetzel, & Ozminkowski (2008), Golaszewski (2001), Hunnicutt & Jahn (2011), McKenzie (1986), Miller & Hendrie (2008), and USDHHS (2003).

| Box 2.4 | METHODS FOR DETERMINING THE VALUES AND BENEFITS THAT SHOULD BE EMPHASIZED |

1. Examine recent or past meeting minutes, decisions, or comments that are relevant to the value placed on health and prevention.
2. Find out from the individuals in a position to know, why past decisions related to budget or employee benefits were made by the managers involved.
3. Review past formal reports or evaluations of health programs and benefits that have been commissioned or carried out on behalf of the decision makers.
4. Conduct an informal survey of the most influential decision makers to get some sense of their own as well as their perception of the value priorities of the other decision makers involved.
5. Conduct a formal survey of all or a portion of the key decision makers involved to determine what is the most important to them.
6. Analyze the implementation questions that have been raised in the past on similar programs or topics.

Source: Art of Health Promotion. L. S. Chapman. Copyright © 1997 by The American Journal of Health Promotion. Reproduced with permission.

Other information and data that are useful in creating a rationale are those that show how the potential outcomes of the proposed program align with what decision makers feel is important. Planners can often get a hint of what decision makers value by reviewing the organization's mission statement and/or annual report. More specific methods of determining the values and benefits that could be included in a rationale are noted in **Box 2.4. Table 2.1** provides a list of values or benefits that can be derived from health promotion programs, while **Table 2.2** provides a list of sources where information about values or benefits could be found.

Table 2.1 Values or Benefits from Health Promotion Programs

Value or Benefit for:	Types of Values or Benefits
Community	Establishing good health as norm; improved quality of life; improve the economic well-being of the community; provide model for other communities
Employee/Individual	Improved health status; reduction in health risks; improved health behavior; improved job satisfaction; lower out-of-pocket costs for health care; increased well-being, self-image, and self-esteem
Employer	Increased worker morale; enhanced worker performance/productivity; recruitment and retention tool; reduced absenteeism and presenteeism; reduced disability days/claims, reduced health care costs; enhanced corporate image

Sources: Adapted from ACS (2009); CDC (2010c); and Chapman (1997).

Table 2.2 Selected Sources of Information About Values or Benefits of Health Promotion Programs

Source	Location of Information
American Cancer Society	
Workplace Solutions	http://www.acsworkplacesolutions.com/index.asp
Centers for Disease Control and Prevention	
National Center for Health Statistics	http://www.cdc.gov/nchs/
Worklife	http://www.cdc.gov/niosh/worklife/
Workplace Health Promotion	http://www.cdc.gov/workplacehealthpromotion/model/index.html
The Community Tool Box	http://ctb.ku.edu/en/tablecontents/index.aspx#partM
National Committee for Quality Assurance	http://www.ncqa.org/Home.aspx
Trust for America's Health (TFAH)	http://healthyamericans.org/reports/
U.S Census Bureau	
Home page	http://www.census.gov/
Statistical Abstract of the United States	http://www.census.gov/prod/www/abs/statab.html
U.S. Department of Health & Human Services	
Office of Assistant Secretary for Planning & Evaluation	http://aspe.hhs.gov/_/index.cfm
Wellness Council of America (WELCOA)	http://www.welcoa.org/wellworkplace/
	http://www.welcoa.org/freeresources/

A fourth source of information for a rationale is a comparison between the proposed program and the health plan for the nation or a state. Comparing the health needs of the priority population with those of other citizens of the state or of all Americans, as outlined in the goals and objectives of the nation (USDHHS, 2010a), should enable planners to show the compatibility between the goals of the proposed program and those of the nation's health plan (see Chapter 6 for a discussion of the *Healthy People 2020* goals and objectives).

A fifth source of information and data is *evidence* that the proposed program will be effective and make a difference if implemented. By **evidence** we mean the body of data that can be used to make decisions when planning a program. Such data can come from needs assessments, knowledge about the causes of a health problem, research that has tested the effectiveness of an intervention, and evaluations conducted on other health promotion programs. When program planners systematically find, appraise, and use evidence as the basis for decision making when planning a health promotion program, it is referred to as **evidence-based practice** (Cottrell & McKenzie, 2011).

Over the years, the number of organizations/agencies that have worked to identify evidence of various types of health-related programs (i.e., health care, disease prevention, health promotion) has increased (see **Table 2.3** for examples). A most useful source for those planning health promotion programs is the *Guide to Community Preventive Services*, referred to simply as *The Community Guide* (Zara, Briss, & Harris, 2005; CDC, 2011). *The Community Guide* summarizes the findings from systematic reviews of

Table 2.3 Examples of Sources of Evidence

Canadian Task Force on Preventive Health Care

Type of evidence: Practice guidelines that support primary care providers in delivering preventive health care.

Website: http://www.canadiantaskforce.ca/

health-evidence.ca

Type of evidence: Public health and health promotion interventions in Canada.

Website: http://health-evidence.ca/

National Caner Institute

Document: *Research-tested Intervention Programs*

Type of evidence: A searchable database of cancer control interventions and program materials that are designed to provide program planners and public health practitioners easy and immediate access to research-tested materials.

Website: http://rtips.cancer.gov/rtips/index.do

Robert Wood Johnson Foundation and the University of Wisconsin Population Health Institute

Document: *County Health Rankings*

Type of Evidence: Fifty state reports, ranking each county within the 50 states according to its health outcomes and the multiple health factors that determine a county's health.

Website: http://www.countyhealthrankings.org/

Substance Abuse and Mental Health Services

Document: *National Registry of Evidence-based Programs and Practices*

Type of Evidence: Searchable online registry of interventions supporting mental health promotion, substance abuse prevention, and mental health and substance abuse treatment.

Website: http://nrepp.samhsa.gov/

Task Force on Community Preventive Services

Document: *Guide to Community Preventive Services*

Type of evidence: Programs and policies to improve health and prevent disease in communities.

Website: http://www.thecommunityguide.org/index.html

U.S. Preventive Services Task Force

Document: *The Guide to Clinical Preventive Services*

Type of evidence: Recommendations on the use of screening, counseling, and other preventive services that are typically delivered in primary care settings.

Website: http://www.ahrq.gov/clinic/pocketgd.htm

World Health Organization

Document: *What is the evidence on school health promotion in improving health or preventing disease and, specifically, what is the effectiveness of the health promoting schools approach?*

Type of evidence: Worth of school health promotion

Website: http://www.euro.who.int/document/e88185

---

public health interventions covering a variety of topics. The systematic reviews are used to answer three questions (CDC, 2011a, para. 1):

- "Which program and policy interventions have been proven effective?
- Are there effective interventions that are right for my community? And,
- What might effective interventions cost; what is the likely return on investment?"

The *Community Guide* was developed and is continually updated by the nonfederal Task Force on Community Preventive Services. The Task Force, which is comprised of public health experts who are appointed by the director of the CDC, is charged with reviewing and assessing the quality of available evidence and developing appropriate recommendations.

Finally, when preparing a rationale to gain the support of decision makers, planners should not overlook the most important resource of any community—the people who make up the community. Promoting, maintaining, and in some cases restoring human health should be at the core of any health promotion program. Whatever the setting, better health of those in the priority population provides for a better quality of life. For those planners who end up practicing in a worksite setting, the importance of protecting the health of employees (i.e., protecting human resources) should be noted in developing a rationale. "Labor costs typically represent 60% to 70% of total annual operating costs for most organizations" (Chapman, 2006, p. 10); thus people are a company's single biggest asset. "Fit and healthy people are more productive, are better able to meet extraordinary demands and deal with stress, are absent less, reflect better on the company or community as exemplars, and so forth" (Chapman, 2006, p. 29).

Step 2: Titling the Rationale

Once planners have identified and are familiar with the sources of information and data that can be used to sell program development, they are ready to begin the process of putting a rationale together. Thus, the next step is giving a title to the rationale. This can be quite simple in nature, such as "A Rationale for (Title of Program): A Program to Enhance the Health of (Name of Priority Population)." Immediately following the title should be a listing of who contributed to the authorship of the rationale.

Step 3: Writing the Content of the Rationale

The first paragraph or two of the rationale should identify the health problem from a global perspective. By global perspective we mean presenting the problem using information and data at the most macro level (whether it be international, national, regional, state, or local) as possible. In other words, begin the rationale by presenting the problem at the most macro level for which supporting data are available. So, if there is international information and data on the problem, say for example HIV/AIDS, then begin describing the problem at that level. If data are not available to present the problem at the international level, say for example people without health insurance, then move down to next level where the presentation can be supported with data. If available, also include the economic costs of such a problem; it will strengthen the rationale. "Much of the decision-making that occurs, for change to take place in an organization is based on financial considerations, and any change within an organization typically must be supported by a positive return on investment. Lacking sound financial support or a firm understanding of the financial implications, a good idea may not be realized in practice" (Gambatese, 2008, p. 153). Most health problems are also present at other levels. Presenting the problem at these higher levels shows decision makers that dealing with the health problem is consistent with the concerns of others.

Showing the relationship of the health problem to the "bigger problem" at the international, national, and/or state levels is the next logical step in presenting the rationale. Thus, the next portion of the rationale is to identify the health problem that is the focus of the rationale. This declaration of the health problem is referred to as the *problem statement* or *statement of the problem*. The problem statement should begin with a concise explanation of the issue that needs to be addressed (WKKF, 2004). The statement should also include *why* it is a problem and *why* it should be dealt with (see **Box 2.5**). If available, the statement should also include supporting data for the problem. Such data may come from a needs assessment if it has already been completed or from related literature.

In presenting the problem statement you may find it useful to use the technique of social math. **Social math** has been defined as "the practice of translating statistics and other data so they become interesting to the journalist, and meaningful to the audience" (Dorfman, Woodruff, Herbert, & Ervice, 2004, p. 112). In other words, data, especially large numbers, are presented in such a way that makes them easier to grasp by putting them in a context that gives instant meaning. "It is critical to select a social math fact that

---

Box 2.5   EXAMPLES OF PROBLEM STATEMENTS

For a local-level program

> The number of children entering kindergarten who have not received two doses of the measles-mumps-rubella (MMR) vaccine in Mitchell County continues to increase. In the 2007–08 school year, 95% of the children who entered kindergarten had received two doses, while only 91% were immunized properly in 2010–11. Because the number of cases of MMR does not seem too high to parents/guardians, many do not feel it is necessary to subject their children to immunizations. Infectious diseases remain a major cause of illness, disability, and mortality. "Vaccines are among the most cost-effective clinical preventive services and are a core component of any preventive services package. Childhood immunization programs provide a very high return on investment" (USDHHS, 2010a, para. 6).

For a state-level program

> Overweight and obesity are critical health threats facing the state of ABC. Between 2008 and 2012, the percentage of overweight adults in ABC increased from 34% to 35%, while the percentage of obese adults increased from 30% to 32%. Overweight and obesity are caused by an imbalance in the calories consumed vs. calories burned ratio. Both overweight and obesity increase the risks for heart disease, stroke, diabetes, and cancer. The annual costs (direct and indirect) of these diseases to the state have been estimated at $15 billion. There is good evidence that shows both the physical and financial costs of overweight and obesity are preventable.

is 100 percent accurate, visual if possible, dramatic, and appropriate for the target audience" (Dorfman et al., 2004, p. 112). For example, $2.3 trillion was spent on health in 2008 in the United States (NCHS, 2011); 2.3 trillion is a large number and hard "to put our heads around." But equating that number with spending $6,400 for every person in the United States (NCHS, 2011) that year makes the number more comprehensible. Or, we could present the $2.3 trillion in social math terms by saying if every dollar equaled one second, then $2.3 trillion would equal 72,932 years! (see **Box 2.6** for other examples)

Box 2.6   EXAMPLES OF SOCIAL MATH

- *Break the numbers down by time.*
  If you know the amount over a year, what does that look like per hour? Per minute? For example, the average annual salary of a childcare worker nationally is $15,430, roughly $7.42 per hour. While many people understand that an annual salary of $15,430 is low, breaking the figure down by the hour reinforces that point—and makes the need for some kind of intervention even more clear.

- *Break down the numbers by place.*
  Comparing a statistic with a well-known place can give people a sense of the statistic's magnitude. For instance, approximately 250,000 children are on waiting lists for childcare subsidies in California. That's enough children to fill almost every seat in every Major League ballpark in California. Such a comparison helps us visualize the scope of the problem and makes a solution all the more imperative.

- *Provide comparisons with familiar things.*
  Providing a comparison to something that is familiar can have great impact. For example, "While Head Start is a successful, celebrated educational program, it is so underfunded that it serves only about three-fifths of eligible children. Applying that proportion to social security would mean that almost a million currently eligible seniors wouldn't receive benefits."

- *Provide ironic comparisons.*
  For example, the average annual cost of full-time, licensed, center-based care for a child under age 2 in California is twice the tuition at the University of California at Berkeley. What's ironic here is how out of balance our public conversation is. Parents and the public focus so much on the cost of college when earlier education is dramatically more expensive.

- *Localize the numbers.*
  Make comparisons that will resonate with community members. For example, saying, "Center-based childcare for an infant costs $11,450 per year in Seattle, Washington," is one thing. Saying, "In Seattle, Washington, a father making minimum wage would have to spend 79 percent of his income per year to place his baby in a licensed care center," is much more powerful because it illustrates why it is nearly impossible.

Source: National Center for Injury Prevention and Control (2008; revised 2010). *Adding Power to Our Voices: A Framing Guide for Communicating About Injury.* Atlanta, GA: Author. Retrieved January 11, 2012, from http://www.cdc.gov/injury/framing/.

At this point in the rationale, propose a solution to the problem. The solution should include the name and purpose of the proposed health promotion program, and a general overview of what the program may include. Since the writing of a program rationale often precedes much of the formal planning process, the general overview of the program is often based upon the "best guess" of those creating the rationale. For example, if the purpose of a program is to improve the immunization rate of children in the community, a "best guess" of the eventual program might include interventions to increase awareness and knowledge about immunizations, and the reduction of the barriers that limit access to receiving immunizations. Following such an overview, include statements indicating what can be gained from the program. Do your best to align the potential values and benefits of the program with what is important to the decision makers.

Next, state why this program will be successful. This is the place to use the results of *evidence-based practice* to support the rationale. It can also be helpful to point out the similarity of the priority population to others with which similar programs have been successful. And finally, using the argument that the "timing is right" for the program can also be useful. By this we mean that there is no better time than now to work to solve the problem facing the priority population.

Step 4: Listing the References Used to Create the Rationale

The final step in creating a rationale is to include a list of the references used in preparing the rationale. Having a reference list shows decision makers that you studied the available information before presenting your idea. (See the examples of rationales presented in the Activities section at the end of the chapter.)

Planning Committee

The number of people involved in the planning process is determined by the resources and circumstances of a particular situation. "One very helpful method to develop a clearer and more comprehensive planning approach is to establish a committee" (Gilmore, 2012, p. 35). Identifying individuals who would be willing to serve as members of the **planning committee** (sometimes referred to as a **steering committee** or **advisory board** or **planning team**) becomes one of the planner's first tasks. Because an effective planning committee is usually composed of interested and well-respected individuals, it is important to establish it carefully (Chapman, 2009). The number of individuals on a planning committee can differ depending on the setting for the program and the size of the priority population. For example, the size of a planning committee for an obesity program in a community of 50,000 people would probably be larger than that of a committee planning a similar program for a business with 50 employees. There is no ideal size for a planning committee, but the following 10 guidelines, which have been presented earlier (McKenzie, 1988) and are given here in a modified form with updates, should be helpful in setting up a committee.

1. The committee should be composed of individuals who represent a variety of subgroups within the priority population. To the extent possible, the committee should have representation from all segments of the priority population (e.g., administrators/students/teachers, age groups, health behavior participants/nonparticipants, labor/management, race/ethnic groups, different genders, socioeconomic groups, union/nonunion members). The greater the number of individuals who are represented by committee members, the greater the chance of the priority population developing a feeling of **program ownership**. With program ownership there will be better planned programs, greater support for the programs, and people who will be willing to help sell the program to others because they feel it is theirs (Strycker et al., 1997).

2. If the program that is being planned deals with a specific health risk or problem, then it would be important that someone with that health risk (e.g., smoker) or problem (e.g., diabetes) be included on the planning committee (Bartholomew, Parcel, Kok, Gottlieb & Fernández, 2011.).

3. The committee should include willing individuals who are interested in seeing the program succeed. Select a combination of **doers** and **influencers**. Doers are people who will be willing to roll up their sleeves and do the physical work needed to see that the program is planned and implemented properly. Influencers are those who with a single phone call or signature on a form will enlist other people to participate or will help provide the resources to facilitate the program. Both doers and influencers are important to the planning process.

4. The committee should include an individual who has a key role within the organization sponsoring the program—someone whose support would be most important to ensure a successful program and institutionalization.

5. The committee should include representatives of other stakeholders (any person or organization with a vested interest in a program) not represented in the priority population. For example, if health care providers are needed to implement a health promotion program they need to be represented on the planning committee.

6. The committee membership should be reevaluated regularly to ensure that the composition lends itself to fulfilling program goals and objectives.

7. If the planning committee will be in place for a long period of time, new individuals should be added periodically to generate new ideas and enthusiasm. It may be helpful to set a term of office for committee members. If terms of office are used, it is advisable to stagger the length of terms so that there is always a combination of new and experienced members on the committee.

8. Be aware of the "politics" that are always present in an organization or priority population. There are always some people who bring their own agendas to committee work.

9. Make sure the committee is large enough to accomplish the work, but small enough to be able to make decisions and reach consensus. If necessary, subcommittees can be formed to handle specific tasks.

10. In some situations there might be a need for multiple layers of planning committees. If the priority population is highly dispersed geographically and/or broken into decentralized subgroups (e.g., various offices of the same corporation, or several different local groups within the same state, or different buildings within a school corporation), these various subgroups may need their own local planning committee that operates with some latitude but maintains and complements the core planning committee as the base of the program (Chapman, 2009).

The actual means by which the committee members are chosen varies according to the setting. Five commonly used techniques are:

1. Asking for volunteers by word of mouth, a newsletter, a needs assessment, or some other widely distributed publication

2. Holding an election, either throughout the community or by subdivisions of the community

3. Inviting/recruiting people to serve

4. Having members formally appointed by a governing group or individual

5. Having an application process then selecting those with the most desirable characteristics

Once the planning committee has been formed, someone must be designated to lead it. This is an important step (Strycker et al., 1997). The leader (chairperson) should be interested and knowledgeable about health promotion programs, and be organized, enthusiastic, and creative (McKenzie, 1988). One might think that most planners, especially health education specialists, would be perfect for the committee chairperson's job. However, sometimes it is preferable to have someone other than the program planners serve in the leadership capacity. For one thing, it helps to spread out the workload of the committee. Planners who are not good at delegating responsibility may end up with a lot of extra work when they serve as the leaders. Second, having someone else serve as the leader allows the planners to remain objective about the program. And third, the planning committee can serve in an advisory capacity to the planners, if this is considered desirable. **Figure 2.2** illustrates the composition of a balanced planning committee.

Once the planning committee has been organized and a leader is selected, for the committee to be effective it needs to be well organized and well run. The committee should meet regularly, have a formal agenda for each meeting, and keep minutes of the meetings (Hunnicutt, 2007a). Further, the committee meetings should be efficient, not long and boring (Johnson & Breckon, 2007). In other words, meetings should be productive and represent a good use of the committee members' time. In addition, it is

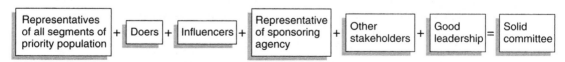

Figure 2.2 Makeup of a Solid Planning/Steering Committee

important for the committee to communicate frequently both with the decision makers and those in the priority population so that all can be kept informed. By communicating regularly, the committee has the unique opportunity to educate and inform others about health and the specific priorities of the program (Hunnicutt, 2007a).

Parameters for Planning

Once the support of the decision makers has been gained and a planning committee formed, the committee members must identify the **planning parameters** within which they will work. There are several questions to which committee members should have answers before they become too deeply involved in the planning process. In an earlier work (McKenzie, 1988), several such questions were presented, using the example of school-site health promotion programs. The questions are modified for presentation here. It should be noted, however, that not all of the questions would be appropriate for every program because of the different circumstances of each setting and the answers to some of the questions may have already been obtained during pre-planning.

1. What is the decision makers' philosophical perspective on health promotion programs? What are the values and benefits of the programs to the decision makers? (Chapman, 1997). Do they see the programs as something important or as "extras"?

2. What type of commitment to the program are decision makers willing to make? Are they interested in the program becoming **institutionalized**? That is, are they interested in seeing that the "program becomes imbedded within the host organization, so that the program becomes sustained and durable" (Goodman et al., 1993, p. 163)? Or are they more interested in providing a one-time or pilot program? (Note: Goodman and colleagues [1993] have developed a scale for measuring institutionalization.)

3. What type of financial support are decision makers willing to provide? Does it include personnel for leadership and clerical duties? Released/assigned time for managing the program and participation? Space? Equipment? Materials?

4. Are decision makers willing to consider changing the **organizational culture**? That is, are decision makers interested in establishing a health supporting culture (Golaszewski, Allen, & Edington, 2008)? Among other things, such a culture might include health-supporting policies, services, and facilities. For example, are they interested in "well" days instead of sick days? Are they as interested in *presenteeism*—that is, showing up for work even if one is too ill, stressed, or distracted to be productive—as much as they are interested in absenteeism? Would they like to create employee nonsmoking and safety belt policies? Change vending machine selections to more nutritious foods? Set aside an employee room for meditation? Develop a health promotion corner in the organization's library?

5. Will all individuals in the priority population have an opportunity to take advantage of the program, or will it be available to only certain subgroups?

6. What type of committee will the planning committee be? Will it be a *permanent* or a *temporary* (*ad hoc*) committee (Hitt, Black, & Porter, 2012)? A permanent committee would indicate that decision makers want the planning committee to be a part of the ongoing structure of the organization.

7. What is the authority of the planning committee? Will it be an advisory group or a programmatic decision-making group? What will the chain of command be for program approval?

After the planning parameters have been defined, the planning committee should understand how the decision makers view the program, and should know what type and number of resources and amount of support to expect. Identifying the parameters early will save the planning committee a great deal of effort and energy throughout the planning process.

SUMMARY

Creating a program rationale to gain the support of decision makers is an important initial step in program planning. Planners should take great care in developing a rationale for "selling" the program idea to these important people. A program rationale can be written using the following four steps: (1) Identify appropriate background information, (2) title the rationale, (3) write the content of the rationale, and (4) list the references used to create the rationale. A planning committee can be most useful in helping with some of the planning activities and in helping to sell the program to the priority population. Therefore, the committee should be composed of interested individuals, doers and influencers, who are representative of the priority population. If the planning committee is to be effective, it will need to work efficiently and to know the planning parameters set for the program by the decision makers.

REVIEW QUESTIONS

1. What is the reason for creating a program rationale?

2. Why is the support of decision makers important in planning a program?

3. What kinds of reasons should be included in a rationale for planning and implementing a health promotion program?

4. How important is selling the idea of a program to decision makers?

5. What items should be addressed when creating a program rationale?

6. What is a problem statement? What does it include?

7. What is social math? Give an example.

8. Who should be selected as the members of a planning committee?

9. What are *planning parameters?* Give a few examples.

10. Why is it important to know the planning parameters at the beginning of the planning process?

ACTIVITIES

1. Write a two-page rationale that sells a program you are planning to decision makers, using the guidelines presented in this chapter.

2. Write a two-page rationale for beginning an exercise program for a company with 200 employees. A needs assessment of this priority population indicates that the number one cause of lost work time in this cohort is back problems and the number one cause of premature death is heart disease.

3. Write a problem statement that could be included in a program rationale for a proposed adult smoking cessation program offered by the local health department in your hometown. The rationale will be given to the members of the County Board of Health. Use information and data from the County Health Rankings (http://www.countyhealthrankings.org/) and *Healthy People 2020* (http://www.healthypeople.gov/2020/default.aspx) to support your problem statement.

4. Select a disease (e.g., diabetes, cancer, heart disease) or a health behavior (e.g., physical inactivity, smoking) and write a paragraph describing the health problem using social math.

5. Visit the Websites of the Task Force on Community Preventive Services (TFCPS) and U.S. Preventive Services Task Force (USPSTF) (see Table 2.3 for URLs of the Websites). At the two sites, find out what the recommendations are for clinical skin cancer screenings and educational programs for skin cancer. Summarize your findings in one to two paragraphs. Based on the recommendations, write another one to two paragraphs describing what advice you would give with regard to future health promotion programming to a community coalition that is trying to reduce the number of cases of skin cancer in its community.

6. For a program you are planning, write a two-page description of the individuals (by position/job title, not name) who will be asked to serve on the planning committee, and provide a rationale for asking each to serve.

7. Provide a list (by position/job title, not name) and a rationale for each of the 10 individuals you would ask to serve on a community-wide safety belt program. Use the town or city in which your college/university is located as the community.

8. Following are two program rationales written by former students at Ball State University. Read each of the rationales and then select one to critique using the guidelines presented in this chapter. Critique by describing the following: (a) the strengths of the rationale, (b) the weaknesses, and (c) how you would change the rationale to make it stronger. Be critical! Closely examine the content, reasoning, and references.

EXAMPLE 1

A rationale for "No Butts About It": A campaign to create a smoke-free ordinance in the restaurants of Delaware County, Indiana.*

The global tobacco use pandemic is responsible for 4.9 million deaths a year worldwide (WHO, 1998). The United States ranks as the second highest consumer of cigarettes in the world with 451 billion consumed each year (WHO, 1998). Tobacco use has been labeled the single most important preventable cause of death and disease in the United States, causing more than 440,000 deaths and resulting in more than $75 billion in direct medical costs annually. Nationally, smoking results in more than 5.6 million years of potential life lost each year.

In the United States, approximately 80% of adult smokers started smoking before the age of 18. That means that each day nearly 5,000 young people under the age of 18 try their first cigarette (USDHHS, 2000). It is clear that years of cigarette smoking vastly increase the risk of developing several fatal conditions. Cigarette smoking is responsible for one-third of all cancers. It is the leading cause of lung cancer contributing to 90% of all lung cancers. It is also associated with cancers of the mouth, pharynx, larynx, esophagus, stomach, pancreas, uteri cervix, kidney, bladder, and colon (USDHHS, 1994). Smoking also increases the risk of cardiovascular disease including stroke, heart attack, vascular disease, and aneurysm (USDHHS, 1994).

Environmental tobacco smoke (ETS) is a mixture of the smoke given off by the burning end of a cigarette (sidestream smoke) and the smoke emitted at the mouthpiece and exhaled from the lungs of smokers (main stream smoke). ETS, also known as second hand smoke, is a major source of indoor air pollution. In the United States, approximately 38,000 deaths are attributable to ETS exposure each year (NCI, 2000). When a cigarette is smoked, only 15% of the smoke is inhaled by the smoker, the other 85% goes directly into the air. Cigarette smoke contains more than 4,000 substances, and 40 of these are classified as carcinogens (cancer causing agents). Nearly nine out of ten nonsmoking Americans are exposed to ETS, as measured by the levels of cotinine, a chemical the body metabolizes from nicotine, in their blood. Eighty-eight percent of all nontobacco users had measurable levels of cotinine in their blood according to a study conducted by the CDC. The presence of cotinine is documentation that a person has been exposed to ETS. Serum cotinine levels can be used to estimate nicotine exposure over the last two to three days.

ETS is estimated to cause approximately 3,000 lung cancer deaths per year among nonsmokers and contributes to 40,000 deaths related to cardiovascular disease (USDHHS, 1994). These deaths are all due to breathing the smoke of others' cigarettes and make ETS the third leading preventable cause of death in the United States. Some of the highest reported exposures to concentrations of ETS are found in food service establishments (EPA, 1992).

Approximately, one out of every four adults in Indiana smokes making it the fourth highest in the nation (27% compared to the U.S. median of 23.3%) (CDC, 2002). The number of adults between ages 18 to 24 who smoke has risen due to the tobacco companies targeting that age group since 1996 (SFI, 2003). The results of the Indiana Youth Tobacco Survey show that 9.8% of middle school students and 31.6% of high school students are current cigarette smokers (SFI, 2000). The smoking attributable mortality

---

*This rationale was written by Peggy Chute, Fariba Mirzaei, and Joe Turner while they were graduate students at Ball State University, Muncie, IN. Reprinted with permission.

rate (SAM) in Indiana is also higher (341.4/100,000) compared to the median for the United States (295.5/100,000) (CDC, 2002).

The five leading causes of death in Delaware County are cardiovascular disease, malignant neoplasm, chronic obstructive pulmonary disease, and unintentional injuries (Synergy, 1998). Lung and bronchial cancer had higher incidence of death when compared to other cancers. "Residents of Delaware County are clearly at risk for cigarette smoking, with 3 in 10 claiming to smoke and having smoked 100 or more cigarettes in their entire lives" (Synergy, 1998, p. 17). Delaware County residents were significantly higher when compared to the national average and the percentage of smokers increased from 1989 (27%) to 1998 (30%). Currently, Delaware County has no ordinance to prohibit smoking in public, including restaurants. This allows ETS to have effects on their nonsmoking clients, smoking clients, and workers of the restaurants.

One of the national health objectives for 2010 is to reduce public exposure to ETS (USDHHS, 2000). Objective 27-13c is specifically related to laws on smokefree air in restaurants. The base line measure for this objective was only 3 states and the target for 2010 is 51 states (50 states and the District of Columbia).

To reduce public exposure to ETS, the Centers for Disease Control and Prevention recommends smoking bans and restrictions in public places to reduce exposure to second-hand smoke. The Task Force on Community Prevention Services, a nonfederal public health panel, which conducted in-depth systematic reviews on selected tobacco interventions concluded that smoking bans and restrictions are the most effective measures to reduce exposure to second-hand smoke (CDC, 2002).

Local ordinances requiring restaurants to be smokefree have spread rapidly. Over 230 U.S. municipalities in different states, among these states Massachusetts, Texas, Colorado, Wisconsin, New York, Oregon, North Carolina, and Arizona, have smokefree ordinances in some of their cities. Fort Wayne is a good example in the state of Indiana, where a smokefree ordinance was passed in 1998. Additionally, the states of California, Maine, Maryland, Vermont, and Utah have smokefree restaurant laws. Several Canadian jurisdictions also have restaurant smoking bans.

Contrary to popular belief, restaurants that implement smokefree policies do not see a decline in profits. Studies in cities that have implemented such policies have shown sales to remain constant and in some cases sales have increased (Americans for Nonsmokers' Rights, 2002).

In addition to stable economic conditions, health care costs decline due to a decrease in worker's compensation claims, decrease in absenteeism, and an increase in worker productivity (CDC, 2002).

After reviewing national, state and local data it is clear that there is a significant health problem in regards to ETS in Delaware County. It is important to "think globally and act locally." This community problem provides a need for action at the local level. In order to succeed in a local campaign to prohibit smoking in restaurants it is important to mobilize grassroots activities. Educating the citizens regarding the health risks of ETS, and mobilizing local advocates will empower the Tobacco Free Coalition of Delaware County's activities in executing a smokefree ordinance campaign. A significant and active grassroots base of support is the most potent weapon to counter the relentless and well-funded opposition from the tobacco industry. Tobacco control advocates have the expertise to draft sound smokefree policies based on successes and lessons learned from other clean indoor air campaigns across the country, while policymakers often lack tobacco control knowledge or expertise.

The above rationale adds up to the conclusion that the Tobacco Free Coalition of Delaware County can succeed in advocating for and passing a smokefree ordinance in

Delaware County if it obtains active grassroots support from the community. Passage of an ordinance in turn will decrease the dangers of ETS exposure in Delaware County. Therefore the *No Butts About It* program can be a means to achieving these goals.

References

Americans for Nonsmoker's Rights Foundation (2002). *Smokefree advertising examples.* Retrieved March 25, 2003, from http://www.no-smoke.org/ads.html

Centers for Disease Control and Prevention (CDC). (2002). Strategies for reducing exposure to environmental tobacco smoke: Increasing tobacco-use cessation, and reducing initiation in communities and health care systems. *Morbidity and Mortality Weekly Report, 49* (RR-12). Retrieved April 6, 2003, from http://www.cdc.gov/mmwr/preview/mmwrhtml/rr4912a1.htm

Centers for Disease Control and Prevention (CDC). (2001). *Clean Indoor Air Regulations, Fact Sheet.* Retrieved March 26, 2003, from http://www.cdc.gov/tobacco/sgr/sgr_2000/factsheets/factsheet_2002clean.htm

Centers for Disease Control and Prevention (CDC). (2002). *Indiana Highlights.* Retrieved April 15, 2003, from http://www.cdc.gov/tobacco/statehi/html_2002/indiana.htm

National Cancer Institute (NCI). (2000). *Cancer Facts, Environmental Tobacco Smoke.* Retrieved April 5, 2003, from http://cis.nci.nih.gov/fact/3_9.htm

Smokefree Indiana (SFI). (2000). *Indiana Youth Tobacco Survey Report.* Retrieved April 5, 2003, from http://www.smokefreeindiana.org/pdf/IYTSExecSumm.pdf

Smokefree Indiana (SFI). (2003, March 3). Indiana smoking rate ranks high. *The Sublink.* Indianapolis, IN: Author.

Synergy. (1998). *Let's Talk Health '98.* Indianapolis, IN: Synergy.

U.S. Department of Health and Human Services (USDHHS). (2000). *Healthy People 2010 (CD-ROM Version).* Washington, DC: Author.

United States Department of Health and Human Services (USDHHS). (1994). *Preventing tobacco use among young people: A report of the Surgeon General.* Atlanta, GA: Author.

World Health Organization (WHO). (1998). *Tobacco Free Initiative.* Retrieved March 26, 2003, from http://www.who.int/tobacco/repsitory/stp84/30%20Map%206%20Cig.%20Consumption.pdf

EXAMPLE 2

A Rationale for "Mind, Body, and Soul": A Health Education Program at First Presbyterian Church, Muncie, IN[*]

The health status of Americans has improved greatly in the last 50 years as evidenced by the decrease in the number of cases of communicable disease, increased life expectancy, and the declining death rates (NCHS, 1997). However, the health status of Americans could be further improved if Americans were willing to make additional changes. We now know that better control of behavioral risk factors alone—such as lack of exercise, poor diet, use of tobacco and other drugs, and alcohol abuse—could prevent between 40% and 70% of all mature deaths, one-third of all acute disabilities, and two-thirds of chronic disabilities (USDHHS, 1990).

---

[*]This rationale was written by the undergraduate students enrolled in the program planning classes at Ball State University, Muncie, Indiana.

Closer to home, recent data also indicate that the health status of Hoosiers has improved but they too could do more to improve their health. In 1996, 32% of the adults (>17 years of age) in Indiana were overweight, 29% were current smokers, and 66% were classified as having a sedentary lifestyle (ISDH, 1998). The data from Indiana are also consistent with the data that were collected from the members of the adult education class, the Mariners, at First Presbyterian Church in Muncie, IN. The data collected using a health risk appraisal (HRA) (Healthier People Software, no date) and a health and spirituality questionnaire (developed by health science students from Ball State University) indicated that the Mariners were interested in educational programs on faith and its relationship to health, humor and healing, and stress management (including prayer as a means of stress reduction). In addition, there appears to be a need for or an interest in programs associated with aging (including Alzheimer's disease), the family, nutrition, weight control, and exercise.

It seems logical to try to address some of the health needs and interests of those in the Mariners class through the Christian Education program of the church. For a long time, religious organizations have functioned as "healing" institutions as evidenced by the mental health issues addressed through pastoral counseling (Ransdell & Rehling, 1996). The idea of addressing the health needs and interests of a priority population in combination with spiritual practices has been encouraged. "In recent years, both the validity of spiritual and religious practices as well as the potential to the overall health and well-being have not only been acknowledged by modern medicine, but encouraged as mechanisms for health enhancement" (Droege, 1996, p. 7). And further, it makes good sense to offer health related programs at church since the Bible "provides a very powerful foundation for the development of health programs within the spiritual framework of the church" (Jackson, 1991, pp. 8–9). In a more practical sense, religious organizations have a number of important potential advantages for involvement in health education/ promotion programs because religious organizations (1) tend to involve large numbers of entire families, (2) are often the center of the neighborhood and a natural gathering place, (3) have a long history of outreach and helping others, (4) often have a talented and multi-disciplinary membership, (5) have been found to be receptive to the efforts of primary prevention, and (6) have the facilities to accommodate such programs (Lasater, Carleton, & Wells, 1991). In addition, religious organizations are good settings for health education/promotion programs because when people attend they do so with the expectation of learning; religious organizations are accepted as educational institutions (Lasater, Carleton, & Wells, 1991). Consequently, the church is a natural community arena for health education/promotion programs that focus on behaviors that are then reinforced by the social support and social networks that exist in churches (Levin, Larson, & Puchalski, 1997; Thomas, Quinn, Billingsley, & Caldwell, 1994).

Several benefits can be anticipated from the Mind, Body, and Soul program offered at First Presbyterian Church. First and foremost, it should be expected that the Mariners class members will increase their knowledge about the topics presented. Such knowledge will be beneficial to both the Mariners class members and the people—family and friends—with whom they come in contact. Second, such a program will introduce participants to topics that have not been addressed before in the class. Third, the program will provide participants with an opportunity to apply spiritual and religious concepts to everyday living. And fourth, such a program may attract other members of the congregation to the Mariners class that have not attended in the past.

The Mind, Body, and Soul program for the First Presbyterian Church Mariners class has great potential for being successful for several reasons. First, as noted earlier, the Bible provides a solid base on which to build a health education/promotion program (Jackson, 1991). A number of the scriptures support the healing power of faith (Lloyd, 1994). Class members are interested in learning more about the Bible. Second, the majority of similar other church-based health promotion programs have been highly successful (Cook, 1993). And finally, the program will be well planned and will meet the needs and interests of the class members. Ransdell and Rehling (1996) have indicated that such programs have a better chance of being successful.

References

Cook, D. A. (1993). Research in African American churches: A mental health imperative. *Journal of Mental Health Counseling, 17:* 320–333.

Droege, T. (1996). Spirituality and healing. *Faith and Health,* Summer: 7.

Healthier People Software. (no date). *Healthier People: Health Risk Appraisal Program.* Memphis, TN: Author.

Indiana State Department of Health (ISDH). (1998). *Indiana Health Behavior Risk Factors.* Indianapolis, IN: Author.

Jackson, C. (1991). Healthy spirits, souls, and bodies. *Spirit of Truth,* June: 8–9.

Lasater, T. M., Carleton, R. A., & Wells, B. L. (1991). Religious organizations and large-scale health related lifestyle change programs. *Journal of Health Education, 22:* 233–239.

Levin, J. S., Larson, D. B., & Puchalski, C. M. (1997). Religion and spirituality in medicine: Research and Education. *The Journal of the American Medical Association, 278:* 792–793.

Lloyd, J. J. (1994). Collaborative health education training for African American health ministers and providers of community services. *Educational Gerontology, 20:* 265–276.

National Center for Health Statistics (NCHS). (1997). *Health, United States, 1996–97 and Injury Chartbook* (DHHS pub. no. PHS 97–1232). Hyattsville, MD: Author.

Ransdell, L. B., & Rehling, S. L. (1996). Church-based health promotion: A review of the current literature. *American Journal of Health Behavior, 20*(4): 195–207.

Thomas, S. B., Quinn, S. C., Billingsley, A., & Caldwell, C. (1994). The characteristics of northern black churches with community outreach programs. *American Journal of Public Health, 84:* 575–579.

U.S. Department of Health and Human Services (USDHHS). (1990). *Prevention '89/'90.* Washington, D.C.: U.S. Government Printing Office.

WEBLINKS

1. http://www.thecommunityguide.org/index.html

   Guide to Community Preventative Services

   This Webpage includes evidence-based recommendations for programs and policies to promote population-based health.

2. http://new.wellsteps.com/

   WellSteps

   This is the home page for WellSteps, a company that helps other companies create worksite wellness programs. At the site you will find a number of different resources that can assist you as you begin the planning process. One tool found at this site is the return on investment (ROI) calculator for health care costs [http://www.wellsteps .com/roi/resources_tools_roi_cal_health.php] that can help you determine if a health promotion for a company would make good economic sense.

3. **http://www.countyhealthrankings.org/**

   County Health Rankings

   At this Website you will find a set of reports that rank the overall health of every county in the United States. If you are planning county-wide programs you will find this to be a valuable resource when creating rationales. The *County Health Rankings* are a part of the Mobilizing Action Toward Community Health (MATCH) project, which is a collaboration between the Robert Wood Johnson Foundation and the University of Wisconsin Population Health Institute.

4. **http://www.astho.org**

   Association of State and Territorial Health Officials (ASTHO)

   ASTHO is the national nonprofit organization representing the state and territorial public health agencies of the United States, the U.S. Territories, and the District of Columbia. This Website has links to all the state and territorial health departments. If you are planning a program for the community setting, this site contains a lot of information that could help you develop a rationale for your program.

5. **http://www.census.gov/compendia/statab**

   U.S. Census Bureau

   This page at the U.S. Census Bureau Website provides information about the national data book called *Statistical Abstract of the United States*. The data book contains a collection of statistics on social and economic conditions in the United States. Selected international data are also included. The *Abstract* is also a guide to sources of other data from the Census Bureau, other federal agencies, and private organizations.

6. **http://www.welcoa.org/**

   Wellness Councils of America (WELCOA)

   WELCOA was established in 1987 as a national nonprofit membership organization dedicated to promoting healthier lifestyles for all Americans, especially through health promotion initiatives at the worksite. If you are planning a program for the worksite setting, this Website contains a lot of information that could help you develop a rationale for your program.

CHAPTER 3

Models for Program Planning in Health Promotion

After reading this chapter and answering the questions at the end, you should be able to:

- Explain the value of using a model in planning a program.
- Explain the value of the Generalized Model in particular.
- Identify key models in planning health promotion programs and briefly describe each.
- Identify the basic components of the planning models presented and how they relate to the Generalized Model.
- Apply a model to a program you are planning.

KEY TERMS

APEX-PH	healthy communities	PRECEDE-PROCEED
ecological framework	Healthy Plan-It	predisposing factors
enabling factors	intervention mapping	reinforcing factors
formative research	MAP-IT	SMART Model
Generalized Model	MAPP	SWOT
Health Communication Model	PATCH	three Fs of program planning
	population-based approach	

A key role, if not the central role, of the health education specialist is planning, implementing, and evaluating programs. **Box 3.1** identifies the responsibilities and competencies for health education specialists that pertain to the material presented in this chapter. Good health promotion programs are not created by chance; they are the product of coordinated effort and are usually based on a systematic planning model or approach. Planning models, which are visual representations and descriptions of steps or phases in the planning process are the means by which structure and organization are given to the successful development and delivery of health promotion programs.

Box 3.1 RESPONSIBILITIES AND COMPETENCIES FOR HEALTH
EDUCATION SPECIALISTS

This chapter covers planning models as well as other considerations and criteria
necessary to develop a planning sequence from start to finish. Responsibilities and
competencies that are connected with the content in this chapter include:

Responsibility II: Plan Health Education

Competency 2.1: Involve priority populations and other
stakeholders in the planning process

Competency 2.2: Develop goals and objectives

Competency 2.3: Select or design strategies and
interventions

Competency 2.4: Develop a scope and sequence for the
delivery of health education

Source: NCHEC, SOPHE, & AAHE (2010).

Models provide planners with direction and a framework from which to build interventions that can improve the health of individuals and communities.

Through the years, an array of planning models has been developed and presented with widely varying degrees of acceptance and use. Although these models tend to share common elements, they often label and describe these elements differently, giving the impression that something unique and useful has been offered. However, when new models emerge and appear novel, keep in mind they are probably more similar to existing models than different and unique. For this reason, we use what we call the *Generalized Model* to teach basic principles of planning and evaluation emphasized in most planning models. With this as a backdrop, it is important to note that the Generalized Model is not a new model either but rather a composite of what is represented in most, if not all other models.

As illustrated in **Figure 3.1**, the Generalized Model consists of five basic elements or steps: (1) assessing needs; (2) setting goals and objectives; (3) developing interventions; (4) implementing interventions; and (5) evaluating results. In addition, pre-planning is a quasi-step in the model but is not included formally since it involves actions that occur before planning technically begins. The first step in the Generalized Model, assessing needs, is the process of collecting and analyzing data to determine the health needs of a population and can include priority setting and the identification of a priority population. Setting goals and objectives identifies *what* will be accomplished while interventions or programs are the means by which the goals and objectives will be achieved (i.e., the how). Implementation is the process of putting interventions into action and evaluation focuses on improving the quality of interventions (formative evaluation) as well as determining their effectiveness (summative evaluation). Collectively, these steps define planning and evaluation at its core. To illustrate how planning models in general are aligned with the steps outlined in the Generalized Model, we briefly describe how certain models have evolved over the last few decades.

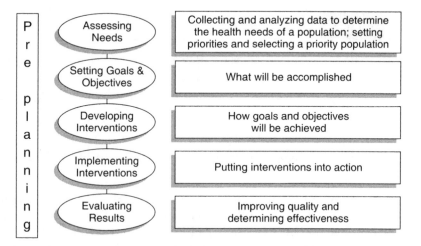

Figure 3.1 The Generalized Model

In 1983, the Centers for Disease Control and Prevention (CDC) introduced **PATCH**, or Planned Approach to Community Health, as its planning model of preference to be used in partnership with state and local health departments and local communities (Lancaster & Kreuter, 2002). **Box 3.2** displays the steps or phases of the PATCH model. Note the similarities between the PATCH model and the Generalized Model. PATCH begins by mobilizing the community and is represented by what we have previously described as pre-planning. Both models collect and organize data (needs assessment), both choose priorities and select priority populations (needs assessment), both select and implement interventions, and both conduct evaluations.

In 1987, a new model, **APEX-PH** (Assessment Protocol for Excellence in Public Health) emerged as a cooperative project among several prominent public health organizations including the CDC, the American Public Health Association (APHA), and the National Association of County and City Health Officials (NACCHO) (NACCHO, 1991). APEX-PH was designed specifically for local health departments to engage in the planning and evaluation process. **Box 3.3** displays the steps/phases of the APEX-PH model. In essence, this model involves data collection (needs assessment), developing and implementing an action plan (interventions), and performing evaluation. APEX-PH does basically the same thing as PATCH and both models do the same thing as the Generalized Model.

Box 3.2   PHASES IN THE PATCH MODEL

Phase 1	Mobilizing the Community
Phase 2	Collecting and Organizing Data
Phase 3	Choosing Health Priorities and Target Groups
Phase 4	Choosing and Conducting Interventions
Phase 5	Evaluating the PATCH Process and Interventions

Box 3.3   PHASES IN THE APEX-PH MODEL

Phase 1	Organizational Capacity Assessment (Internal Assessment of Strengths)
Phase 2	The Community Process:
	Collection and Analysis of Community Health Status Data
	Collection and Analysis of Community Opinion Data
	Development of an Action Plan with Goals and Objectives
Phase 3	Completing the Cycle (Implementation Plan and Evaluation Plan)

Beginning in 1997, the CDC and NACCHO collaborated on the development of a new model and in 2000 released the **MAPP** model—Mobilizing for Action through Planning and Partnerships (NACCHO, 2001). In essence, the MAPP model replaced APEX-PH as a foundational approach to planning and evaluation. **Box 3.4** displays steps in the MAPP process. Starting with organizing for success and visioning (i.e., pre-planning), the MAPP model guides planners through four needs assessments, which lead to the identification of strategic issues, then formulation of goals and objectives, and finally the action cycle (implementing interventions and evaluation) (see Figure 3.4 later in the chapter). Again, these steps are very consistent with the Generalized Model.

More recently, in December 2010, *Healthy People 2020*, a national planning framework, was released to help guide public health and health promotion planning efforts for the next decade (USDHHS, 2011c). **Box 3.5** displays a planning guide entitled **MAP-IT**

Box 3.4   PHASES OF MAPP

Phase 1	Organizing for Success and Partnership Development
Phase 2	Visioning
Phase 3	Four MAPP Assessments
Phase 4	Identify Strategic Issues
Phase 5	Formulate Goals and Strategies
Phase 6	Action Cycle

Box 3.5   PHASES IN MAP-IT

Phase 1	Mobilize
Phase 2	Assess
Phase 3	Plan
Phase 4	Implement
Phase 5	Track

(mobilize, assess, plan, implement, and track), introduced as a way to assist communities in implementing their own adaptations of *Healthy People 2020*. The steps in MAP-IT are nearly identical to the other models that have been introduced over the last 30 years as well as the Generalized Model.

As you can see, the Generalized Model represents what is displayed in all of these other models. PATCH, APEX-PH, MAPP, and MAP-IT are all theoretically good models and can each be used to successfully plan, implement, and evaluate programs. The same could be said for dozens of other models, some of which are presented later in this chapter. However, if the disciplines of health education and health promotion could streamline the planning process with a model that establishes a common framework with universally accepted labels and definitions, practitioners could consistently engage in the same process regardless of place or setting. This might allow for better measurement and reporting of the key steps associated with planning and evaluation, and more importantly, improvement in our ability to engage in the process. For these reasons, we promote the use of the Generalized Model.

In practice, most planners will encounter situations where it is not feasible to use a model in its entirety or when it is necessary to combine parts of different models to meet specific needs. What is most critical for any student, practicing health education specialist, or planner is a working knowledge of the basic steps that guide any model or planning approach. The two most significant challenges you will face in planning efforts are: (1) the preferences of stakeholders for a planning model or approach; and (2) interpersonal conflicts among stakeholders. Careful study of the Generalized Model will help you address the first challenge.

Understanding the Generalized Model will help you adapt and respond to complex planning tasks you will experience in professional practice. With planning expertise associated with your working knowledge of the Generalized Model, you will be able to both lead planning processes and educate other stakeholders about the basic sequence of the planning process. Even though at first glance most models look linear (i.e., one step leads to the next), in practice, the steps outlined in the Generalized Model get blended as practitioners skip back and forth between tasks. Thus, knowledge and familiarity with the Generalized Model and the basic principles of planning and evaluation will help you quickly assimilate and interpret varying or competing stakeholder preferences for planning into a guiding paradigm that will generally keep you on track. Although there is nothing unique about the Generalized Model itself, its principles are the building blocks for all other models and actually represent the foundation of health education and health promotion practice.

Another benefit of understanding the Generalized Model is an increased ability to apply an important process closely related to program planning—grant writing. Requirements listed in *requests for applications* (RFAs) or *requests for proposals* (RFPs) related to grant announcements will be developed by the funding agency/organization and include their preferences for language and terminology. But the steps or requirements related to requests for health funding almost always relate back to the steps displayed in the Generalized Model.

For example, funding requests from the CDC and other federal or national organizations generally require applicants to organize proposals with the following types of sections: background and statement of need; work plan; management plan; evaluation; and budget. These sections parallel closely with the Generalized Model: the background and statement of need relate to the needs assessment; the work plan includes goals and objectives as well as a description of interventions; and the management plan generally includes requirements for program implementation. The Community Tool Box (see Weblinks at the end of this chapter), a Website designed to assist health professionals with various tasks, outlines the standard components of a grant proposal. Sections include the statement of the problem/ needs assessment; project description (goals and objectives and methods/activities); the evaluation plan; and the budget request and justification (University of Kansas, 2011b).

Clearly, understanding the basic steps of program planning as presented in the Generalized Model or the other planning models used in health promotion have broader benefit than just understanding principles related to program planning. A serious study of program planning models in general will help prepare you with key skills necessary to perform your work in health promotion.

Pay particular attention to the models presented in this chapter and see how they integrate the basic elements from the Generalized Model in one form or another. With an understanding and appreciation for the steps presented in this chapter, all planning models will become much easier to use in health promotion settings. Then, when you need to make adjustments in the middle of a planning process, you will be able to identify and preserve the critical planning components.

In practice, selecting a specific planning model to apply will be based on many factors: (1) the preferences of stakeholders (e.g., decision makers, program partners, consumers); (2) how much time and funding are available for planning purposes; (3) how many resources are available for data collection and analysis; (4) the degree to which clients are actually involved as partners in the planning process or the degree to which your planning efforts will be consumer oriented (i.e., planning is largely based on the wants and needs of consumers or the planning process is owned by the community itself); and (5) preferences of a funding agency (in the case of a grant or contract award). Planners must have the capacity to not only lead a planning process, but also negotiate these important issues with and among a diverse set of stakeholders.

Three important criteria, or the **three Fs of program planning:** *fluidity, flexibility,* and *functionality,* should also help guide the selection of your model and govern the application of its use. *Fluidity* suggests that steps in the planning process are sequential, or that they build on one another. It is usually a problem if certain steps in the planning process are performed out of sequence as diagrammed in the Generalized Model. For example, a planner cannot develop goals and objectives until a needs assessment has been performed and a priority health problem has been identified.

Flexibility means that planning is adapted to the needs of stakeholders. Due to various circumstances, planning is usually modified as the process unfolds. For example, some health problems, such as an outbreak of influenza, require a rapid assessment and scan of the environment. Strict adherence to a model in light of unique and pressing circumstances will generally lead to frustration among partners and a less-than-desirable outcome. *Functionality* means that the outcome of planning is improved health conditions, not the production of a program plan itself. A model is only a tool to help planners accomplish their real work—to enhance health and decrease disease and disability.

In addition to the *three Fs,* when deciding on a planning model, it is also important to ensure that the model is conducive to planning a **population-based approach** and that it uses an **ecological framework**. Whereas systematic and strategic planning efforts can address smaller populations such as those found in a small community or worksite, many planning processes, due to costs and other resources, usually pertain to large population segments of even larger populations—thus the term *population-based approach.*

Planners must also understand the interaction between a priority population and the communities in which they live. The ecological framework helps planners better appreciate that families, schools, employers, social networks, organizations, communities, and societies exert an influence on individuals and priority populations as they attempt to change health behaviors and improve their health (Bartholomew et al., 2011). Thus, planners must work with priority populations within the context of broad environments.

In addition, during pre-planning, planners need to determine the extent to which members of the priority population will be involved in the planning process and in decision making. This varies widely in practice and may range from no community involvement on one end of a continuum to an approach like community-based partici- patory research where the community itself owns the program and is the unit of iden- tity, solution, and practice involved in all aspects of program development and delivery (Trickett, 2011). Ideally, planning efforts in health promotion should use a partnership- based approach in the context of community empowerment and mobilization where professionals work in unison with community members in taking actions to improve health and reduce disease.

The remainder of this chapter will provide an example of how the Generalized Model could hypothetically operate in practice and also present a few other prominent models used by planners in health promotion settings including PRECEDE-PROCEED; MAPP and MAP-IT (as previously introduced); and SMART. These models represent a wide range of planning approaches even though they share elements displayed in the Generalized Model. Still other models, each of which may be just as good from theoretical or practical perspec- tives, will be briefly presented and referenced.

Generalized Model

To help you better understand how the Generalized Model might work in practice, we will use a hypothetical example to walk you through its five steps. Of course, in practice, stakeholders may choose a different approach than what is presented here. But at least you can see how the steps in the model build upon each other.

Let's assume Jane Doe, CHES, a recent health promotion graduate, has just been hired by a medium-sized county health department in California. She has been asked to lead a planning process to identify a health problem that will become the health department's key priority for the next three years. As daunting as this might seem to a new professional, it is not out of the realm of possibility.

The first thing Jane decides to do is some pre-planning. She sets out to identify key stakeholders who can help guide the process as well as partners who will actually help her carry out the work. She organizes a few meetings with stakeholders to discuss the collec- tive vision for the process including purpose, scope, and deliverables as well as the leader- ship structure (i.e., authority, roles, and responsibilities). She ensures that five partners are community residents who have volunteered previously with the health department and can help represent the community in general. Jane begins discussions with her partners to identify and secure resources to be able to implement a program once a priority health problem and priority population have been identified. Although Jane realizes she does not need to spend months or even weeks pre-planning, she also understands the value of getting all stakeholders on the same path with respect to vision, leadership, and resources. This will help ensure a more positive and successful planning approach.

The actual planning and evaluation process begins with a *needs assessment*. Stakeholders determine together that they will collect data in three main categories: chronic diseases, infectious diseases, and injuries. Three teams are assembled to address each of the categories and each team is charged with identifying 8–10 leading health problems or diseases within the three categories. Teams agree to use a recent data report produced by the California Department of Health Services (organized by county) that describes leading causes of mortality, morbidity, and hospitalizations to select the 8–10 health problems for each of the categories. Stakeholders further determine that they will collect the following types of data for each of the 8–10 health problems: county-specific mortality and morbidity data; hospital discharge data; economic data; years of potential life lost; disability data; data on disparities; social determinants and risk factors for each health problem; and evidence of successful interventions that relate to the preventable nature of each health problem. The planning team decides on a presentation template for each health problem that includes graphs as well as brief descriptions for each of the predetermined criteria. The three planning teams decide to allow two months to collect and organize all the data.

After two months have passed, all three teams come together to compile all of their work in a single report and to make an oral presentation of their findings. Afterward, Jane and the five community residents are given the assignment to use the basic priority rating (BPR) model (Neiger, Thackeray, & Fagen, 2011) to narrow the list of health problems within each category to five (see Chapter 4 for BPR). Jane serves as the moderator of priority setting to make sure everyone understands the process. Within a week, five chronic diseases (heart disease, breast cancer, lung cancer, diabetes, and arthritis), five infectious diseases (HIV/AIDS, pneumonia, chlamydia, E.coli, and meningitis), as well as five unintentional injuries (falls, drownings, motor vehicle injuries, bicycle crashes, and auto-pedestrian injuries) surface as leading health problems in the county.

After preliminary priority setting, the group of stakeholders decides it would like to supplement its needs assessment with a series of focus groups throughout the county to determine what community residents feel are the most significant health problems among the initial priorities. Stakeholders decide to hire an evaluation firm to conduct 20 focus groups across the county and prepare a report. The final bid for services is $8,500, which the community outreach office of a local hospital agrees to pay.

As the evaluation firm begins to organize and conduct focus groups, stakeholders use the BPR model to further prioritize the remaining 15 health problems. Jane leads all discussions but is assisted by a program coordinator from the local chapter of the American Cancer Society who has years of experience in health promotion and some experience with the BPR model. It takes the group two additional meetings to develop a list of their top five priorities: (1) motor vehicle injuries; (2) heart disease; (3) breast cancer; (4) chlamydia; and (5) diabetes.

Within a month, the contracted evaluation team returns with its findings from the focus groups. Data indicate that the community believes effective prevention should start with children and adolescents and that the county should focus on childhood obesity as a risk factor for heart disease as well as the prevention of sexually transmitted diseases (i.e., chlamydia) among adolescents.

With these findings, Jane and her stakeholders are faced with a difficult decision. The BPR model and process produced a convincing case that motor vehicle injuries should be the county's top priority. But community residents are not in agreement. After thoughtful deliberation, stakeholders decide to develop a safe driving program among high school students throughout the county as well as a childhood obesity prevention program among elementary and junior high students. They further decide to create two planning teams for each of the priorities, with each team taking responsibility for grant writing and funding in general. The teams are also tasked to identify appropriate partners with specific expertise and resources in each of the two priority areas.

With health problems and priority populations identified, each newly formed team develops *goals and objectives* for each of the two priorities. Using *Healthy People* 2020 as a starting point, the teams develop general goals for each of the priorities as well as process, impact, and outcome objectives. The teams carefully develop their baseline measurements (i.e., starting points) for each objective based on the data collected in the needs assessment. Again, using the targets in *Healthy People 2020*, each team develops its own targets for each objective, ensuring that each one is specific, measurable, achievable, realistic, and time-phased.

With goals and objectives developed, the planning teams turn to *developing the interventions*, the third step in the Generalized Model. Here, planners need to determine if they will use existing programs and tailor them to their priority population or develop their own programs. Jane remembers from her undergraduate coursework that interventions need to be evidence-based. She works with both teams to ensure that the interventions selected will offer a high probability of success. In the end, the childhood obesity team decides to adapt a program from Utah entitled *Gold Medal Schools*. This program is selected for its successful track record and its multifaceted approach combining educational components with policies leading to healthy school environments. The safe driving team selects a program called *Driving School Home*, a successful defensive driving course involving high school students from Illinois. Both teams then begin the process of fully understanding their programs and drafting budgets, including an analysis of how many staff members and volunteers would be required to implement each program, how much funding would be required to purchase program materials or capital equipment, and how much money might be required for consultants. Program protocols are available for each program and in a matter of weeks, both teams feel they understand the basic sequence of tasks and activities required to implement each program.

The fourth phase of the Generalized Model, *implementing interventions*, is focused on delivering interventions to the community. Before implementation occurs however, both teams begin to lay the necessary groundwork with school personnel to establish partnerships and to receive approval to proceed as planned. This becomes more complicated than Jane had anticipated. However, protocols and policies previously developed by the various school districts need to be observed. For example, one thing all school districts require is that each program be implemented on a pilot basis first to determine whether the likelihood of success is high enough to justify full implementation of the programs on a broader basis. In total, this process takes three months. But afterward, strong partnerships are established and implementation is approved for each program.

Implementation is equivalent to program management. In this phase, program partners ensure that programs are implemented as per predetermined protocol. Regular meetings are held to ensure that everyone is doing his/her job as planned. Managers follow up with their staff and make sure that timelines are carefully followed and that monies from approved budgets are accessible for program support. Implementation also focuses on marketing and communication. It is important that an adequate number of members from the priority population is reached and that enough people actually participate in the programs. Jane and her teams conduct in-depth interviews with school administrators to understand how to best communicate the purpose of the programs to potential participants (e.g., schools, students, and parents).

Jane helps to coordinate all the work of implementation and discovers that it takes a great deal of assertiveness and diplomacy to keep people moving forward on schedule. She also learns that certain aspects of both programs need to be modified in the process of implementation in order to increase the likelihood of their success. Toward the end of year one of implementation, Jane realizes that while neither program was implemented perfectly, both programs are running smoothly with continued enthusiasm and support.

During program implementation, Jane, along with two colleagues from the county health department conduct formative evaluation to ensure that the quality of program components and implementation are being presented as planned and that modifications are made continually to improve the likelihood of success. This also proves to be a challenge for Jane. During the course of implementing the *Driving School Home* program, she has to replace an ineffective teacher. As the *Gold Medal Schools* program is evaluated, Jane discovers that the kick-off assembly is too long and that both teachers and students are losing attention. As the assembly is shortened by 20 minutes and more incentives and small prizes are distributed, everyone feels more energized. These come to represent just a few of the many program improvements that are made during year one.

In addition, both teams had decided prior to implementation that outcome evaluation, which would measure both changes in behavior as well as decreases in the actual health problems, would be conducted by faculty and graduate students from a nearby university. University personnel were willing to conduct the research at no cost, providing they could use all data for publications in scientific journals. While the researchers required certain things of Jane and her partners, it became a win-win situation in the end. The researchers collected data immediately after the programs concluded and then again at three months after the conclusion of the programs. Data indicated that the *Gold Medal Schools* program was moderately effective and that the *Driving School Home* program was moderately to highly effective. Jane communicated to stakeholders that the programs were more likely to experience higher levels of success in future implementations based on continual improvements as part of formative and process evaluation. After data had been collected and analyzed, Jane made several presentations to stakeholders reporting on what went well and what went poorly. These presentations helped ensure continued funding for both programs.

To reiterate, the preceding example could have played out in many different ways based on the vision and competency of those leading the planning efforts. The purpose of the example was to describe how the phases in the Generalized Model might unfold. As you now read about other key planning models, it may be easier for you to see how these same phases are evident in the other models.

PRECEDE-PROCEED

"PRECEDE is an acronym for *p*redisposing, *r*einforcing, and *e*nabling *c*onstructs in *e*ducational/*e*cological *d*iagnosis and *e*valuation" (Green & Kreuter, 2005, p. 9). "PROCEED stands for *p*olicy, *r*egulatory, and *o*rganizational *c*onstructs in *e*ducational and *e*nvironmental *d*evelopment" (Green & Kreuter, 2005, p. 9).

The first half of the model, PRECEDE, "consists of a series of planned assessments that generate information that will be used to guide subsequent decisions" (Green & Kreuter, 2005, p. 8). The second half of the model, PROCEED, "is marked by the strategic implementation of multiple actions based on what was learned from the assessments in the initial phase" (Green & Kreuter, 2005, p. 9).

The Eight Phases of PRECEDE-PROCEED

As displayed in **Figure 3.2**, PRECEDE-PROCEED is composed of eight phases or steps. The underlying approach **of this model is to begin by** identifying the desired outcome, to determine what causes it, and finally to design an intervention aimed at reaching the desired outcome. In other words, PRECEDE-PROCEED begins with the final consequences and works backward to the causes. Once the causes are known, an intervention can be designed.

Phase 1 in the model is called *social assessment and situational analysis* and seeks to subjectively define the quality of life (problems and priorities) of those in the priority population while involving individuals in the priority population in an assessment of their own needs and aspirations. Some of the social indicators of quality of life include achievement, alienation, comfort, crime, discrimination, happiness, self-esteem, unemployment, and welfare.

Phase 2, *epidemiological assessment*, is the step in which the planners use data to identify and rank the health goals or problems that may contribute to or interact with problems identified in Phase 1. These data include traditional vital indicators (e.g., mortality, morbidity, and disability data) as well as genetic, behavioral, and environmental factors (Green & Kreuter, 2005) and represent a traditional needs assessment. It is important to note that ranking the health problems in this phase is critical, because there are rarely, if ever, enough resources to deal with all or multiple problems. Also, this phase of the model is used to plan health programs. Note that in Figure 3.2, arrows connect the genetics, behavior, and environment boxes of Phase 2 with the health box of Phase 2 and with Phase 1.

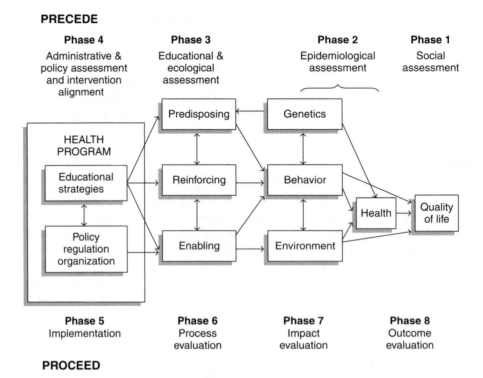

Figure 3.2 PRECEDE-PROCEED Model for Health Promotion Planning and Evaluation

Source: Health Promotion Planning. Lawrence W. Green and Marshall W. Kreuter. Copyright © 2005 by McGraw-Hill. Reprinted with permission.

Once identified, the risk factors or conditions related to broader health problems need to be prioritized. This can be accomplished by first ranking these factors by importance and changeability and then using the 2 × 2 matrix presented in **Figure 3.3**.

Phase 3, *educational and ecological assessment*, identifies and classifies the various factors that have the potential to influence a given behavior into three categories: predisposing, reinforcing, and enabling. **Predisposing factors** include knowledge and many affective traits such as a person's attitude, values, beliefs, and perceptions. These factors can facilitate or hinder a person's motivation to change and can be altered through direct communication. Barriers or facilitators created mainly by societal forces or systems make up **enabling factors,** which include access to health care facilities or other health-related services, availability of resources, referrals to appropriate providers, transportation, negotiation and problem-solving skills, among others. **Reinforcing factors** involve the different types of feedback and rewards that those in the priority population receive after behavior change, which may either encourage or discourage the continuation of the behavior. Reinforcing behaviors can be delivered by, but not limited to, family, friends, peers, teachers, self, and others who control rewards. "Social benefits—such as recognition, appreciation, or admiration; physical benefits such as convenience, comfort,

	More important	Less important
More changeable	High priority for program focus (Quadrant 1)	Low priority except to demonstrate change for political purposes (Quadrant 3)
Less changeable	Priority for innovative program; evaluation crucial (Quadrant 2)	No program (Quadrant 4)

Figure 3.3 Prioritization Matrix

Source: Health Promotion Planning. Lawrence W. Green and Marshall W. Kreuter. Copyright © 1999 by McGraw-Hill. Reprinted with permission.

relief of discomfort, or pain; tangible rewards such as economic benefits or avoidance of cost; and self-actualizing, imagined, or vicarious rewards such as improved appearance, self-respect, or association with an admired person who demonstrates the behavior—all reinforce behavior" (Green & Kreuter, 2005, p. 15).

Phase 4 comprises two parts: (1) *intervention alignment*; and (2) *administrative and policy assessment.* The intent of intervention alignment is to match appropriate strategies and interventions with projected changes and outcomes identified in earlier phases (Green & Kreuter, 2005). In administration and policy assessment, planners determine if the capabilities and resources are available to develop and implement the program. It is between Phases 4 and 5 that PRECEDE (the assessment portion of the model) ends and PROCEED (implementation and evaluation) begins. However, there is no distinct break between the two phases; they really run together, and planners can move back and forth between them.

The four final phases of the model—Phases 5, 6, 7, and 8—make up the PROCEED portion. In Phase 5—*implementation*—with appropriate resources in hand, planners select the interventions and strategies and implementation begins. Phases 6, 7, and 8 focus on the *process, impact,* and *outcome evaluation,* respectively, and are based on the earlier phases of the model, when objectives were outlined in the assessment process. Whether all three of these final phases are used depends on the evaluation requirements of the program. Usually, the resources needed to conduct evaluations of impact (Phase 7) and outcome (Phase 8) are much greater than those needed to conduct process evaluation (Phase 6).

Mobilizing for Action through Planning and Partnerships (MAPP)

As described earlier, Mobilizing for Action through Planning and Partnerships *(MAPP)* was developed by the National Association of County and City Health Officials (NACCHO). As such, it represents a planning approach especially appropriate for city or county health departments (e.g., local health departments). The vision for implementing the MAPP approach involves improving health and quality of life through mobilized partnerships and taking strategic action (NACCHO, 2001). **Figure 3.4** displays the six phases of MAPP as well as the four MAPP assessments.

MAPP is composed of multiple steps in six general phases. In the first phase of MAPP, *Organizing for Success and Partnership Development,* core planners assess whether the MAPP process is timely, appropriate, or even possible. This involves assessing resources (including budgets), the expertise of available personnel, support of key decision makers and other stakeholders, and general interest of community members. If resources are not in place, the process is not undertaken. If the decision is made to proceed with a MAPP process, the following work groups are created: (1) a core support team, which prepares most, if not all of the material needed for the process; (2) the MAPP committee, composed of key sponsors (usually influential figures from the private sector who lend support and other resources) and stakeholders who guide and oversee the process; and (3) the community itself, which provides input, representation, and decision making. This phase answers basic questions about the general feasibility, resources, and appropriateness of the MAPP process.

Phase 2 of the MAPP process, *Visioning,* guides the community through a process that results in a shared vision (what the ideal future looks like) and common values (principles and beliefs that will guide the remainder of the planning process) (NACCHO, 2001). Generally, a facilitator conducts the visioning process and involves anywhere

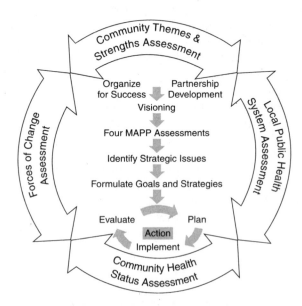

Figure 3.4 Display of the Six Phases of MAPP as Well as the Four MAPP Assessments

Source: Achieving Healthier Communities through MAPP: A User's Handbook. Copyright © 2009 by the National Association of County and City Health Officials. Reprinted with permission.

from 50 to 100 participants including the advisory committee, the MAPP committee, and key community leaders. This process is typical of what should occur in pre-planning.

Phase 3, the *Four MAPP Assessments,* represent the defining characteristic of the MAPP model. The four assessments include (1) the community themes and strengths assessment (community or consumer opinion), (2) the local public health assessment (general capacity of the local health department), (3) the community health status assessment (measurement of the health of the community by use of epidemiologic data), and (4) the forces of change assessment (forces such as legislation, technology, and other environmental or social phenomena that do or will impact the community). Collectively, the MAPP assessments provide insight on the gaps that exist between current status in the community and what was learned in the visioning phase as well as strategic direction for goals and strategies (NACCHO, 2001). The MAPP assessments provide an excellent framework for the types of data collection that should be part of any comprehensive needs assessment.

In Phase 4 of MAPP, *Identify Strategic Issues,* a prioritized list of the most important issues facing the health of the community is developed. Only issues that jeopardize the vision and values of the community are considered. Important tasks in this phase include consideration of what would happen if certain issues were not addressed, understanding why an issue is strategic, consolidating overlapping issues, and identifying a prioritized list. Phase 5, *Formulate Goals and Strategies,* creates goals related to the vision and priority strategic issues. It also selects and adopts strategies. This phase is not unlike similar phases in the models that have already been discussed in this chapter. Finally, Phase 6, the *Action Cycle,* is similar to implementation and evaluation phases in the Generalized Model and other planning models. In this phase, implementation details are considered, evaluation plans (gathering credible evidence) are developed, and plans for disseminating results are made (NACCHO, 2001).

MAP-IT

As briefly described earlier, MAP-IT is a planning guide or model used to assist communities in adapting *Healthy People 2020* at the state or local level (see Box 3.5). As mentioned, the five phases of MAP-IT are nearly identical to the Generalized Model.

MAP-IT starts by mobilizing key individuals and organizations into a coalition that can work together to improve the health of the community (USDHHS, 2011c). Once partners are identified and the coalition is organized, roles are established for each partner and responsibilities are assigned. These responsibilities may include facilitating community input through meetings and other events, developing and presenting educational and/or training programs, leading fundraising or policy initiatives, and providing technical assistance in planning or evaluation (U.S. Department of Health and Human Services, 2011a). In essence, the *mobilize* phase of MAP-IT is the same thing as pre-planning.

The second phase of MAP-IT is *assess* which is the equivalent of a needs assessment. This phase directs planners to ask and answer questions such as: (1) who is affected by key health problems in our community? (2) what resources do we have to address the problems that we identify?; and (3) what resources are required to have a meaningful impact? This phase of the model examines both the problems as well as the assets within a community to help planners focus on what the community can do versus what it would like to do (U.S. Department of Health and Human Services, 2011a).

In the *assess* phase both state and local data are collected and analyzed to help coalition members set priorities. In addition, the MAP-IT model directs planners to examine the social determinants, or root causes of the problems associated with the data collected. This might include an investigation of how the physical or social environments affect the health of the community, how a lack of access to health services contributes to death and illness, and how individual behavior as well as biology and genetics affect the health issues identified as priorities.

The third phase of MAP-IT, *plan*, involves developing goals and objectives, measures, baselines, and targets. This means that as part of the objectives that are developed, planners will determine what will be measured (e.g., a decrease in smoking among adults), the baseline (e.g., percent of adults who currently smoke in the community), and the targeted decrease (e.g., a decrease of three percent in five years). In this phase, planners also identify the specific interventions that will be used to accomplish the identified goals and objectives. This means addressing the following questions: (1) "what do we need to do to reach our goals?" and (2) "how will we know when we have reached our goals?" This phase is the equivalent of developing goals and objectives and interventions in the Generalized Model.

The fourth phase in MAP-IT, *implement*, involves organizing the coalition so it can put the plan into action. Here, a detailed work plan, including all of the information developed in Phase 3, is assembled to identify clear action steps, describe who is responsible for completing the action steps, and display a timeline with related deadlines. A communication plan is also produced in this phase to outline how program partners will reach and recruit participants and communicate the benefits of engaging in the program.

The final phase of MAP-IT, *track*, is the equivalent of evaluation. Here, coalition partners ask and answer specific questions such as: Are we evaluating our work appropriately (i.e., formative evaluation)? Did we follow the plan (i.e., process evaluation)? What did we change (i.e., impact evaluation)? And, did we reach our goal (i.e., outcome evaluation) (USDHHS, 2011c)? MAP-IT encourages regular evaluations to measure and track progress over time and draws special attention to the quality of data being collected, the limitations of self-reported data, and the validity and reliability of data collected (USDHHS, 2011c). Progress on the impact of related interventions is shared often with stakeholders (USDHHS, 2011c).

SMART

Although most planning models try to involve members of the priority population in the planning process at some level and some go so far as to incorporate consumer data (see MAPP for a good example), planning models such as **SMART** (Social Marketing Assessment and Response Tool (Neiger & Thackeray, 1998), with a social marketing focus, generally do a better job of orienting program interventions to the preferences of consumers throughout the entire planning process (see Chapter 11 for more information on marketing/social marketing). Consumer data are collected continually, first to understand the wants and needs of consumers and then to test all aspects of intervention and

Box 3.6 THE SMART MODEL

Phase 1: Preliminary Planning

- Identify a health problem and name it in terms of behavior.
- Develop general goals.
- Outline preliminary plans for evaluation.
- Project program costs.

Phase 2: Consumer Analysis

- Segment and identify the priority population.
- Identify formative research methods.
- Identify consumer wants, needs, and preferences.
- Develop preliminary ideas for preferred interventions.

Phase 3: Market Analysis

- Establish and define the market mix (4Ps).
- Assess the market to identify competitors (behaviors, messages, programs, etc.), allies (support systems, resources, etc.), and partners.

Phase 4: Channel Analysis

- Identify appropriate communication messages, strategies, and channels.
- Assess options for program distribution.
- Identify communication roles for program partners.
- Determine how channels should be used.

Phase 5: Develop Interventions, Materials, and Pretest

- Develop program interventions and materials using information collected in consumer, market, and channel analyses.
- Interpret the marketing mix into a strategy that represents exchange and societal good.
- Pretest and refine the program.

Phase 6: Implementation

- Communicate with partners and clarify involvement.
- Activate communication and distribution strategies.
- Document procedures and compare progress to time lines.
- Refine the program.

Phase 7: Evaluation

- Assess the degree to which the priority population is receiving the program.
- Assess the immediate impact on the priority population and refine the program as necessary.
- Ensure that program delivery is consistent with established protocol.
- Analyze changes in the priority population.

Source: Adapted from Walsh et al. (1993) by Neiger & Thackeray (1998).

communication strategies. There is some evidence to suggest that this planning approach may be more effective than traditional approaches used in health promotion (Neiger & Thackeray, 2002).

The SMART model, influenced primarily by Walsh and colleagues (1993), is also a composite of several social marketing planning frameworks but differs from most planning models used in health promotion settings due to its multistep focus on the consumer. Unlike some social marketing planning models, SMART has been used from start to finish in successful social marketing interventions (Neiger & Thackeray, 2002).

As displayed in **Box 3.6**, SMART is composed of seven phases. Like other social marketing planning models, the central focus of SMART is consumers. The heart of this model, composed of Phases 2 through 4, pertains to acquiring a broad understanding of the consumers who will be the recipients of a program and its interventions. These three phases seek to understand consumers before interventions are developed or implemented. Though these phases (2–4) are displayed in linear fashion, and for clarity will be described in sequence, they are typically performed simultaneously with members of the priority population.

The Phases of SMART

Preliminary Planning is critical for any type of health promotion program and in this model includes the planning elements of pre-planning and needs assessment as described earlier. Preliminary planning allows program planners to objectively assess all health problems and determine which one is most appropriate to address. This is most often accomplished through analysis of epidemiologic data, including various mortality and morbidity rates and associated risk factor data. It also includes objective priority setting with predetermined criteria. Sometimes planners do not undergo a process to select a priority health problem because the decision has already been made or the organization is dedicated to a specific health problem (e.g., the American Heart Association). Once a single health problem is determined, it is defined in terms of behaviors. Risk factors, or contributing factors, then become the focus of the social marketing process. This is similar to most health promotion programs.

Some social marketing practitioners and those who engage in community-based participatory research would argue that the priority population itself should determine the focus of an intervention or program. Good arguments can be made for this approach, including the idea that priority populations are capable of identifying their own problems and solutions and that they will be more vested in long-term involvement if they have ownership in the process. The SMART model suggests that planners, as trained health professionals, have both the expertise and responsibility to use various data sets to oversee and determine priority health problems within a community in partnership with members of the priority population. Once a priority or priorities are identified, the remainder of the process becomes almost exclusively consumer driven.

While health professionals may determine initial program direction, the SMART model directs that consumers drive the development and implementation of interventions. This is not unlike most ventures in commercial marketing where a product or service is developed internally then tested with consumers and modified prior to distribution. For example, a company such as Coca Cola develops its own identity and mission and creates the basic essence of its products (e.g., soft drinks). But it engages in complex marketing campaigns to better understand how to modify, improve, position, and deliver these products to its consumers in a way that offers benefits at reasonable costs.

Although goals are outlined in Phase 1, objectives are not. This makes sense from a social marketing perspective, since consumer research has not yet been performed. The goals are general statements of intent or direction, but they do not specify program components or direct the planner into specific courses of action.

Another task in Phase 1 is to develop preliminary plans for evaluation. Theoretically, it will make sense to most planners to consider evaluation early in the planning process. In reality, evaluation is too often an afterthought. Preliminary decisions regarding evaluation outcomes must be made early in the planning process in order to account for personnel, time, and budget requirements. Therefore, it is also important to determine how baseline and post-program (posttest) data will be collected and to identify valid survey or data collection instruments. Planners can also control for various kinds of bias or error in data collection if these basic evaluation concepts are considered before the program is implemented.

Finally, program costs need to be projected before the social marketing project begins. Social marketing can be an expensive proposition in terms of staff costs and direct expenses. When performed correctly, a social marketing project can take several months or up to a year before implementation even begins. Program planners and organizations must decide if they are ready to make these kinds of time and financial commitments.

At the end of Phase 1, the social marketing planners have (1) identified the focus of interest in terms of modifiable behaviors, (2) developed goals that provide general direction, (3) outlined preliminary plans for evaluation, and (4) estimated total project costs. Based on this information, the planners and organizations can make an informed decision about the potential costs and benefits of the project.

Phase 2 of SMART is *Consumer Analysis*. In social marketing language, the process of performing consumer analysis is formative research. **Formative research**, as defined in social marketing, is a process that identifies differences among subgroups within a population, identifies a subgroup, determines the wants and needs of the subgroup, and identifies factors that influence its behavior, including benefits, barriers, and readiness to change (Bryant, 1998).

It is important to remember that no single type of data collection technique is necessarily best in performing formative research. To the contrary, it is helpful to use multiple methods to gain a better perspective of the priority population. It is a mistake for those who engage in social marketing to perform one or two focus groups in the name of consumer analysis and claim they understand their consumers. Ordinarily, however, formative research will involve the use of focus groups, in-depth interviews, and surveys, and so on, to understand consumer preferences.

At the conclusion of Phase 2, a priority population is also identified. Adequate formative research has been performed yielding data about major themes, directions, and consumer preferences related to the health problem and related interventions. Although Phases 2 through 4 are often performed simultaneously, information collected in Phase 2 can provide context for the other two phases. For example, knowing about consumer preferences related to some type of behavior change allows planners to more effectively understand consumer preferences related to the market mix and communication strategies.

Phase 3, *Market Analysis,* examines the fit between the focus of interest (desired behavior change) and important market variables within the priority population. *Marketing mix* is a term that is often used in both commercial and social marketing. It is composed of four components, also known as the 4Ps: product, price, place, and promotion (see Chapter 11 for more on the 4Ps).

At the conclusion of this phase, consumer analysis is enriched by a better understanding of important market variables that influence consumers. Combined with consumer analysis and channel analysis, market analysis provides a powerful combination of useful information about consumers, the environment they live in, and strengths and weakness associated with potential social marketing interventions.

The fourth phase of SMART is *Channel Analysis.* Although communication may not be the focal point of a social marketing campaign, it will play a secondary role in communicating important messages about the product. In addition to messages and related strategies, formative research includes specific questions about the type of communication channels consumers believe are most appropriate for the behavior change being addressed.

Finally, Phase 4, *Channel Analysis,* which considers which potential partners, if any, might collaborate in sharing the responsibility for communication. For example, if mass media is an appropriate channel, and consumer-oriented public service announcements are used in the communication strategy, television and radio stations may be willing to donate air time. One problem frequently experienced in social marketing is that multiple organizations with similar missions communicate competing, albeit only slightly different messages. In extreme cases, the messages can be nearly polar opposites. For this reason alone, it is important to develop communication partners. At the conclusion of Phase 4, communication channels are identified that are consistent with preliminary messages, and product distribution points and potential communication and intervention partners are identified.

Phase 5 of SMART consists of *Develop Interventions, Materials, and Pretesting.* Once formative research is performed, it is critical that the data are transferred or infused adequately into the design of programs, interventions, and communication strategies. To do this, data must be analyzed and categorized appropriately to assure that planners understand what they have seen, heard, and observed. As planners meet to design programs and materials, they should keep formative research data in front of them and refer to them often. Discussion and decisions should reflect all data and represent a consensus among all planners. In other words, materials and methods should represent what was learned in formative research.

Once a program prototype is developed, it is imperative to return to the priority population and test the concepts before implementing a widespread campaign. In fact, social marketing represents a process of continually returning to the consumers until the program and all its support mechanisms are consistent with their views and preferences. Several mechanisms are available to perform pretesting. One example is a pilot test where the program can be implemented with the priority population on a smaller, less expensive scale. Phase 6 of SMART is *Implementation.* This phase is concerned with clarifying everyone's role, including external partners. This means that procedures are communicated and documented, and that time lines are developed and followed. In this phase, the communication and distribution plans are activated and the actual program and its interventions are offered. In addition, the program is refined continually, based on consumer feedback.

The seventh and final phase of SMART is *Evaluation*. The preliminary evaluation strategies that were identified in Phase 1 now take effect. Evaluation always has at least two major objectives: improve the quality of the program and determine the effectiveness of the program. With respect to quality, program planners assess the degree to which the priority population, within the larger population, is actually receiving the program or interventions. Planners also assess the immediate impact the program is having and whether the interventions and related support strategies are acceptable and engaging to the priority population. In addition, planners ensure that program delivery is consistent with program protocol or at least consistent with developed timelines.

Ultimately, social marketing, and all its related work, is of little value unless behavior change occurs and health is improved. Evaluation also concerns itself with measuring these outcomes. Effective planners and evaluators also make sure that evaluation results are folded back into the program so that it can be improved before it is too late. This requires communicating evaluation results effectively to stakeholders.

Other Planning Models

As noted, other planning models are available to planners in addition to the PRECEDE-PROCEED, MAPP, MAP-IT, and SMART models. If you are interested in learning more about these models, check the original sources provided in the reference section at the back of the book.

SWOT (Strengths, Weaknesses, Opportunities, Threats) Analysis

The **SWOT** analysis has historically been associated with strategic planning efforts in the business and marketing sectors. In simple terms, it is an analysis of an organization's internal strengths and weaknesses, as well as opportunities and threats in the operating environment. Technically, its use should be limited to the preliminary stages of decision making in preparation for more comprehensive strategic planning (Bartol & Martin, 1991; Johnson, Scholes, & Sexty, 1989).

In health promotion practice, SWOT analyses are common among planners who want to minimize planning time and move quickly to action steps. Generally, a facilitator helps a planning group identify issues or problems, set or clarify goals, and create a plan. Common to SWOT analyses is the use of a 2 × 2 matrix that lists strengths and weaknesses along the horizontal axis and opportunities and threats along the vertical axis. The organization can then decide if it prefers to build upon strengths or improve on weaknesses in context of environmental opportunities and threats.

A SWOT analysis requires planners to examine their organization's strengths. This may include an assessment of what the organization does well or what it does differently or better than similar organizations, existing resources (i.e., funds, equipment, supplies, materials), expertise of personnel, quality of partnerships in the community, or track record of successful working relationships. Conversely, the SWOT analysis also examines weaknesses that may pertain to the same factors cited under strengths. In addition, weaknesses may involve a poor reputation among stakeholders, including clients. It may involve an inability to address certain health problems or determinants because of codes, regulations, policy, or management decisions that give authority or opportunity to another entity.

Whereas strengths and weaknesses assessed in a SWOT analysis pertain to an organization's internal environment, opportunities and threats relate to the external environment. Opportunities may involve unfulfilled consumer needs, loosening or removal of administrative or legislative barriers that finally allow the development of a new program, a new funding stream made available by a government agency or other granting agency, or a newly organized coalition formed to address an emerging health problem. Threats may involve shifts in consumer trends, organizational or ideological competition, or private industry that promotes products or services that are harmful to the health of a community (e.g., the tobacco or alcohol industries, fast food corporations), or changing technology.

The SWOT analysis differs substantially from other models discussed in this chapter. It truly represents rapid internal and external scans that allow planners to implement interventions in a much shorter time frame. Building upon strengths or addressing specific weaknesses while taking advantage of opportunities in the environment is an advantage of the SWOT analysis. Certainly, this approach can lead to challenges if consumer input is not received, problems are not analyzed thoroughly, relevant determinants are not addressed, or interventions are identified and implemented without adequately understanding the underlying theory or rationale. In fact, poorly planned programs can be more harmful than no programs at all. However, the SWOT analysis has its place in planning methodology and its simplicity is appealing to many planners.

Healthy Communities

Healthy Communities (or Healthy Cities) is a movement that began in the 1980s in Canada and, with the assistance of the World Health Organization, spread to various locations throughout Europe. As a result, organizations like California Healthy Cities and Indiana Healthy Cities were created in the United States. The movement is characterized by community ownership and empowerment and driven by the values, needs, and participation of community members with consultation from health professionals. Another characteristic of Healthy Communities is diverse partnership. It is not uncommon to see partners from business or labor, transportation, recreation, public safety, or even politicians participate in the Healthy Communities process.

The Healthy Communities Program at the CDC has created what it calls the CHANGE tool (Community Health Assessment and Group Evaluation) to assess community needs; action guides to assist in the development of interventions and strategies; and technical assistance with program evaluation (CDC, 2011a). This represents a viable planning framework for organizations and communities engaging in the Healthy Communities approach.

Although many of the steps associated with Healthy Communities appear quite similar to the Generalized Model, this approach is characterized by community ownership more so than any other planning approach. While organizing community groups and getting people involved requires patience, the model has been implemented widely throughout the world. Lessons learned from Healthy Communities include the idea that the pursuit of shared values in the context of ownership and empowerment is a viable approach to improving health in the community.

The Health Communication Model

The National Cancer Institute (NCI) has produced a document that is essential to any planner engaged in health communication planning entitled, *Making Health Communications Work* (NCI, 2002). The NCI model for health communication is presented in four phases: (1) Planning and Strategy Development; (2) Developing and Pretesting Concepts, Messages, and Materials; (3) Implementing the Program; and (4) Assessing Effectiveness and Making Refinements.

Planning and Strategy Development involves several steps including assessing the health issue or problem and identifying potential solutions; defining communication objectives; defining potential audiences and learning about them; investigating appropriate settings, channels, and activities best suited for the identified audiences; and developing a communication strategy for each potential audience (NCI, 2002). *Developing and Pretesting Concepts, Messages, and Materials* direct planners to review existing materials for appropriateness. At times, print material, public service announcements, and other resources may be available and appropriate with few, if any, modifications. Still, it may be necessary to create new concepts, messages, and materials to meet the needs of a specific audience. In this phase, *message concepts* (messages or visuals in early stages) are developed and tested. These will eventually evolve into messages and materials that become the basis of the communication campaign. In this phase, planners develop and pretest the finished messages and materials as per the process generally followed in social marketing campaigns. The exception to these rules is the introduction and increasing use of social media where consumers themselves are generating their own messages and content.

The third phase, *Implementing the Program,* usually begins with a kickoff event that draws positive attention to the campaign and related programs and interventions. This is generally associated with a press conference that brings partners together to formally introduce a new program. Appropriate spokespeople are selected and special attention is given to framing issues to maximize coverage, interest, and participation. Developing strategies for ongoing media relationships and coverage are also designed in this phase. As with other planning models, communication, reinforcement of partnerships, and adherence to planned timelines are characteristics of this phase. Again, with the advent of social media, traditional press conferences and press coverage are being increasingly replaced or supplemented with more timely and accessible platforms (e.g., blogs, Facebook, Twitter).

Finally, *Assessing Effectiveness and Making Refinements* involves refining the communication plan as immediate feedback is received through *process evaluation* and evaluating the effectiveness of the campaign in terms of changes in determinants and health status. Planners must determine what information the evaluation must provide, define the data to collect, decide upon data collection methods, collect and process the data, analyze the data, write an evaluation report, and disseminate the evaluation report (NCI, 2002).

Intervention Mapping

Intervention mapping was designed to fill a gap in health promotion practice by translating data collected in the PRECEDE phases of PRECEDE-PROCEED (i.e., social, epidemiological, educational, ecological, administrative, organizational, and policy assessments) into theoretically based and otherwise appropriate interventions (Green & Kreuter, 2005). Once planners identify program objectives, they are guided by diagrams and matrices that incorporate outputs of the assessment process with relevant theory (Green & Kreuter, 2005). These diagrams and matrices are perhaps the defining strength of intervention mapping.

Intervention mapping is comprised of six steps. The first step, *Needs Assessment*, is conducted by using the PRECEDE phases of the PRECEDE-PROCEED model and includes establishing a participatory planning group, assessing community capacity, and linking the needs assessment to health outcomes and quality of life goals (Bartholomew et al., 2011). Step 2, *Matrices of Change Objectives*, specifies who and what will change as a result of the intervention (Bartholomew et al., 2011). Although the identification of goals and objectives is common to all planning models, intervention mapping makes a unique contribution in this regard. In this step, planners create a matrix of change objectives for each level of intervention planning (individual, interpersonal, organizational, community, and societal) by crossing performance objectives with determinants and writing change objectives (Bartholomew et al., 2011, p. 21).

Step 3, *Theory-Based Methods and Practical Applications*, guides the planner through a process of selected theory-based interventions and strategies that hold the greatest promise to change the health behavior(s) of individuals in the priority population. Step 4, *Program Production*, describes the scope and sequence of the intervention, the completed program materials, and program protocols (Bartholomew et al., 2011). In addition, program materials are pretested with the priority population prior to implementation.

Step 5 of intervention mapping is *Adoption and Implementation*. This step requires the same development of matrices as in Step 2, except in these matrices, the focus is on adoption and implementation of performance objectives (Bartholomew et al., 2011). In other words, instead of focusing on who and what will change within the priority population, the focus is on what will be done by whom among planners or program partners. Finally, Step 6 is *evaluation planning*. In this step, planners decide if determinants were well specified, if strategies were appropriately matched to methods, what proportion of the priority population was reached, and whether or not implementation was complete and executed as planned (Bartholomew et al., 2011).

Healthy Plan-It

Healthy Plan-It was developed by the Sustainable Management Development Program at the Centers for Disease Control and Prevention (CDC, 2000) to strengthen in-country management training capacity in the health sector of developing countries. The Health Analysis for Planning Prevention Services (HAPPS), a planning model that was commonly used in the 1980s prior to the development of PATCH, is the basis for Healthy Plan-It (CDC, 2000). The model itself consists of six steps: (1) priority setting, (2) establishing goals, (3) outcome objectives, (4) strategy, (5) evaluation, and (6) budget.

The first step, *Priority Setting,* involves participatory planning and consensus building, as well as priority setting, using the Basic Priority Rating Process (Neiger, Thackeray, & Fagen, 2011). Participatory planning and consensus building requires broad representation from the community, a facilitation process that promotes empowerment, and nurturing respect for all those involved in the planning process. This phase builds a foundation of trust within an atmosphere of flexibility (CDC, 2000). Priority setting examines the size and seriousness of health problems, effectiveness of interventions, and the propriety, economic feasibility, acceptability, resources, and legality associated with all potential health problems. The result is a ranked list of priorities.

The second step, *Establishing Goals,* follows the pattern outlined in previous models. Goals are generalized statements of the result or achievement to which the planning effort is directed (CDC, 2000). The third step in Healthy Plan-It develops *Outcome Objectives.* These are related to the program goal(s), are usually long-term in nature, and are always measurable. Outcome objectives also relate to the actual health problem (the specific disease or injury). The basis for program success is generally linked to the degree to which objectives are accomplished. The fourth step, *Strategy*, involves developing the methods or interventions that will be implemented to accomplish outcome objectives. Strategies are designed to affect the determinants and contributing factors that lead to the health problem and will vary depending on program goals and objectives.

The final phases, *Evaluation* and *Budget,* identify ways to measure the success of outcome objectives as well as program impacts related to determinants and contributing factors (impact objectives). The process of evaluating program delivery, as well as changes in behaviors and actual health problems, is designed and implemented. Development of program budgets involves planning for physical resources, personnel, facilities, and equipment. Although initial budgetary planning may be performed prior to step one to identify planning parameters, actual project costs are analyzed and distributed in the final step.

SUMMARY

A model can provide the framework for planning a health promotion program. Several different planning models have been developed and revised over the years. The planning models for health promotion presented in this chapter are the following:

1. The Generalized Model
2. PRECEDE-PROCEED
3. MAPP
4. MAP-IT

5. SMART (Social Marketing Assessment and Response Tool)

6. SWOT (Strengths, Weaknesses, Opportunities, Threats)

7. Healthy Communities (or Healthy Cities)

8. The Health Communication Model

9. Intervention Mapping

10. Healthy Plan-It

The Generalized Model is recommended as the template for learning the basic principles of planning and evaluation: (1) assessing needs; (2) setting goals and objectives; (3) developing interventions; (4) implementing interventions; and (5) evaluating results. Several other models used in health promotion also continue to make valuable contributions typically using these same elements.

REVIEW QUESTIONS

1. How does an understanding of the Generalized Model help you understand other planning models?

2. What are the elements or steps in the Generalized Model that are common in most, if not all other planning models?

3. Why is it important to use a model when planning?

4. How does pre-planning relate to most of the models presented in this chapter?

5. Explain the degree to which you believe consumers or members of the community should be involved in the planning process. Do you believe they should own or control the process?

ACTIVITIES

1. After reviewing the models presented in this chapter, create your own model by identifying what you think are the common components of the models. Provide a rationale for including each component. Then draw a diagram of your model so that you can share it with the class. Be prepared to explain your model.

2. In a one-page paper, defend what you believe is the best planning model presented in this chapter.

3. Using a hypothetical health problem for a specific priority population, write a paper explaining the steps/phases for one of the models presented in this chapter.

4. Identify a public service announcement on television or radio, or obtain a copy of one from a nearby health agency. Analyze factors such as messages, settings, and channels. Based on your analysis, was the public service announcement developed appropriately for the intended audience? Summarize your comments in a one-page paper.

WEBLINKS

1. **http://www.healthypeople.gov/2020/default.aspx**

   Healthy People

   At this Website, *Healthy People 2020* is outlined with several helpful links including: (1) About Healthy People (background and general information); (2) *Healthy People 2020* topics and objectives; (3) Implementing *Healthy People 2020* (MAP-IT); (4) a list of the *Healthy People 2020* consortium and partners; and (5) Staying Connected (ongoing links to the process). It is a site with which planners in health promotion should be familiar.

2. **http://healthypeople.gov/2020/implementing/default.aspx**

   MAP-IT: A Guide to Using *Healthy People 2020* in Your Community

   This Website provides a valuable resource to assist health promotion professionals in implementing *Healthy People 2020*. The site includes field notes for each of the phases in MAP-IT with examples or case studies from various health organizations, as well as other resources and tool kits for each planning phase.

3. **http://ctb.ku.edu/**

   Community Tool Box

   This Website is an indispensable tool for all planners in health promotion. According to the site, "The Tool Box offers more than 7,000 pages of practical guidance in creating change and improvement" related to planning steps and phases discussed in this chapter. "Topic sections include step-by-step instruction, examples, checklists, and related resources."

4. **http://www.naccho.org/topics/infrastructure/mapp/index.cfm**

   National Association of County and City Health Officials

   At this Website, the MAPP model is comprehensively diagrammed and explained. The four MAPP assessments are described, including how they are implemented, how to use subcommittees for each assessment, and how to make linkages between assessments.

5. **http://www.communityhlth.org/communityhlth/resources/hlthycommunities.html**

   Association for Community Health Improvement

This Website provides helpful information on the Healthy Communities Initiative including current projects and links.

6. **http://www.cdc.gov/healthcommunication/**

Gateway to Health Communication and Social Marketing Practice, Centers for Disease Control and Prevention

This Website provides an overview of health communication and social marketing practice including how to develop programs, segmenting an audience, and selecting appropriate channels and tools for program delivery.

7. **http://www.cancer.gov/cancertopics/cancerlibrary/pinkbook**

Making Health Communications Work (National Cancer Institute, 2002)

At this Website, the entire 2002 edition is available, including the Health Communication model. This is arguably the most comprehensive document available on health communication planning

Assessing Needs

After reading this chapter and answering the questions at the end, you should be able to:

- Define *need* and *needs assessment*.
- Define *capacity*, *community capacity*, and *capacity building*.
- Explain why a needs assessment is an important part of the planning process.
- Explain what should be expected from a needs assessment.
- Differentiate between primary and secondary data sources.
- List the various methods for collecting primary data.
- Locate secondary data sources that are in print and on the World Wide Web.
- Explain how a needs assessment can be completed.
- Explain what is meant by health impact assessment.
- Conduct a needs assessment within a given population.

action research
basic priority rating (BPR)
BPR model 2.0
bias
capacity
capacity building
categorical funds
community capacity
community forum
Delphi technique
focus group
health assessments (HAs)
health impact assessment (HIA)

HIPAA
key informants
mapping
need
needs assessment
networking
nominal group process
observation
obtrusive observation
opinion leaders
participatory data collection
participatory research
photovoice

primary data
proxy measure
random-digit dialing (RDD)
secondary data
self-assessments
self-report
significant others
single-step survey
unobtrusive observation
walk-through
windshield tour

Once the planning committee is in place and a planning model has been selected, the next step in the planning process is to identify the needs of those in the priority population. Gilmore (2012) has defined **need** as "the difference between the present situation and a more desirable one" (p. 8). These needs can be expressed in many different ways. For example, there may be a need for better health, or a need for more knowledge, or a need to possess a certain skill, to name a few. Whether a need of the priority population is actual (*true* need) or perceived (*reported* need) does not matter (Gilmore, 2012). What matters is being able to identify all needs, actual and perceived, so that they can be addressed through appropriate program planning.

The process of identifying, analyzing, and prioritizing the needs of a priority population is referred to as a **needs assessment.** Other terms that have been used to describe the process of determining needs include *community analysis, community diagnosis,* and *community assessment.* Conducting a needs assessment may be the most critical step in the planning process because it "provides objective data to define important health problems, sets priorities for program implementation, and establishs a baseline for evaluating program impact" (Grunbaum et al., 1995, p. 54).

There are many reasons why a needs assessment should be completed before the other steps of the planning process begin. First, it is a logical place to start (Gilmore, 2012). Before a need can be met, it first must be identified and measured. Second, a needs assessment can help ensure the appropriate use of planning resources. Without determining and prioritizing needs, resources can be wasted on unsubstantiated programming. Third, failure to perform a needs assessment may lead to a program focus that prevents or delays adequate attention directed to a more important health problem. For example, a health problem that tends to create a high emotional response, particularly among parents, is the trauma associated with bicycle injuries in children. Of course, it is a tragedy when a preventable death occurs. In 2009, 13% of the 630 bicyclists killed in the United States were children age 16 and under (NHTSA, n.d.). But an even more significant determinant of childhood injury and death in the United States is the inadequate use of safety belts or car seats involved with motor vehicle crashes. In fact, motor vehicle injuries are the leading cause of death among children at every age after their fourth birthday and are the greatest public health threat to children in the United States today (Miniño, Xu, & Kochanek, 2010). A needs assessment that examined both bicycle and motor vehicle crashes would lead planners to determine in most locations, in most instances, that restraining children in motor vehicles with safety belts or approved car seats is an even more important issue.

Fourth, a needs assessment can determine the capacity of a community to address specific needs. **Capacity** refers to the individual, organizational, and community resources, such as leadership, relationships, operations, structures, infrastructure, politics, and systems, to name a few, that can enable a community to take action (Brennan Ramirez, Baker, & Metzler, 2008; Gilmore, 2012). In other words, when related to health promotion **community capacity** is the "characteristics of communities that affect their ability to identify, mobilize, and address social and public health problems" (Goodman et al., 1998, p. 259) (see Chapter 9 for mapping community capacity). "Assessing community capacity helps you think about existing community strengths that can be mobilized to address social, economic, and environmental conditions affecting health inequities. In general, you should look at the places (e.g., parks, libraries) and organizations (e.g., education, health care, faith-based groups, social services, volunteer groups, businesses, local government, law enforcement) in various sectors of the community" (Brennan Ramirez et al., 2008, p. 54). "It is also important to identify the nature of the relationships across these sectors (e.g., norms, values), with the community (e.g., civic participation), and among various subgroups within the community (e.g., distribution of power and authority, trust, identity)" (Sampson & Raudenbush, 1999, and Trachim, 1989, as cited in Brennan Ramirez et al., 2008, p. 54).

Fifth, a needs assessment can provide a focus for developing an intervention to meet the needs of the priority population. And finally, knowing the needs of a priority population provides a reference point to which future assessments can be compared.

Having just stated several reasons why a needs assessment should be completed, it may seem odd that there are a few planning scenarios in which a needs assessment would not be used. The first would be if another needs assessment had been conducted recently, possibly for another related program, and the funding or other resources to conduct a second needs assessment in such a short period of time were not available. A second scenario in which a needs assessment may not be used is one where the program planners are employed by an agency that deals only with a specific need that is already known (e.g., cancer and the American Cancer Society), or the agency for which they work has received **categorical funds** that must be used for dealing with a specific disease (e.g., HIV/AIDS) or program (e.g., immunization) (Bartholomew et al., 2011).

The remaining portions of this chapter will present discussions on what to expect from a needs assessment, the types and sources of data used to conduct a needs assessment, and a suggested process for conducting a needs assessment. **Box 4.1** identifies

---

Box 4.1 RESPONSIBILITIES AND COMPETENCIES FOR HEALTH EDUCATION SPECIALISTS

The content of this chapter is associated with a single area of responsibility. That responsibility and related competencies include:

Responsibility I: Assess Needs, Assets, and Capacity for Health Education

Competency 1.1: Plan Assessment Process

Competency 1.2: Access Existing Information and Data Related to Health

Competency 1.3: Collect Quantitative and/or Qualitative Data Related to Health

Competency 1.4: Examine Relationships among Behavioral, Environmental, and Genetic Factors That Enhance or Compromise Health

Competency 1.5: Examine Factors That Influence the Learning Process

Competency 1.6: Examine Factors That Enhance or Compromise the Process of Health Education

Competency 1.7: Infer Needs for Health Education Based on Assessment Findings

Source: NCHEC, SOPHE, & AAHE (2010).

the responsibilities and competencies for health education specialists that pertain to the material presented in this chapter.

What to Expect From a Needs Assessment

By examining the needs assessment definitions presented by others, planners can get an idea of what to expect from a needs assessment. Gilmore (2012) defined needs assessment as "a planned process that identifies the reported needs of an individual or group" (p. 9). The National Commission for Health Education Credentialing, Inc., along with two professional health education organizations, have defined needs assessment as a "process by which health education specialists gather information regarding health needs and desires of a population" (NCHEC, SOPHE, & AAHE, 2010, p. 20). A third definition of needs assessment states that it is the process of collecting and analyzing information to develop an understanding of the issues, resources, and constraints of the priority population, as related to the development of health promotion programs (Anspaugh et al., 2000). Altschuld and Witkin (2000) provided a more encompassing definition when they defined a needs assessment as a "process of determining, analyzing, and prioritizing needs, and in turn, identifying and implementing solution strategies to resolve high-priority needs" (p. 253).

Other authors have indicated that a needs assessment should answer certain questions. Peterson and Alexander (2001) have suggested that a needs assessment should answer the following questions: (1) Who is the priority population? (2) What are the needs of the priority population? (3) Which subgroups within the priority population have the greatest need? (4) Where are these subgroups located geographically? (5) What is currently being done to resolve identified needs? (6) How well have the identified needs been addressed in the past? Indirectly, getting answers to the latter two questions, numbers 5 and 6, provides some information about the community capacity and whether part of the identified needs may include the need to build capacity. **Capacity building** refers to activities that enhance the resources of individuals, organizations, and communities to improve their effectiveness to take action.

No matter how needs assessment is defined, the concept embedded in the definitions is the same: identifying the needs of the priority population and determining the degree to which the needs are being met. If needs are not being met, is there also a need to enhance capacity to do so?

Acquiring Needs Assessment Data

Two types of data are generally associated with a needs assessment: primary data and secondary data. **Primary data** are those data you collect yourself (via a survey, a focus group, in-depth interviews, etc.) that answer unique questions related to your specific needs assessment. Most methods of collecting primary data are ones in which those collecting the data interact with (e.g., interviewing) those from whom the data are being collected. Such methods have been labeled as *interactive contact methods* (Marti-Costa & Serrano-Garcia as cited in Minkler, 2005). **Secondary data** are those data already collected by somebody else and available for your use. Thus, the methods to collect these data have been labeled as *no contact methods* (Marti-Costa & Serrano-Garcia as cited in Minkler, 2005). The advantages of using secondary data are that (1) they already exist, and thus collection time is minimal, and (2) they are usually fairly inexpensive to access. Both of these advantages are important to planners because programs are often planned when both time and money are limited. However, a drawback of using secondary data is that the information might not identify the true needs of the priority population—perhaps because of how the data were collected, when they were collected, what variables were considered, or from whom the data were collected. A good rule is to move cautiously and make sure the secondary data are applicable to the immediate situation before using them.

Primary data have the advantage of directly answering the questions planners want answered by those in the priority population. However, collecting primary data can be expensive and when done correctly, take a great deal of time.

An overview of the means of acquiring primary and secondary data are presented in the following pages.

Sources of Primary Data

Primary data can be collected using a variety of methods. Those most commonly used in planning health promotion programs are presented in **Table 4.1**.

Single-Step or Cross-Sectional Surveys Single-step surveys, or as they are often called *cross-sectional* (point-in-time) *surveys,* are a means of gathering primary data from

Table 4.1 Sources of Primary Data

Single-Step or Cross-Sectional Surveys
From priority population—self-report
written questionnaires
telephone interviews
face-to-face interviews
electronic interviews
group interviews
Proxy measures
From significant others
From opinion leaders
From key informants
Multistep Survey: Delphi Technique
Community Forum (Town Hall Meeting)
Meetings
Focus Group
Nominal Group Process
Observation
Direct observation
Indirect observation (proxy measures)
"Windshield" or walk-through (walking tours)
Photovoice and videovoice
Self-Assessments

individuals or groups with a single contact—thus, the term *single-step*. Such surveys often take the form of written questionnaires and interviews. When individuals or groups (also sometimes called *respondents* or *participants*) are answering questions about themselves, the information that is provided is referred to as **self-report** data. Thus, respondents are asked to recall ("When was your last visit to your dentist?") and report accurate ("On average, how many minutes do you exercise each day?") information. Self-report measures are essential for many needs assessments and evaluations because of the need to obtain subjective assessments of experiences (e.g., feelings about available programs, self-assessments of health status, and health behavior, such as eating patterns) (Bowling, 2005). Even marketing data (e.g., the best location for a program, the best time to offer a program, and willingness to pay for a program) and capacity data ("What resources are needed to make this change?) can be collected through these assessments. In addition, self-report measures have a broad appeal to those who need to collect data, because "they are often quick to administer and involve little interpretation by the investigator" (Bowling, 2005, p. 15). However, planners should be aware that self-report data do have limitations. One such limitation is **bias**—those data that have been distorted because of the way they have been collected. (See the section in Chapter 5 on bias free data.) To overcome some of these limitations and to maximize the usefulness of self-report, Baranowski (1985) has developed eight steps to increase the accuracy of this method of data collection:

1. Select measures that clearly reflect program outcomes.

2. Select measures that have been designed to anticipate the response problems and that have been validated.

3. Conduct a pilot study with the priority population. (See Chapter 5 for pilot studies.)

4. Anticipate and correct any major sources of unreliability.

5. Employ quality-control procedures to detect other sources of error.

6. Employ multiple methods.

7. Use multiple measures.

8. Use experimental and control groups with random assignment to control for biases in self-report.

By following these steps, planners can enhance the accuracy of self-report, making this a more effective method of data collection.

   For a variety of reasons, there are times when those in the priority population cannot respond for themselves or do not want to respond. In such situations, planners will have to collect data indirectly. Such a method is referred to as a proxy (or indirect) measure. A **proxy measure** is an outcome measure that provides evidence that a behavior has occurred. Or as Dignan (1995) states, "indirect measures are unmistakable signs that a specific behavior has occurred" (p. 103). Examples of proxy measures include (1) lower blood pressure for the behavior of medication taking, (2) body weight for the behaviors of exercise and dieting, (3) cotinine in the blood for tobacco use, (4) empty alcoholic beverages in the trash for consumption of alcohol, or (5) another person reporting on the compliance of his/her partner (Cottrell & McKenzie, 2011). Proxy measurements of skills or behavior usually require more resources and cooperation to obtain than self-report or direct observation

(Dignan, 1995). The greatest concern associated with proxy measures is making sure that the measure is both valid and reliable (Cottrell & McKenzie, 2011).

In addition to surveying the priority population, there are other groups of individuals who are commonly asked to respond to single-step surveys for the purpose of collecting primary needs assessment data. They include significant others of the priority population, community opinion leaders, and key informants. **Significant others** may include family members and friends. Collecting data from the significant others of a group of heart disease patients is a good example. Program planners might find it difficult to persuade heart disease patients themselves to share information about their outlook on life and living with heart disease. A survey of spouses or other family members might help elicit this information so that the program planners could best meet the needs of the heart disease patients.

Opinion leaders are individuals who are well respected in a community and who can accurately represent the views of the priority population. These leaders are:

1. Discriminating users of the media

2. Demographically similar to the priority group

3. Knowledgeable about community issues and concerns

4. Early adopters of innovative behavior (see Chapter 11 for an explanation of these terms)

5. Active in persuading others to become involved in innovative behavior

Opinion leaders include political figures, chief executive officers (CEOs) of companies, union leaders, administrators of local school districts, and other highly visible and respected individuals. (See **Figure 4.1** for a form for tallying opinion leader survey data.)

Key informants are strategically placed individuals who have the knowledge and ability to report on the needs of those in the priority population. They may or may not be in positions with formal authority, but they are often respected by others in the community and thus possess informal authority. Because they may be biased, planners need to be careful not to base an entire needs assessment on the data generated from a key informant survey.

Single-step surveys of those in the priority population, significant others, opinion leaders, and key informants can be administered, as noted earlier, several different ways. The primary means of collecting data from these individuals include written questionnaires, telephone interviews, face-to-face interviews, electronic interviews, and group interviews. A discussion of each follows.

Written Questionnaires.   Probably the most often used method of collecting self-reported data is the written questionnaire. It has several advantages, notably the ability to reach a large number of respondents in a short period of time, even if there is a large geographic area to be covered. This method offers low cost with minimum staff time needed. However, it often has the lowest response rate.

With a written questionnaire, each individual receives the same questions and instructions in the same format, so that the possibility of response bias is lessened. The corresponding disadvantage, however, is the inability to clarify any questions or confusion on the part of the respondent.

Data collection method _____			Number of interviewers _____
Total number of people interviewed _____			From: _____ To: _____ Date Collected _____

Rank	Health Problem	Number of Persons Identifying Problem	Percentage of Persons Identifying Problem
1.			
2.			
3.			
4.			
5.			
6.			
7.			
8.			
9.			
10.			

Figure 4.1 Form to Tally Opinion Leader Survey Data

Source: U.S. Department of Health and Human Services, Centers for Disease Control and Prevention (no date), p. A3–12.

As mentioned, the response rate for mailed questionnaires tends to be low especially if respondents cannot remain anonymous, but there are several ways to overcome this problem. One way is to include with the questionnaire a postcard that identifies the person in some way (such as name or identification number). The individual is asked to return the questionnaire in the envelope provided and to send the postcard back separately. Anonymity is thus maintained, but the planner/evaluator knows who returned a questionnaire. The planner/evaluator can then send a follow-up mailing (including a letter indicating the importance of a response and another copy of the questionnaire with a return envelope) to the individuals who did not return a postcard from the first mailing. The use of incentives also can increase the response rate. For example, some hospitals offer free health risk appraisals to those who return a completed needs assessment instrument.

The appearance of the questionnaire is also extremely important when collecting data. It should be attractive, easy to read, and offer ample space for the respondents' answers. It should also be easy to understand and complete, because written questionnaires provide no opportunity to clarify a point while the respondent is completing the questionnaire. In addition, all mailed questionnaires should be accompanied by a cover letter, to help clarify directions for completion.

Short questionnaires that do not take a long time to complete and questionnaires that clearly explain the need for the information are more likely to be returned. Planners/evaluators should give thought to designing a questionnaire that is as easy to complete and return as possible.

Face-to-Face Interviews. At times, it is advantageous to administer the instrument to the respondents in a face-to-face interview setting. This method is time consuming, since it may require not only time for the actual interview but also travel time to the interview site and/or waiting time between interviews. The interviewer must be carefully trained to conduct the interview in an unbiased manner. It is important to explain the need for the information in order to conduct the needs assessment/evaluation and to accurately record the responses. Methods of probing, or eliciting additional information about an individual's responses, are used in the face-to-face interview, and the interviewer must be skilled at this technique.

This method of self-report allows the interviewer to develop rapport with the respondent. The flexibility of this method, along with the availability of visual cues, has the advantage of gaining more complete data from respondents. Smaller numbers of respondents are included in this method, but the rate of participation is generally high. It is important to establish and follow procedures for selecting the respondents. There are also several disadvantages to the face-to-face interview. It is more expensive, requiring more staff time and training of interviewers. Variations in the interviews, as well as differences between interviewers, can influence the results.

Telephone Interviews. Compared to mailed surveys or face-to-face interviews, the telephone interview offers a relatively easy method of collecting self-reported data at a moderate cost. But it is not as easy and inexpensive as it once was "due in part to the increasing use of cell phones" (SHADAC, 2009, p. 1). The number of households in the United States that do not have landline telephone service, known as *wireless-only households*, continues to grow. It has been estimated that more than one out of four American homes (26.6%) have only wireless telephones and another 2.0% do not have any phone service (Blumberg & Luke, 2010). "The prevalence of such 'wireless-only' households now markedly exceeds the prevalence of households with only landline telephones (12.9%), and this difference is expected to grow" (Blumberg et al., 2011, p. 1). Those most likely to live in wireless-only households are younger, living with other nonrelated adults, renting their residence, and being non-white (Blumberg & Luke, 2010). Therefore, depending on whom planners/evaluators are trying to interview and how they plan to select the participants for interviews, some individuals may not have a chance of being selected and/or contacted.

Prior to so many people living in wireless-only households participants who were to be interviewed by telephone were selected using some type of random process. One method was to randomly select people from a "list." For example, a program participants' list, a local telephone book, student directory, church directory, or employee directory. However, selecting people randomly from a list misses people with unlisted telephone numbers and/or cell phones. One way to overcome this problem is a method known as **random-digit dialing (RDD)**, in which telephone number combinations are chosen at random. This method would include businesses as well as residences and nonworking as well as valid numbers, making it more time consuming. The numbers may be obtained from a table of random numbers or generated by a computer. The advantage of random-digit dialing is that it includes the entire survey population with a telephone in the area, including people with unlisted numbers and cell phones. However, there are several drawbacks to using RDD. The first is that those with cell phones may not have a telephone number with an area code in which they live. This is a problem because in order to use the RDD technique both the area codes and the exchanges (i.e., the first three digits of the seven-digit telephone number) must be known. Another drawback is some peoples' resistance to answering questions over the telephone or resentment about being interrupted with an unwanted call. And finally, those conducting the interviews may also have difficulty reaching individuals because of unanswered phones or answering machines.

Like face-to-face interviews, telephone interviewing requires trained interviewers; without proper training and use of a standard questionnaire, the interviewer may not be consistent during the interview. Explaining a question or offering additional information can cause a respondent to change an initial response, thus creating a chance for interviewer bias. The interviewer does have the opportunity to clarify questions, which is an advantage over the written questionnaire, but does not have the advantage of visual cues that the face-to-face interview offers.

Electronic Interviews.   With more and more individuals having access to the Internet and email ["74% of American adults go online, 57% of American households have broadband connections, and 61% of adults look online for health information" (Fox & Jones, 2009, para. 1)], it was only a matter of time until planners/evaluators used them to conduct interviews. Advantages to using this type of interviewing compared to using a written questionnaire include the reduced response time, cost of materials, ease of data collection, flexibility in the design and format of the questionnaire, control over the administration such as distribution to the recipients all at the same time on the same day, and recipient familiarity with the format and technology (Granello & Wheaton, 2003). In addition, responses received can be formatted to enter directly into a spreadsheet/statistical package eliminating manual data entry or scanning (Cottrell & McKenzie, 2011). However, there are several drawbacks to using the Internet for interviewing: not everyone has access to the Internet, obtaining email addresses of the possible respondents can be difficult, and some people's lack of comfort in using a computer. As such, studies in the literature to date on the response rate to electronic interviews has been mixed, with some studies reporting good results and others reporting lower rates similar to written questionnaires sent via the U.S. mail (Cottrell & McKenzie, 2011).

With the expanded use of the Internet has come an increase in the number of commercial companies (e.g., Qualtrics, SurveyMonkey, Zoomerang) that offer services to assist those in using this method of interviewing. This is how they work. Customers sign up and pay a fee. For the most part, the fee is based on the amount of service provided and the length of time the service is used. Typical services offered include design and preparation of the questionnaire, translation of the questionnaire into another language, customizing the questionnaire with organization logo/branding, personalized email cover letter introducing the questionnaire, personalized email thank-you letters for those who complete the instrument, data tallying and analysis, various trainings, and customer support. The costs of the services vary depending on the type of customer, but most companies provide a discount for not-for-profit and educational organizations.

Group Interviews. Interviewing individuals in groups provides for economy of scale. That is, data can be collected from several people in a short period of time. But there are some drawbacks of such data collection that primarily revolve around one or more group members' influencing the response of others. A specific form of group interview discussed later in this chapter is focus groups. Focus groups are useful in collecting information for a needs assessment, but can also be used to determine if programs are being implemented effectively or determine program outcomes.

Multistep Survey   As its title suggests, a multistep survey is one in which those collecting the data contact those who will provide the data on more than one occasion. The technique that uses this process is called the **Delphi technique.** It is a process that generates consensus through a series of questionnaires, which are usually administered via the mail or electronic mail. The process begins with those collecting the data asking the priority population to respond to one or two broad questions. The responses are analyzed, and a second questionnaire, with more specific questions based on responses to the first questionnaire, is developed and sent to the priority population. The answers to these more specific questions are analyzed again, and another new questionnaire is created and sent out, requesting additional information. If consensus is reached, the process may end here; if not, it may continue for another round or two (Gilmore 2012). Most often, this process continues for five or fewer rounds.

Community Forum   The **community forum,** also sometimes referred to as a *town hall meeting,* approach brings together people from the priority population to discuss what they see as their group's problems/needs. It is not uncommon for a community forum to be organized by a group representing the priority population, in conjunction with the program planners. Such groups include labor, civic, religious, or service organizations, or groups such as the Parent Teacher Association (PTA). Once people have arrived, a moderator explains the purpose of the meeting and then asks those from the priority population to share their concerns. One or several individuals from the organizing group, called *recorders,* are usually given the responsibility for taking notes or taping the session to ensure that the responses are recorded accurately. However, when moderating a community forum, it is important to be aware that the silent majority may not speak out and/or a vocal minority may speak too loudly. For example, an individual parent's view may be wrongly interpreted to be the view of all parents.

At a community forum, participants may also be asked to respond in writing (1) by answering specific questions or (2) by completing some type of instrument. **Figure 4.2** is an example of an instrument that could be used to collect data from participants in a community forum.

Meetings   Meetings are a good source of information for a preliminary needs assessment or various aspects of evaluation. For example, if a health department is planning to conduct a needs assessment and would like some direction on what health topics to key in on, planners may meet with a small group from the priority population to find out what they see as health issues in the community.

Directions: Please rank the need for each program in the community by placing a number in the space to the left of the programs. Use 1 to rank the program of greatest need, 2 for the next greatest need, and so forth, until you have ranked all seven programs. The program with the highest number next to it should be the one that, in your opinion, is least needed. If you feel that a program should not be considered for implementation in our community, please place an X in the space to the left of the program instead of a number. Please note that the number you place next to each program represents its need in the community, not necessarily your desire to participate in it. After ranking the program, place an X to the right of the program in the column(s) that represent the age group(s) to which you feel the program should be targeted.

Program	All ages	Children 5–12	Teens 13–19	Adults 20–64	Older adults 65+
_____ Alcohol education:	_____	_____	_____	_____	_____
_____ Exercise/fitness:	_____	_____	_____	_____	_____
_____ Nutrition education:	_____	_____	_____	_____	_____
_____ Safety belt use:	_____	_____	_____	_____	_____
_____ Smoking cessation:	_____	_____	_____	_____	_____
_____ Smoking education:	_____	_____	_____	_____	_____
_____ Weight loss:	_____	_____	_____	_____	_____

Figure 4.2 Instrument for Ranking Program Need

Source: Instrument for Ranking Program Need. Amy L. Bernard. Copyright © 2011 by Amy L. Bernard. Reprinted with permission.

The meeting structure can be flexible to avoid limiting the scope of the information gained. The cost of this form of data collection is minimal. Possible biases may occur when meetings are used as the sole source of data collection. Those involved may give "socially acceptable" responses to questions rather than discussing actual concerns. There also may be limited input if relatively few participants are included, or if one or two participants dominate the discussion.

Focus Group   The **focus group** is a form of qualitative research that grew out of group therapy. Focus groups are used to obtain information about the feelings, opinions, perceptions, insights, beliefs, misconceptions, attitudes, and receptivity of a group of people concerning an idea or issue. Focus groups are rather small, compared to community forums, and usually include only 8 to 12 people. If possible, it is best to have a group of people who do not know each other so that their responses are not inhibited by acquaintance. Participation in the group is by invitation. People are invited about one to three weeks in advance of the session. At the time of the invitation, they receive general information about the session but are not given any specifics. This precaution helps ensure that responses will be spontaneous yet accurate.

Once assembled, the group is led by a skilled moderator who has the task of obtaining candid responses from the group to a set of predetermined questions. In addition to eliciting responses to the questions, the moderator may ask the group to prioritize the different responses. As in a community forum, the answers to the questions are recorded through either written notes and/or audio or video recordings, so that at a later date the interested parties can review and interpret the results.

Focus groups are not easy to conduct. Special care must be given to developing the questions that will be asked. Poorly written questions will yield information that is less than useful. In addition, the moderator should be one who is skilled in leading a group. As might be surmised, the level of skill needed to conduct a focus group increases as the topic of discussion becomes more controversial.

Although focus groups have been shown to be an effective way of gathering data, they do have one major limitation. Participants in the groups are usually not selected through a random-sampling process. They are generally selected because they possess certain attributes (e.g., individuals of low income, city dwellers, parents of disabled children, or chief executive officers of major corporations). Participants may not be representative of the priority population. Therefore, the results of the focus group are not generalizable. "Findings [of focus groups] should be interpreted as suggestive and directional rather than as definitive" (Schechter, Vanchieri, & Crofton, 1990, p. 254). For more detail and information about preparing for and conducting focus groups, see Gilmore (2012) and National Cancer Institute (2002 & 2004).

Nominal Group Process   The **nominal group process** is a highly structured process in which a few knowledgeable representatives of the priority population (five to seven people) are asked to qualify and quantify specific needs. Those invited to participate are asked to record their responses to a question without discussing it among themselves. Once all have recorded a response, participants share their responses in a round-robin fashion. While this is occurring, the facilitator is recording the responses on a chalkboard or flip-chart for all to see. The responses are clarified through a discussion. After the discussion, the participants are asked to rank-order the responses by importance to the priority population. This ranking may be considered either a preliminary or a final vote. If it is preliminary, it is followed with more discussion and a final vote.

Observation   Observation, defined as "notice taken of an indicator" (Green & Lewis, 1986, p. 363), can also be an effective means of collecting data. Not only can people be observed, but the environment (i.e., those things around the priority population) can be observed as well. Because those doing the observation can "see" but do not interact with those in the priority, observation has been labeled a *minimal-contact method of data collection.*

Observation can be direct or indirect. *Direct observation* means actually seeing a situation or behavior. For example, direct observation may include watching the eating patterns of children in a school lunchroom, observing workers on an assembly line to see if they are wearing their protective glasses, checking the smoking behavior of employees on break, and observing drivers for safety belt use. This method is somewhat time consuming, but it seldom encounters the problem of people refusing to participate in the data collection, resulting in a high response rate.

Observation is generally more accurate than self-report, but the presence of the observer may alter the behavior of the people being observed. For example, having someone observe smoking behavior may cause smokers to smoke less out of self-consciousness due to their being under observation. When people know they are being observed it is referred to as **obtrusive observation. Unobtrusive observation** means just the opposite; the persons being studied are not aware they are being measured, assessed, or tested. Typically, unobtrusive observation provides less biased data, but some question whether unobtrusive observation is ethical.

Differences among observers may also bias the results, because different observers may not observe and report behaviors in the same manner. Some behaviors, such as safety belt use, are very easy to observe accurately. Others, such as a person's degree of tension, are more difficult to observe. This method of data collection requires a clear definition of the exact behavior to observe and how to record it, in order to avoid subjective observations. Observer bias can be reduced by providing training and by determining rater reliability. If the observers are skilled, observation can provide accurate evaluation data at a moderate cost.

As noted earlier in this chapter, *indirect observation* (or proxy measure) can also be used to determine whether a behavior has occurred. This can be completed by either "observing" the outcomes of a behavior or by asking others (e.g., spouse) to report on such outcomes (see the earlier discussion on proxy measures). In addition, these measures can be used to verify self-reports when observations of the actual changes in behavior cannot be observed.

Some specific methods of observation that have been useful in collecting data for health promotion programs are *windshield tours* or *walk-throughs* and *photovoice*. When using a **windshield tour** or **walk-through**, the person(s) doing the observation "walks or drives slowly through a neighborhood, ideally on different days of the week and at different times of the day, on the lookout for a variety of potentially useful indicators of community health and well-being" (Hancock & Minkler, 2005, p. 150). Potentially useful indicators may include: "(A) Housing types and conditions, (B) Recreational and commercial facilities, (C) Private and public sector services, (D) Social and civic activities, (E) Identifiable neighborhoods or residential clusters, (F) Conditions of roads and distances most travel, (G) Maintenance of buildings, grounds and yards" (Eng & Blanchard, 1990–1991, p. 96–97).

Photovoice (formerly called photo novella) is the creation of Wang and Burris (1994, 1997). It is a form of **participatory data collection** (i.e., those in the priority population participate in the data collection) in which those in the priority population are provided with cameras and skills training (on photography, ethics, data collection, critical discussion, and policy), then use the cameras to convey their own images of the community problems and strengths (Kramer et al., 2010; Minkler & Wallerstein, 2005). "Photovoice has 3 main goals: (1) to enable people to record and reflect their community's strengths and concerns; (2) to promote critical dialogue and enhance knowledge about issues through group discussions of the photographs; and (3) to inform policy makers" (FYVPC, 2006, para. 2).

Photovoice has been used a lot with "marginalized groups of various ages that want their perspective seen and heard by those in power" (WCPH, 2009, p. 1). More recently it has been receiving increased attention because of its application to health promotion. There are a number of reports of its use in the literature that have resulted in successful policy and environmental changes (e.g., Goodhard et al., 2006; Kramer et al., 2010; Wang, Morrel-Samuels, Hutchinson, Bell, & Pestronk, 2004).

The process for using photovoice involves the following steps: (1) defining the goals and objectives of the project; (2) identifying the community participants; (3) providing participants with the purpose and philosophy behind photovoice; (4) providing participants with training to carry out the project; (5) providing a theme for taking the pictures (e.g., "show what is unhealthy about our community"); (6) letting the participants take the pictures; (7) selecting the photographs that reflect the concerns of the project; (8) in groups, engaging in meaningful dialogue about the significance of each photograph; (9) contextualizing the photographs by writing captions based on the mnemonic SHOWeD created by Wallerstein (1987) (i.e., What do you See here? What's really Happening here? How does this relate to Our lives? Why does this problem or this strength exist? What can we Do about this?); (10) codifying the results by identifying the issues, themes, or theories that emerge; (11) identifying the stakeholders and venues to present the results; (12) making the presentation(s) to the community stakeholders (e.g., policy makers, decision makers) and the public; and (13) taking action based on results of the photovoice process (Downey, Ireson, Scutchfield, 2009; Kramer et al., 2010; Wang & Burris, 1997; Wang, Morrel-Samuels, et al., 2004; Wang, Yi, Tao, & Carovano, 1998; WCPH, 2009).

For those interested in learning more about photovoice please see reviews by Catalani and Minkler (2010) and Hergenrather, Rhodes, and Bardhoshi (2009).

Self-Assessments   Data can also be collected by those in the priority population through **self-assessments**. "A majority of these approaches address primary prevention issues, such as the assessment of risk factors and protective factors in one's lifestyle pattern, and the secondary prevention process of the early detection of disease symptoms" (Gilmore, 2012, p. 179). Examples of such assessments include breast self-examination (BSE), testicular self-examination (TSE), self-monitoring for skin cancer, and **health assessments (HAs)**. "Health assessments include instruments known as health risk appraisals or health risk assessments (HRAs), health status assessments (HSAs), various lifestyle-specific (e.g., nutrition, stress, and physical activity) assessment instruments, wellness and behavioral/habit inventories" (SPMBoD, 1999, p. xxiii), and disease/condition status assessments (e.g., chances of getting heart disease or diabetes).

Of the different self-assessments, it is the HAs that have been most useful in the needs assessment process, because from such assessments planners can obtain "group data which summarize major health problems and risk factors" (Alexander, 1999, p. 5). And of the HAs, it is the HRAs that are most often included in the needs assessment process. HRAs are instruments that estimate "the odds that a person with certain characteristics will die from selected causes within a given time span" (Alexander, 1999, p. 5). Even though HRAs are used as part of needs assessments, this was not their original intent. The original purpose of HRAs was to engage family physicians and their patients in conversation about risks of premature death and preventive health behaviors (Robbins & Hall, 1970).

To use an HRA as part of a needs assessment, planners would have those in the priority population complete a questionnaire. The instruments include questions about health behavior (e.g., smoking, exercise), personal or family health history of diseases (e.g., cancer, heart disease), demographics (e.g., age, sex), and usually some physiological data (e.g., height, weight, blood pressure, cholesterol). The resulting risk appraisals, in most cases, are calculated by computers, but some HRAs are hand-scored by the participant or health professional (Alexander, 1999). Most HRAs generate both individual and group reports. Thus planners can use the individual reports as part of an educational program for the priority population and use the group reports as another source of primary needs assessment data.

There are many HA instruments on the market. Before using one, you need to review information about the instruments that are available. Hunnicutt (2008a) created 10 critical questions that need to be asked when a health risk appraisal is purchased from a vendor: (1) How long has the vendor been in business? (2) How many other clients have used the instrument? (3) Who was behind the development of the HRA? (4) What is the best price? (5) Is the vendor willing to share the names of other clients who have used the HRA? (6) Is there any litigation pending against the vendor? (7) Is the vendor HIPAA (Health Insurance Portability and Accountability Act) compliant? (8) Will the vendor store the HRA data at a site outside the United States? (9) Is customer service/technical assistance included with the purchase of the HRA? (10) Who is the key contact within the company of the vendor and what is his/her emergency number?

Although this discussion has revolved around the use of HRAs as means of providing information for a needs assessment, they have also been used to help motivate people to act on their health, to increase awareness, to serve as cues to action, and to contribute to program evaluation (see Hunnicutt, 2008b, for benefits of using personal health assessments in a worksite). However, the reliability, validity, and effectiveness in predicting risk and prompting behavior change is questionable (Edington, Yen, & Braunstein, 1999).

The following conclusions relative to HRAs can be made:

1. The reliability of HRA risk scores can vary greatly from one instrument to another.

2. Reliability scores decrease when users calculate their own score, as opposed to computer scoring.

3. There is a great variance in the self-reporting of specific risk factors and clinical physiologic measurements.

4. Only those HRAs for which reliability can be demonstrated should be used for evaluating the effectiveness of health education.

Table 4.2 summarizes the advantages and disadvantages of the various methods of collecting primary data.

Sources of Secondary Data

Several sources of secondary needs assessment data are available to planners. The main sources include data collected by government agencies at multiple levels (federal, regional, state, or local), data available from nongovernment agencies and organizations, data from existing records, and data or other evidence that are presented in the literature (see **Table 4.3**).

Data Collected by Government Agencies   Certain government agencies collect data on a regular basis. Some of the data collection is mandated by law (e.g., census, births, deaths, notifiable diseases, etc.), whereas other data are collected voluntarily (e.g., usage rates for

Table 4.2   Methods of Collecting Primary Data

Method	Advantages	Disadvantages
Self-Report		
Written questionnaire via mail	Large outreach	Possible low response rate
	No interviewer bias	Possible problem of representation
	Convenient	No clarification of questions
	Low cost	Need homogenous group if response is low
	Minimum staff time required	No assurance addressee was respondent
	Easy to administer	
	Quick	
	Standardized	
Telephone interview	Moderate cost	Possible problem of representation
	Relatively easy to administer	Possible interviewer bias
	Permits unlimited callbacks	Requires trained interviewers
	Can cover wide geographic areas	Wireless-only households
		Unlisted number households
Face-to-face interview	High response rate	Expensive
	Flexibility	Requires trained interviewers
	Gain in-depth data	Possible interviewer bias
	Develop rapport	Limits sample size
		Time-consuming
Electronic interview	Low cost	Must have Internet access
	Ease and convenience	Self-selection
	Almost instantaneous	May lack anonymity
	Commercial companies' services	
Group interview	High response rate	May intimidate and suppress individual differences
	Efficient and economical	Fosters conformity
	Can stimulate productivity of others	Group pressure may influence responses
Delphi technique[*]	Pooled responses	
	Spans time and distance	High cost and time commitment
	High motivation and commitment	Reduced clarification opportunities
	Reduced influence of others	Reduced immediate reinforcement
	Enhanced response quality and quantity	
	Equal representation	
	Consistent participant contact	

(Table 4.2 continues)

Table 4.2 *(continued)*

Method	Advantages	Disadvantages
Community forum (town hall meeting)*	Relatively straightforward to conduct	Often difficult to achieve good attendance
	Relatively inexpensive	Participants in the community forum may tend to represent special interests
	Access to a broad cross-section of the community	
	People participate on own terms	The forum could degenerate into gripe session
	Can identify most interested	Data analysis can be time consuming
Meetings	Good for formative evaluation	Possible result bias
	Low cost	Limited input from participants
	Flexible	
Focus groups*	Low cost	Qualitative information
	Convenience	Limited representativeness
	Creative atmosphere	Dependence on moderator skill
	Ease of clarification	Preliminary insights
	Flexibility	Participant involvement
Nominal group process*	Direct involvement of priority groups	Time commitment
	Planned interactivity	Competing issues
	Diverse opinions	Participant bias
	Full participation	Segmented planning involvement
	Creative atmosphere	
	Recognition of common ground	
Observation	Accurate behavioral data	Requires trained observers
	Can be obtrusive	May bias behavior
	Moderate cost	Possible observer bias
		May be time-consuming
Self-assessments	Convenient	Possible low response rate
	No interviewer bias	Possible problem of representation
	Moderate cost	Self-selection
	Minimum staff time required	
	Easy to administer	
	Flexibility	

*From Gilmore (2012).

Table 4.3   Sample Sources of Secondary Data Available from Governmental and Nongovernmental Agencies and Organizations

Type of Agency/ Organization	Type of Data	URL (Web Address)
Government Agencies		
U.S. Bureau of Census	Demographic	
	U.S. Census	http://www.census.gov/
	Statistical Abstract of the United States	http://www.census.gov/ compendia/statab/
Centers for Disease Control and Prevention (CDC)	Health and Vital Statistics	
	National Center for Health Statistics (NCHS)	http://www.cdc.gov/nchs/
	Morbidity Mortality Weekly Report (MMWR)	http://www.cdc.gov/mmwr/
	CDC WONDER	http://wonder.cdc.gov/ welcome.html
	Behavioral Risk Factors	
	Behavioral Risk Factor Surveillance System (BRFSS)	http://www.cdc.gov/brfss/
	Youth Risk Behavior Surveillance System (YRBSS)	http://www.cdc.gov/ healthyyouth/yrbs/index.htm
Food & Drug Administration (FDA)	Food, Drugs and Medical Device Data	http://www.fda.gov/
Environmental Protection Agency (EPA)	Environmental Data and Statistics	http://www.epa.gov/
Substance Abuse & Mental Health Services Administration (SAMHSA)	Substance & Mental Health Statistical Information	http://www.samhsa.gov/
National Cancer Institute	Cancer Statistics	http://www.cancer.gov/
Nongovernmental Agencies and Organizations		
American Cancer Society	Cancer Information and Statistics	http://www.cancer.org/
American Heart Association	Heart Disease and Stroke Information and Statistics	http://www.heart.org/ HEARTORG
County Health Rankings	Health Data by U.S. Counties	http://www.countyhealthrank-ings.org
Henry J. Kaiser Family Foundation	Health Data by States	http://www.statehealthfacts.org

safety belts). Because the data are collected by the government, program planners can gain free access to them by contacting the agency that collects the data, or by finding them on the Internet, or in a library that serves as a United States government depository. Many college and university libraries and large public libraries serve as such depositories.

Data Available from Nongovernment Agencies and Organizations   In addition to the data available from government agencies, planners should also consult with nongovernment agencies and groups for data. Included among these are health care systems, voluntary health agencies, business, civic, and commerce groups. For example, most of the national voluntary health agencies produce yearly "facts and figures" booklets that include a variety of epidemiological data. In addition, local agencies and organizations often have data they have collected for their own use. For example, it is not unusual for a local United Way to have performed a needs assessment in the community before distributing funds.

Data from Existing Records   These are health data that are often "collected as a by-product of a service effort, such as managing a clinic, an immunization program, or a water pollution control program" (Pickett & Hanlon, 1990, p. 151). These data can also serve as useful secondary needs assessment data. Using such data may be an efficient way to obtain the necessary information for a needs assessment (or an evaluation) without the need for additional data collection. The advantages include low cost, minimum staff needed, and ease in randomization. The disadvantages include difficulty in gaining access to the necessary records and the possible lack of availability of all the information needed for a needs assessment or program evaluation.

Examples of the use of existing records include checking medical records to monitor blood pressure and cholesterol levels of participants in an exercise program, reviewing insurance usage of employees enrolled in an employee health promotion program, and comparing the academic records of students engaging in an after-school weight loss program with those who are not. In these situations, as with all needs assessments using existing records, the cooperation of the agencies that hold the records is essential. At times, agencies may be willing to collect additional information to aid in the needs assessment for (or an evaluation of) a health promotion program. Keepers of records are concerned about confidentiality and the release of private information. The importance of privacy for those planners working in health care settings was further emphasized in 2003 with the enactment of the *Standards for Privacy of Individually Identifiable Health Information* section (The Privacy Rule) of the Health Insurance Portability and Accountability Act of 1996 (officially known as Public Law 104-191 and referred to as **HIPAA,** pronounced "hip-a"). The rule sets national standards that health plans, health care clearinghouses, and health care providers who conduct certain health care transactions electronically must implement to protect and guard against the misuse of individually identifiable health information. Failure to implement the standards can lead to civil and criminal penalties (USDHHS, OCR, n.d.). Planners can deal with these privacy issues by getting permission from all participants to use their records or by using only anonymous data.

Data from the Literature   Planners might also be able to identify the needs of a priority population by reviewing any available current literature about that priority population. An example would be a planner who is developing a health promotion program for individuals infected by the human immunodeficiency virus (HIV). Because of the seriousness of this disease and the number of people who have studied and written about it, there is a good chance that present literature could reflect the need of a certain priority population.

The best means of accessing data from the literature is by using the available literature databases. Most literature databases today are available in several different forms, including computer databases and the Internet. Depending on the database used, planners can expect to find comprehensive listings of citations for journal articles, book chapters, and books, and, in some databases, abstracts of the literature. Within the listings, most databases cite sources by both author and subject/title. **Figure 4.3** provides an example of what planners might find when searching a database.

Many literature databases are available to planners. Next is a short discussion of those databases that have proved helpful to health promotion planners.

PsycINFO PsycINFO®, which is produced by the American Psychological Association (APA), is an abstract (not full-text) "that provides systematic coverage of the psychological literature from the 1800s to the present" (APA, 2011, para. 1). In addition to the abstracts, it also contains bibliographic citations, cited references, and descriptive information (APA, 2011). The database is divided into several major categories, but two of particular interest to planners are (1) behavioral science and (2) mental health.

Medline Medline, the primary component of and accessed through PubMed®, is the U.S. National Library of Medicine's® (NLM) premier bibliographic database that contains over 18 million references from more than 5,500 journals covering the life sciences with a concentration on biomedicine. "A distinctive feature of Medline is that the records are indexed with NLM's Medical Subject Headings (MeSH®)" (NLM, 2011, para. 1).

Education Resource Information Center (ERIC) ERIC is an online digital library of education literature sponsored by the Institute of Education Sciences (IES) of the U.S.

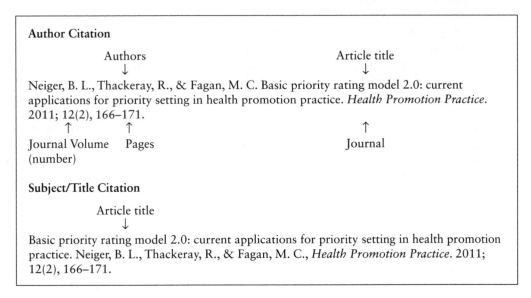

Figure 4.3 Sample Citations

Department of Education. ERIC provides free access to more than 1.3 million bibliographic records of journal articles and other education-related materials that have been indexed from 1966 to the present (ERIC, n.d.).

Cumulative Index to Nursing & Allied Health Literature (CINAHL)   The CINAHL grew out of the work of a hospital librarian in the 1940s who created an index for nursing journals. Demand for this work grew over the years until in 1961 the first volume of *Cumulative Index to Nursing Literature (CINL)* was published. In order to keep pace with the trend toward a multidisciplinary approach to health care, the scope of coverage was expanded in 1977 to include allied health journals. That is the year its name changed to CINAHL. This database went online in 1984.

ETHXWeb   ETHXWeb, which originates from the Bioethics Research Library at Georgetown University, is a database that "covers ethical, legal, and public policy issues surrounding health care and biomedical research. Citations are derived from the literature of law, religion, ethics, social sciences, philosophy, the popular media, and the health sciences" (Cottrell et al., 2012, p. 304).

Steps for Conducting a Literature Search

General Search Procedures   The process of searching a database is not difficult, and with the exception of a few individual differences, most indexes are arranged in a similar format. As Figure 4.3 indicated, most indexes include both an author and a subject/title index. An item that is specific to each index is its thesaurus (or in the case of Medline, Medical Subject Headings), a listing of the key words the indexes used to index the subject/titles. Planners can find the thesauri online or in a separate volume with or near a hard copy of the indexes.

Figure 4.4 provides planners with a literature search strategy in the form of a flowchart. The chart begins by identifying the need of the priority population or topic to be searched. At this point, planners can search either by subject/title or by author. If planners know of an author who has done work on their topic, they can search the database using the author's last name. If they do not have information on authors, they will need to match their topic with the key words presented in the thesaurus. Since there are times when a topic is not expressed in the same terms used in the thesaurus, planners will need to look for related terms. Once they have a list of key words, they need to search the database for possible matches. In conducting this search, they need to ensure that they are using the database that covers the years of literature in which they are interested. This search should identify possible sources and citations.

Once sources are identified, planners may review abstracts (or entire documents) online or locate a hard copy of the document. Then, planners must determine the quality and usefulness of the publication in the needs assessment process. One means by which planners can judge the quality of the literature is to examine the references at the end of the publications. First, this reference list may lead planners to other sources not identified in the original search. Second, if the sources found in the database include all those commonly cited in the literature, this can verify the exhaustiveness of the search.

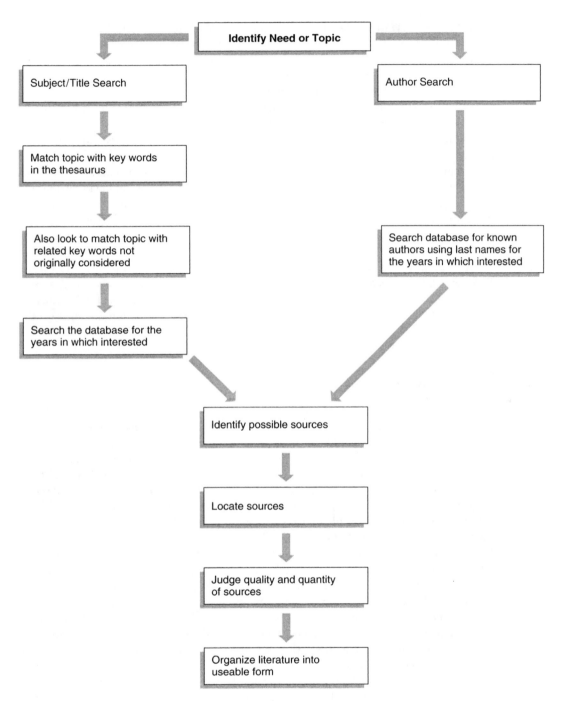

Figure 4.4 Literature Search Strategy Flowchart

Source: Adapted from Deeds (1992) and Marcarin (1995).

Searching via the World Wide Web   The continued development of the World Wide Web (WWW) has enhanced the opportunities for planners to obtain a variety of needs assessment data with the "touch of a button" from their home or office. Many of the government and nongovernment agencies and organizations, as well as the databases, discussed in this chapter have Websites that planners can access if they have the Web address, also known as the uniform resource locator (URL). If the Web address is unknown, planners can use a search engine to identify appropriate Websites.

Popular search engines include Yahoo, Google, and bing. Planners can experiment with and select the sites that best fit their needs. If planners are using a term that has more than one word (i.e., *heart disease*), it is best to use quotation marks around the term when entering it on the search engine. "This will let the search engine know that the exact phrase, as contained in the quotation marks, is to be used when seeking sites that match. If the quotation marks are not used, the search engine will find sites that contain any of the words in the query" (Cottrell et al., 2012, p. 307) and thus many of the sites found may not be of use.

As with any data source, planners need to be aware that not all data found via the Web are valid and reliable. Thus planners need to scrutinize sources just as they would data found in hard copies. Several authors (e.g., Kotecki & Chamness, 1999; Pealer & Dorman, 1997) have published useful guides for evaluating information obtained via the Internet.

Using Technology to Map Needs Assessment Data

As has already been mentioned in this chapter, more and more needs assessment data are being obtained through the use of technology (i.e., electronic interviews, computerized searchers of the World Wide Web and databases).

One other process that is being used more frequently is the use of geographic information systems (GIS) to help provide meaning to collected data. Being able to "map" the data provides this meaning. **Mapping** is the visual representation of data by geography or location, linking information to a place (Kirschenbaum & Russ, 2005). "Mapping is a powerful tool for two reasons: (1) it makes patterns based on place much easier to identify and analyze, and (2) it provides a visual way of communicating those patterns to a broad audience, quickly and dramatically" (Kirschenbaum & Russ, 2005, p. 450). The process of mapping involves (1) identifying the geographic area that the map will cover, (2) collecting the necessary data, (3) importing the data into GIS software so that the data can be placed on maps, and (4) analyzing what is found in the maps. In more technical terminology, "with GIS, digital maps and databases are stored with linked geo-referenced identifiers to facilitate rapid computer manipulation, analysis, and spatial display of information" (Riner, Cunningham, & Johnson, 2004, p. 57). The use of GIS in the needs assessment process will continue to grow as the development of such software becomes more widely available and easier to use. Some examples of how GIS has been used in health education programs are available in a document titled *Approaches to GIS Programs in Health Education* (available from ESRI at http://www.esri.com/library/brochures/pdfs/health-education.pdf).

Conducting a Needs Assessment

A number of different approaches can be used to determine the needs of the priority population. "Need assessments range from informal approaches, using educated and informed observations to formal, comprehensive research projects. However, the informal approaches are less reliable than a planned and scientifically developed research approach" (Timmreck, 2003, p. 89). Oftentimes, informal approaches are used because of limited time, personnel, and money. However, as noted in the beginning of this chapter, needs assessment may be the most critical step in the planning process and should not be taken lightly. Resources used on need assessments usually pay dividends many times over. Therefore the authors present a six-step process that is more formal in nature: (1) determining purpose and defining the scope of the needs assessment, (2) gathering data, (3) analyzing the data, (4) identifying the risk factors linked to the health problem, (5) identifying the program focus, and (6) validating the need before continuing on with the planning process (see **Figure 4.5**).

Step 1: Determining the Purpose and Scope of the Needs Assessment

The initial step in the needs assessment process is to determine the purpose and the scope of the needs assessment. In other words, what is the goal of the needs assessment? What does the planning committee hope to gain from the needs assessment? How extensive will the needs assessment be? What kind of resources will be available to conduct the needs assessment? In reality, the first challenge associated with conducting a needs assessment is determining whether an assessment should even be performed, and if so, what type of needs assessment is appropriate. For example, a great deal of health promotion today is driven by **categorical funding**. This means that the funding that supports programs is earmarked or dedicated to a specific health problem or determinant (e.g., risk factor). If this is the case, planners will not assess needs related to what health problem they should address since this is already predetermined by the funding agency. Likewise, if a planner works for the American Heart Association, he or she will not assess needs to determine a priority health problem—that has already been identified as heart disease.

Even if a health problem is already identified, it may be necessary to identify which determinants are most significant or which intervention strategies demonstrate the most promise in addressing the problem at hand. For example, heart disease may be the priority health problem, but it may be critical to assess the comparative importance of smoking, high blood pressure, and high blood cholesterol to identify appropriate

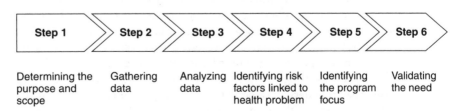

Figure 4.5 Steps in Conducting a Needs Assessment

interventions. The extent to which a needs assessment is necessary and appropriate should be determined by stakeholders, including key decision makers.

Some times, it is important to perform a needs assessment even if the health problem or determinant has been identified. For example, if the priority health problem is breast cancer, it is still necessary to collect current information on the degree to which women are either dying or suffering from the disease. It will be important to know how prevalent breast cancer is and where it is most prevalent in the population, as well as the high-risk subpopulations, economic costs, and general trends over time. Stakeholders will want continual status reports on the extent of the problem.

In other cases, a planner may be in a situation where a community needs assessment has not been performed for a long period of time or where categorical funding does not dictate what health problem(s) should be addressed. This will require planners and their partners to collect a wide range of data, compare the importance of multiple health problems, and set priorities. In a general sense, this is the process that is often referred to as *community assessment*. This implies that all significant health problems are examined to assess their relative significance. Stakeholders and planning groups will also usually determine how many health problems will be analyzed in the needs assessment. This will be influenced by how much time, and how many resources, can be directed to the needs assessment.

Another important decision that must be made is the extent to which actual consumers or clients will be involved in the needs assessment. The term **participatory** or **action research** has gained popularity in recent years, though it is often misunderstood or used inappropriately. *Participatory research* has been "defined as systematic inquiry, with the collaboration of those affected by the issue being studied, for the purposes of education and of taking action or effecting change" (Mercer et al., 2008, p. 409).

Once the basic purpose and scope of the needs assessment is identified, planners may proceed to data collection. However, planners must not take this first step too lightly. Although a natural tendency is to move forward quickly, an understanding of why a needs assessment is being performed will give proper direction to all other steps that follow.

Step 2: Gathering Data

The second step in the needs assessment process is gathering data. As noted earlier in this chapter, there are many different sources of needs assessment data. A part of the art of conducting a needs assessment is to be able to identify the most relevant data possible. By *relevant data,* we mean those data that are most applicable to the planning situation and that will do the best job of helping planners to identify the actual needs of the priority population. Because of the cost and availability, it is recommended that planners begin the data-gathering process by trying to locate relevant secondary data. For example, if a national program is being planned, then national secondary data should be sought from appropriate national government and nongovernment agencies. If a local program is being planned, then appropriate local data should be sought. When planning a local program, it is not unusual to find that local data do not exist. If that is the case, planners may need to use state, regional or national data (in that order) and apply them to the local area. For example, let's assume diabetes mellitus mortality data are needed for local planning and the only data available are national level data. Planners could use national data (e.g., 21.8 per 100,000 people died of diabetes in 2008) to estimate the number of deaths in a local community. If the population of a local city is 250,000, planners could infer that the number of deaths due to diabetes in the city during 2008 totaled 55 (i.e., 21.8×2.5). If the city's population were older, 55 deaths could be viewed as a low estimate since diabetes deaths are more prevalent in older populations. Conversely, if the population were younger, 55 deaths could be viewed as a high estimate. Obviously, as noted at the beginning of this chapter, there are disadvantages of using secondary data, but good planners use and interpret them in light of their limitations (McDermott & Sarvela, 1999).

Once relevant secondary data have been identified, planners need to turn their attention to gathering the appropriate primary data in order to fill in the "data gaps" to better understand the needs of the priority population. For example, if secondary data show that there is a need for cancer education programming, but does not specifically identify the type of cancer or segment the priority population by useful demographic characteristics (e.g., age or sex), then efforts should be made to collect such data. Or, it may be that all the secondary data are *quantitative data* such as how frequently a service is used, and thus it might be very useful to collect primary data that are *qualitative* in nature such as detailed explanations of why a service was not used. It should be noted that primary data collection could have a dual purpose. Not only do primary data collections provide valuable information about the specific planning situation that cannot be obtained from secondary data, they also provide an opportunity to get those in the priority population actively involved and contributing to the program planning process. Thus, planners need to decide what primary data are needed, from whom they should be collected (e.g., All? Some? Just certain demographic groups?), and what methods (e.g., Interviews? Questionnaires? Focus groups?) would be best for not only collecting the needed information but also in getting active participation from the priority population.

It should also be noted that the planning model used to develop a program might also drive the types of data collected for the needs assessment. For example, when the SMART (Social Marketing Assessment and Response Tool) model is used planners would be interested in collecting data that would assist with Consumer Analysis (Phase 2), Market Analysis (Phase 3), and Channel Analysis (Phase 4). When the Mobilizing for Action through Planning and Partnerships (MAPP) model is being used planners should be collecting data that would provide information for the Assessments (Phase 3) which yield a list of challenges and opportunities in a community (see **Box 4.2** for the four assessments found in Phase 3 of MAPP).

As planners conclude the second step in the needs assessment process, they must remember that each planning situation is different. It is desirable to have both primary and secondary needs assessment data in order to gain a clear picture of needs; however, depending on the resources and circumstances, planners may have access to only one or the other. In addition, there is usually a trade-off between quality and quantity of data. Planners must use the best data available under the challenges and constraints facing them.

Step 3: Analyzing the Data

At this point in the needs assessment process, planners must analyze all the data collected, with the goal of identifying and prioritizing the health problems. The goal of data analysis is easily stated, but this step may be the most difficult to complete. There are those rare

> **Box 4.2** THE FOUR MAPP ASSESSMENTS
>
> - The **Community Themes and Strengths Assessment** provides a deep understanding of the issues that residents feel are important by answering the questions: "What is important to our community?" "How is quality of life perceived in our community?" and "What assets do we have that can be used to improve community health?"
> - The **Local Public Health System Assessment** (LPHSA) focuses on all of the organizations and entities that contribute to the public's health. The LPHSA answers the questions: "What are the components, activities, competencies, and capacities of our local public health system?" and "How are the Essential Services being provided to our community?"
> - The **Community Health Status Assessment** identifies priority community health and quality of life issues. Questions answered include: "How healthy are our residents?" and "What does the health status of our community look like?"
> - The **Forces of Change Assessment** focuses on identifying forces such as legislation, technology, and other impending changes that affect the context in which the community and its public health system operate. This answers the questions: "What is occurring or might occur that affects the health of our community or the local public health system?" and "What specific threats or opportunities are generated by these occurrences?"
>
> *Source:* "The Four MAPP Assessments" in *The Assessments.* Copyright © 2011 by National Association of County and City Health Officials. Reprinted with Permission.

occasions when the data analysis is not very complicated because the need is obvious. For example, the data may clearly show that breast cancer rates have continued to rise in a community, while the number of breast screenings has dropped, and those in the priority population recognize the problem. Or, in another setting the data analysis shows a very clear correlation between the health status of the priority population and the lack of primary health care received. However, not all analyses of data yield such obvious needs. More often than not, planners are faced with trying to compare data that are not easily compared. The data may be mixed (i.e., apples and oranges) or confusing. For example, they may have mortality data for one health problem, morbidity data for another, and perhaps behavioral risk factor data for yet another. Or, if planners are working with a multicultural priority population, data analysis may even be more confusing, because health concepts held by one culture may be very different than the health concepts held by the planners. These cultural differences "often involve family, community, and/or supernatural agents in cause and effect, placation, and treatment rituals to prevent, control, or cure illness. A failure to understand and appreciate these 'differences' can have serious implications for success of any health promotion/disease prevention effort" (Kline & Huff, 1999, p. 106).

One systematic way to analyze the data is to use the first few phases of the PRECEDE-PROCEED model for guidance. Start by asking and answering the following questions:

1. What is the quality of life of those in the priority population?

2. What are social conditions and perceptions shared by those in the priority population?

3. What are the social indicators (e.g., absenteeism, crime, discrimination, performance, welfare, etc.) in the priority population that reflect the social conditions and perceptions?

4. Can the social conditions and perceptions be linked to health promotion? If so, how?

5. What are the health problems associated with the social problems?

6. Which health problem is most important to change?

The last question in this list is really asking the question, Which problem/need should get priority? The problems/needs must be prioritized not because the lowest-priority problems/needs are not important, but because organizations have limited resources to deal with all identified problems/needs. Thus, "priority setting is critical in narrowing the scope of activity to reflect the availability of resources within the context of stakeholders' values and preferences. In addition, priority setting helps health promotion practitioners stay focused on problems that actually affect the health status of the population" (Neiger, Thackeray, & Fagen, 2011, p. 166). Therefore, in setting priorities, the planners should seek answers to these questions:

1. What is the most pressing need?

2. Are there resources adequate to deal with the problem?

3. Can the problem best be solved by a health promotion intervention, or could it be handled better through another means?

4. Are effective intervention strategies available to address the problem?

5. Can the problem be solved in a reasonable amount of time?

The actual process of setting priorities can take many different forms and can range from subjective approaches such as simple voting procedures, forced rankings, and the nominal group process with stakeholders to more objective but time-consuming processes such as the Delphi technique (Gilmore, 2012) and the **basic priority rating (BPR)** model. The BPR model, which was first known as the "priority rating process," was introduced more than 50 years ago (Hanlon, 1954) in an attempt to prioritize health problems in developing countries. During this span of time, the BPR has been most useful to program planners. Although the BPR model has provided basic direction in priority setting, it does not represent the broad array of data available to decision makers today (Neiger et al., 2011). In addition, "elements in the model give more weight to the impact of communicable diseases as compared to chronic diseases" (Neiger et al., 2011, p. 166). As such, Neiger and his colleagues have proposed changes to the BPR model and suggested a new name for the model; **BPR Model 2.0.** To provide both background and currency, both the BPR model (Pickett & Hanlon, 1990) and the BPR model 2.0 (Neiger et al., 2011) are presented here.

BPR model The BPR model requires planners to rate four different components of the identified needs and insert the ratings into a formula in order to determine a priority rating between 0 and 100. The components and their possible scores (in parenthesis) are:

A. size of the problem (0 to 10)

B. seriousness of the problem (0 to 20)

C. effectiveness of the possible interventions (0 to 10)

D. propriety, economics, acceptability, resources, and legality (PEARL) (0 or 1)

The formula in which the scores are placed is:

$$\text{Basic Priority Rating (BPR)} = \frac{(A + B)C}{3} \times D$$

Component *A*, size of the problem, can be scored by using epidemiological rates or determining the percentage of the priority population at risk. The higher the rate or percentage, the greater the score. Pickett and Hanlon (1997) offer the scale noted in **Table 4.4** for scoring the size of the problem when using incidence and prevalence rates.

Component *B*, seriousness of the problem, is examined using four factors: economic loss to community, family, or individuals; involvement of other people who were not initially affected by the problem, as with the spread of an infectious disease; the severity of the problem measured in mortality, morbidity, or disability; and the urgency of solving the problem because of additional harm. Because the maximum score for this component is 20, raters can use a 0 to 5 score for each of the four factors.

Component *C*, effectiveness of the interventions, is often the most difficult of the four components to measure. The efficacy of some intervention strategies is known, such as immunizations (close to 100%) and smoking cessation classes (around 30%), but for many, it is not. Planners will need to estimate this score based upon the work of others or their own expert opinions. In scoring this component, planners should consider both the effectiveness of intervention strategies in terms of behavior change, as well as the degree to which the priority population will demonstrate interest in the intervention strategy.

Component *D*, PEARL, consists of several factors that determine whether a particular intervention strategy can be carried out at all. The score is 0 or 1; any need that receives a zero will automatically drop to the bottom of the priority list because a score of zero (a multiplier) for this component will yield a total score of zero in the formula. Examples of when a zero may result are if an intervention is economically impossible, unacceptable to the priority population or planners, or illegal. Ideally, some of these assessments will be made before a health problem is considered in the priority setting process.

Once the score for the four components is determined, an overall priority rating for each need can be calculated, and the prioritizing can take place.

Table 4.4 Scoring the Size of the Problem

Incidence or Prevalence per 100,000 Population	Score
50,000 or more	10
5,000 to 49,999	8
500 to 4,999	6
50 to 499	4
5 to 49	2
0.5 to 4.9	0

Source: Public Health: Administration and Practice. George E. Pickett and John J. Hanlon. Copyright © 1997 by McGraw Hill Education. Adapted with permission.

BPR model 2.0   Building on the BPR model, Neiger and his colleagues (2011) offered the following adaptations to the model and suggested calling the revised model the BPR model 2.0.

A. Size of the problem. "Depending on the availability of data and preferences of the stakeholders use one of the following:

1. Use incidence *and* prevalence data and score each on a scale of 0 to 5 for a total of 10 points (it is recognized that incidence represents a proportion of prevalence).
2. Use incidence *or* prevalence data and score each health problem on a scale of 0 to 10 points.
3. Use age-adjusted cause-specific mortality rates *and* proportional mortality ratios for each health problem and score each on a scale of 0 to 5 for a total of 10 points.
4. Use age-adjusted cause-specific mortality rates *or* proportional mortality ratios and score each health problem on a scale of 0 to 10 points" (p. 168).

B. Seriousness of the problem. Both the definitions for the components of "seriousness" and the scoring for the components be changed as follows:

1. Urgency—defined "as the degree to which a health problem is increasing, stabilizing, or decreasing and that 5-year mortality trend data be used to score it" (p. 168). Scores should be assigned as follows: increasing trend data (5 or 4 points); stabilized trend data (3 or 2 points); and decreasing trend data (1 or 0 points).
2. Severity—expand the definition of the criterion to include: (a) the lethality of a health problem (as measured by five-year survival rate), (b) premature mortality (as measured by years of potential life lost or years of productive life lost), and (c) disability (as measured by disability-adjusted life years [DALYs]). Scores should be assigned as follows: 0- to 5-point scale (i.e., 5–4 is high, 3–2 is medium, and 1–0 is low).
3. Economic loss—defined as the accumulation of costs (direct and indirect) borne by society associated with the health problem. Scores should be assigned as follows: 0- to 5-point scale (i.e., 5–4 is high, 3–2 is medium, and 1–0 is low).
4. Impact on others—expand the definition of the criterion to include: "(a) as the communicable nature of the health problem (particularly when analyzing communicable diseases); (b) the behavioral effects related to the health problem on others (e.g., secondhand smoke, driving while under the influence of alcohol or other drugs, violence perpetrated on others, etc.); or (c) the emotional and physical impact the health problem (with attendant disabilities) has on others with respect to care giving" (p. 169). Scores should be assigned as follows: 0- to 5-point scale (i.e., 5–4 is high, 3–2 is medium, and 1–0 is low).

C. Effectiveness of the possible interventions. Limit the definition of "effectiveness" to evidence of successful intervention and not rate the "reach" of the intervention. The scoring of effectiveness should be based on the typology of evidence developed by Brownson, Fielding, and Maylahn (2009). Scores should be assigned as follows: 0- to 10-point scale (i.e., 10–9 reflect evidence-based interventions, 8–7 reflect effective programs, 6–5 reflect promising interventions, 4–3 reflect emerging interventions, and 2–0 reflect unproven interventions).

D. PEARL. The calculation of PEARL should remain the same. However, if secondary data are available to calculate the PEARL it should be calculated prior to collecting primary data so that the needs assessment may be more focused.

For an example application of the BPR model 2.0 readers should refer to Neiger et al. (2011).

Finally, how will planners know when they have completed Step 3 (Analyzing the Data) of the needs assessment process? Planners should be able to list in rank order the problems/needs of the priority population.

Step 4: Identifying the Risk Factors Linked to the Health Problem

Step 4 of the needs assessment process is parallel to the second part of Phase 2 of the PRECEDE-PROCEED model: epidemiological assessment. In this step, planners need to identify the determinants of the health problem identified in the previous step. That is, what genetic, behavioral, and environmental risk factors are associated with the health problem? Because most genetic determinants either cannot be changed or interact with the behavior and/or environment, the task in this step is to identify and prioritize the behavioral and environmental factors that, if changed, could lessen the health problem in the priority population. Also, it should be noted that the term *environmental factors* applies to more than just the physical environment (e.g., clean air and water, proximity to facilities). Environment is multidimensional and can include economic environment (e.g., affordability, incentives, disincentives); service environment (e.g., access to health care, equity in health care, barriers to health care); social environment (e.g., social support, peer pressure); psychological environment (e.g., emotional learning environment); and the political environment (e.g., health policy). In essence then, modifying behavioral and/or environmental factors or determinants is the real work of health promotion. Thus, if the health problem is lung cancer, planners should analyze the health behaviors and environment of the priority population for known risk factors of lung cancer. For example, higher than expected smoking behavior may be present in the priority population, and the people may live in a community where smokefree public environments are not valued. Once these risk factors are identified, they too need to be prioritized (see Figure 3.3 for a means of prioritizing these risk factors).

Step 5: Identifying the Program Focus

The fifth step of the needs assessment process is similar to the third phase of the PRECEDE-PROCEED model: educational and ecological assessment. With behavioral, environmental, and genetic risk factors identified and prioritized, planners need to identify those predisposing, enabling, and reinforcing factors that seem to have a direct impact on the risk factors. In the lung cancer example, those in the priority population may not have (1) the skills necessary to stop smoking (predisposing factor), (2) access to a smoking cessation program (enabling factor), or (3) people around them who support efforts to stop smoking (reinforcing factor). "Study of the predisposing, enabling, and reinforcing factors automatically helps the planner decide exactly which of the factors making up the three classes deserve the highest priority as the focus of the intervention. The decision is based on their importance and any evidence that change in the factor is possible and cost-effective" (Green & Kreuter, 1999, p. 42).

In addition, when prioritizing needs, planners also need to consider any existing health promotion programs to avoid duplication of efforts. Therefore, program planners should seek to determine the status of existing health promotion programs by trying to answer as many questions as possible from the following list:

1. What health promotion programs are presently available to the priority population?

2. Are the programs being utilized? If not, why not?

3. How effective are the programs? Are they meeting their stated goals and objectives?

4. How were the needs for these programs determined?

5. Are the programs accessible to the priority population? Where are they located? When are they offered? Are there any qualifying criteria that people must meet to enroll? Can the priority population get to the program? Can the priority population afford the programs?

6. Are the needs of the priority population being met? If not, why not?

There are several ways to seek answers to these questions. Probably the most common way is through **networking** with other people working in health promotion and the health care system—that is, communicating with others who may know about existing programs. (See Chapter 9 for a more detailed discussion of networking.) These people may be located in the local or state health department, in voluntary health agencies, or in health care facilities, such as hospitals, clinics, nursing homes, extended care facilities, or managed care organizations.

Planners might also find information about existing programs by checking with someone in an organization that serves as a clearinghouse for health promotion programs or by using a community resource guide. The local or state health department, a local chamber of commerce, a coalition, the local medical/dental societies, a community task force, or a community health center may serve as a clearinghouse or produce such a guide. Another avenue is to talk with people in the priority population. Although they may not know about all existing programs, they may be able to share information on the effectiveness and accessibility of some of the programs. Finally, some of the information could be collected in Step 2 through separate community forums, focus groups, or surveys.

Step 6: Validating the Prioritized Needs

The final step in the needs assessment process is to validate the identified need(s). *Validate* means to confirm that the need that was identified is the need that should be addressed. Obviously, if great care were taken in the needs assessment process, validation should be a perfunctory step. However, there have been times when a need was not properly validated; much energy and many resources have thereby been wasted on unnecessary programs.

Validation amounts to "double checking," or making sure that an identified need is the actual need. Any means available can be used, such as (1) rechecking the steps followed in the needs assessment to eliminate any bias, (2) conducting a focus group with some individuals from the priority population to determine their reaction to the identified need (if a focus group was not used earlier to gather the data), and (3) getting a "second opinion" from other health professionals.

Application of the Six-Step Needs Assessment Process

In the previous sections, a six-step approach for conducting a needs assessment was presented. Now we would like to present an example of how this process may be applied. Let's assume that a committee has been appointed by the health administrator of a local health department to plan a cancer prevention program for the county, and that the composition of the committee closely represents the greater community. Let's also assume that the parameters for the authority of the planning committee have also been set. Here is how this needs assessment may be carried out.

Step 1: Determining the Purpose and Scope of the Needs Assessment—After an organizational meeting and a couple subsequent meetings, the planning committee decided that the purpose of the needs assessment was fourfold. To determine (1) what types of cancers were of greatest concern in the county, (2) which subpopulations within the county were at the greatest risk for the cancers identified, (3) what the most common risk factors were for the cancer(s) and subpopulation(s) identified, and (4) the focus of the proposed program. The committee members also decided that the scope of the needs assessment would be defined by the collection of both primary and secondary data, and that they wanted part of the primary data collection to be participatory in nature. That is, they wanted some of those in the priority population to participate in the data collection process.

Step 2: Gathering Data—Because of the costs and resources associated with primary data collection, the committee members decided to begin data collection by identifying available sources of secondary data. Initially they gathered secondary data for the past five years for both the state and the county in which they lived from the state health department for the incidence of invasive cancer; cancer mortality rates (i.e., crude and age-adjusted); mortality rates for various types of cancer broken down by sex, age, and race/ethnicity; and behavioral risk factors that were known to contribute to or cause the various types of cancer. In addition, committee members were able to get secondary data from the state environmental agency regarding the levels of air and water pollution in all 92 counties of the state.

The secondary data were good but they did not present a complete picture of the cancer issue in their county. What was not available in the secondary data were information and data related to cancer education programs, cancer screening programs, access to health care providers that specialized in cancer care, and the county residents' interest in taking part in activities that would reduce the incidence and prevalence in their community. Therefore, the committee created three different questionnaires to be administered via single-step surveys. The three questionnaires dealt with cancer prevention activities (i.e., education and screenings), cancer treatment, and attitudes toward and willingness to participate in cancer programs if offered in the community.

To make part of the primary data collection a participatory process the committee sought out two groups of volunteers from the county who were interested in cancer control. The first group was asked to assist in data collection by administering the surveys to various individuals in the county by visiting places where residents were likely to gather such as service group meetings, religious organizations (i.e., churches, mosques, and synagogues), services, worksites, and neighborhood meetings. The second group of volunteers was asked to collect data via a photovoice process with a theme of "identify those unhealthy areas of the county that contribute to cases of cancer."

Step 3: Analyzing the Data—The committee members decided to analyze the data comparing their county data versus the state data using the informal technique of eye-balling the data. To help make sense of some of the data they created a few cross-tabulation tables. The analysis of the secondary cancer data from the state health department, the County Health Rankings (see Weblinks at the end of the chapter), and the Kaiser Family Foundation's state health facts (see Weblinks at the end of the chapter) showed:

- higher county incidence rate for invasive cancers (501/100,000 vs. 426/100,000)
- both higher county cancer crude mortality rates (208/100,000 vs. 195/100,000) and age-adjusted (199/100,000 vs. 183/100,000)
- higher county prevalence rates for colorectal, lung, and pancreas cancers
- lower county prevalence rates for breast, cervix, and prostate cancers

The analysis of the secondary behavior risk data from the state's Behavior Risk Factor Surveillance System data showed:

- higher percentage of county residents who had not had either a sigmoidoscopy or colonoscopy in the recommended time period
- higher percentage of county women who had either a clinical breast examination (77.1% vs. 74.5%) or mammogram (76.3% vs. 73.1%) in the recommended time period
- higher percentage of county women who had a Papanicolaou smear (82.6% vs. 77.4%) in the recommended time period
- higher percentage of county residents who were physically inactive (55.7% vs. 48.9%)
- higher prevalence of county residents who smoked (28.3% vs. 23.0%)

The analysis of the primary data from the three surveys conducted by the committee showed county residents:

- would participate in free and/or inexpensive cancer screenings if they were convenient
- were in favor of creating more smokefree public areas
- felt, and the data showed, that there were too few health care providers in the county that dealt with cancer.

The analysis of the photovoice process identified two major themes in the county:

- many of the county residents were physically inactive and appeared to be either overweight or obese, and
- there were few smokefree public places in the county

Based on all the available primary and secondary data the committee prioritized the list of cancers using the BPR model 2.0. Those calculations yielded the following BPR scores: breast (38.7), colorectal (56.8), lung (51.8), cervix (30.4), pancreas (24.0), and prostate (41.7). Therefore, the committee decided to work to reduce the incidence of colorectal and lung cancers in the county.

Step 4: Identifying the Risk Factors Linked to the Health Problem—The risk factors associated with colorectal cancer include age (> 50 years), personal history of colorectal polyps or cancer, personal history of inflammatory bowel disease, family history of colorectal cancer, diets high in red meats, physical inactivity, obesity, smoking, heavy alcohol use, and type 2 diabetes (ACS, 2011). The risk factors associated with lung cancer include smoking, exposure to radon, exposure to asbestos, high levels of arsenic in the drinking water, personal or family history of lung cancer, and air pollution (ACS, 2011).

Step 5: Identifying the Program Focus—Based on the analysis of the data and the risk factors associated with identified priority cancers the planning committee decided to focus the cancer prevention program on two areas: working to offer more cancer screening programs in the county, and working toward a nonsmoking ordinance in the county in order to create smokefree public places.

Step 6: Validating the Prioritized Needs—Before moving forward with the planning for the cancer prevention programs to deal with colorectal and lung cancer, the committee had representatives from both the state department of health's cancer prevention program and the American Cancer Society review their needs assessment to validate their findings. Both groups agreed with the program focus.

Health Impact Assessment

Before leaving the topic of needs assessment we need to introduce the term **health impact assessment (HIA)**. It is an important topic because an HIA could impact the focus of a needs assessment and it is "a rapidly emerging practice" (CDC, 2009b, para. 6) in the United States (see Dannenberg et al., 2008, for examples of its use). A HIA has been defined as "a combination of procedures, methods, and tools by which a policy, program, or project may be judged as to its potential effects on the health of a population, and the distribution of those effects within the population" (ECHP, 1999, p. 4). In other words, an HIA is an "approach that can help to identify and consider the potential—or actual—health impacts of a proposal on a population. Its primary output is a set of evidence-based recommendations geared to informing the decision making process. These recommendations aim to highlight practical ways to enhance the positive aspects of a proposal, and to remove or minimise [sic] any negative impacts on health, well-being and health inequalities that may arise or exist" (Taylor & Quigley, 2002, pp. 2–3).

The World Health Organization (2011) has noted that HIAs are based on four values. They include:

1. Democracy—allowing people to participate in the development and implementation of policies, programmes or projects that may impact on their lives.

2. Equity—HIA assesses the distribution of impacts from a proposal on the whole population, with a particular reference to how the proposal will affect vulnerable people (in terms of age, gender, ethnic background, and socio-economic status).

3. Sustainable development—that both short and long term impacts are considered, along with the obvious, and less obvious impacts.

4. Ethical use of evidence—the best available quantitative and qualitative evidence must be identified and used in the assessment. A wide variety of evidence should be collected using the best possible methods (para. 1.).

There are a number of different frameworks (i.e., guides) that can be used to conduct a HIA (see Mindell, Boltong, & Forde 2008 for a review of guides) and they "can range from simple, fairly easy-to-conduct analyses to more in-depth, complex analyses" (Brennan Ramirez et al., 2008, p. 46), but most of these guides include the following major steps:

1. Screening (identify projects or policies for which an HIA would be useful)
2. Scoping (identify which health effects to consider)
3. Assessing risks and benefits (identify which people may be affected and how they may be affected)
4. Developing recommendations (suggest changes to proposals to promote positive or mitigate adverse health effects)
5. Reporting (present the results to decision makers)
6. Evaluating (determine the effect of the HIA on the decision) (CDC, 2009a, para. 3)

As planners prepare for a needs assessment they must also consider whether an HIA should be a part of the process.

SUMMARY

This chapter presented several definitions of needs assessment and a discussion of primary and secondary data. The sources of these data were discussed at length. Also, presented in this chapter was a six-step approach that planners can follow in conducting a needs assessment on a given group of people. It is by no means the only way of conducting an assessment, but it is one viable option. No matter what procedure is used to conduct a needs assessment, the end result should be the same. Planners should finish with a clearly defined program focus. Finally, the term health impact assessment was introduced.

REVIEW QUESTIONS

1. What is a need? What does *needs assessment* mean?
2. What is meant by the terms *capacity*, *community capacity*, and *capacity building*?
3. What should program planners expect from a needs assessment?
4. What is the difference between primary and secondary data?
5. Name several different sources of both primary and secondary data.

6. What advice might you give to someone who is interested in using previously collected data (secondary data) for a needs assessment?

7. What is the difference between a single-step (cross-sectional) and a multistep survey?

8. Explain the difference between a community forum and a focus group.

9. What are the steps in the photovoice process?

10. What is a health assessment (HA)?

11. Describe the steps used to conduct a literature search.

12. What are the six steps in the needs assessment process, as identified in this chapter? What is the most difficult step to complete?

13. What is the difference between BPR model and the BPR model 2.0?

14. What is health impact assessment (HIA) and how could it affect a needs assessment?

ACTIVITIES

1. Assume a local health department (LHD) that serves a rural population of about 100,000 people has hired you. After a few months on the job, your supervisor has given you the task of conducting a needs assessment. The last one completed by this LHD was 15 years ago. Based on the annual reports of the LHD over the past 5 years, it has been determined that the needs assessment should focus on the needs of the elderly. For the purpose of this needs assessment, the LHD has defined elderly as those 65 years of age and older. Working with the six-step approach to needs assessment presented in this chapter, complete the first two steps. Complete Step 1 by writing a purpose and scope for the needs assessment. Complete the first part of Step 2 by identifying at least four sources of relevant secondary data. Also, describe what you think would be the best way to go about collecting primary data and defend your choice. Then complete this activity by creating a list of things you would like to find out by gathering primary data.

2. Visit the Website of a commercial company (e.g., Zoomerang, SurveyMonkey, and Qualtrics) that is in the business of helping others collect primary data via the Internet. Once at the site, find out as much as you can about using the service. What specific services does the company offer? How much do the services cost? What group of program planners do you think would most benefit from using the services? Summarize the results of your fact-finding experience in a one-page paper.

3. Using secondary data provided by your instructor or obtained from the World Wide Web (such as data from a Behavioral Risk Factor Surveillance System, state or local secondary data, or data from the National Center for Health Statistics), analyze the data and determine the health problems of the priority population.

4. Using data from the County Health Rankings Website (http://www.county healthrankings.org/), examine the data presented for the county in which you grew up or currently live. After reviewing the data, prepare a written response that summarizes the general health status of the county.

5. Visit the Community Tool Box Website (http://ctb.ku.edu/en/tablecontents/sub_ tools_1165.aspx) and review the information presented in the sample informed consent forms. After reviewing the information, create a consent form that could be used with the collection of primary data via a written questionnaire for a program you are planning.

6. Administer an HHA/HRA to a group of 25 to 30 people. Using the data generated, identify and prioritize a collective list of health problems of the group.

7. Plan and conduct a focus group on an identified health problem on your campus. Develop a set of questions to be used, identify and invite people to participate in the group, facilitate the process, and then write up a summary of the results based on your written notes and/or an audiotape of the session.

8. Using the data (paper-and-pencil instruments, clinical tests, and health histories) generated from a local health fair, identify and prioritize a collective list of health problems of those who participated.

WEBLINKS

1. **http://ctb.ku.edu/**

   The Community Tool Box

   This site provides excellent resources on community assessment, conducting surveys, identifying problems, and assessing community needs and resources. Topic sections include step-by-step instruction, examples, checklists, and related resources.

2. **http://www.countyhealthrankings.org/**

   County Health Rankings

   This Website is a result of collaboration between the Robert Wood Johnson Foundation and the University of Wisconsin Population Health Institute to develop a collection of county health rankings for each state.

3. **http://www.cdc.gov/nchs/surveys.htm**

   National Center for Health Statistics

   This Webpage of the National Center for Health Statistics (NCHS) provides an overview of all of the surveys and data collections systems of the NCHS. In addition, it provides the results of many of the surveys and examples of the questionnaires used to collect the data.

4. http://www.statehealthfacts.org

   Kaiser Family Foundation State Health Facts Online

   This site contains current state-level data on demographics, health, and health policy, including health coverage, access, financing, and state legislation. Planners can access information as tables, bar graphs, or color-coded maps.

5. http://wonder.cdc.gov/

   CDC WONDER

   This is the home page for the Centers for Disease Control and Prevention's (CDC) Wide-ranging Online Data for Epidemiologic Research (WONDER). CDC WONDER is an easy-to-use, menu-driven system that provides access to a wide array of secondary public health information. It also has a link to the latest data to support the *Healthy People 2020* objectives.

CHAPTER 5

Measurement, Measures, Measurement Instruments, and Sampling

After reading this chapter and answering the questions that follow, you should be able to:

- Define measurement.
- Explain the difference between quantitative and qualitative measures.
- Explain why measurement is such an important process as it relates to program planning and evaluation as well as research.
- Briefly describe the four levels of measurement.
- List the variables that are often measured by health education specialists.
- List the four desirable characteristics of data.
- Explain the various types of validity.
- Define *reliability* and explain why it is important.
- Define *bias* in data collection and discuss how it can be reduced.
- Explain why measurement instruments must be fair.
- Briefly describe the steps to identify, obtain, and evaluate existing measurement instruments.
- Briefly describe the process for creating a data collection instrument.
- Describe how a sample can be obtained from a population.
- Differentiate between probability and nonprobability samples.
- Describe how a pilot test is used.

bias	construct validity	culture
census	content validity	cultural competence
cluster sampling	convergent validity	discriminant validity
concurrent validity	criterion-related validity	face validity

Key Terms, continued

fairness	pilot testing	sample
field study	population	sampling
instrumentation	predictive validity	sampling frame
internal consistency	preliminary review	sampling unit
inter-rater reliability	pre-pilots	sensitivity
interval level measures	probability sample	simple random sample
intra-rater reliability	proportional stratified	(SRS)
levels of measurement	random sample	specificity
measurement instrument	psychometric qualities	strata
nominal level measures	public domain	stratified random sample
nonprobability samples	qualitative measures	survey population
nonproportional stratified	quantitative measures	systematic sample
random sample	random selection	test–retest reliability
ordinal level measures	rater reliability	universe
parallel forms reliability	ratio level measures	validity
pilot test	reliability	

In this chapter, we will examine critical concepts necessary to maximize the quality of data, whether for a needs assessment or a program evaluation. Specifically, we will examine the (1) term *measurement*, (2) types of data generated from measurement, (3) importance of measurement, (4) levels of measurement, (5) types of measures, (6) desirable characteristics of measures, (7) measurement instruments, (8) sampling, and (9) the importance of pilot testing in the data collection process.

Box 5.1 identifies the responsibilities and competencies for health education specialists that pertain to the material presented in this chapter.

Measurement

Measurement can be defined as the process of applying numerical or narrative data from an instrument (e.g., a questionnaire) or other data-yielding tools to objects, events, or people (Windsor, Clark, Boyd, & Goodman, 2004). For example, if researchers collect data on height and weight from a group of people then translate those data to body mass index (BMI) values (weight in kilograms divided by height in meters squared), they can classify participants as either underweight (usually a BMI of < 18.50), normal (18.50–24.99), overweight (25–29.99) or obese (> 30). In order to measure something then, planners/evaluators need to identify what instrument or tool will be used to collect data, how data will be categorized using numbers or words, and how these categories of data will be classified (e.g., high risk, medium risk, low risk or excellent health, good health, poor health, etc.).

The data generated by measurements can be classified into two broad categories, depending on the method by which they are collected. **Quantitative measures** "are

Box 5.1	Responsibilities and Competencies for Health Education Specialists

Because of the importance of measurement to program planning and evaluation, the content of this chapter cuts across two different areas of responsibility. Those responsibilities and related competencies include:

Responsibility I: Assess Needs, Assets, and Capacity for Health Education

Competency 1.2: Access existing information and data related to health

Competency 1.3: Collect quantitative and/or qualitative data related to health

Competency 1.4: Examine relationships among behavioral, environmental, and genetic factors that enhance or compromise health

Competency 1.6: Examine factors that enhance or compromise the process of health education

Competency 1.7: Infer needs for health education based on assessment findings

Responsibility IV: Conduct Evaluation and Research Related to Health Education

Competency 4.2: Design instruments to collect evaluation/research data

Competency 4.3: Collect and analyze evaluation/research data

Competency 4.4: Interpret results of the evaluation/research

Competency 4.5: Apply findings from evaluation/research

Source: NCHEC, SOPHE, & AAHE (2010).

numerical data collected to understand individuals' knowledge, understanding, perceptions, and behavior" (Harris, 2010, p. 208). Examples of quantitative data could include the mortality rates for diabetes over the last five years, the aforementioned BMIs of participants in a weight loss program, the prevalence of cigarette smoking among adolescents, the ratings on a patient satisfaction survey, and the pretest and posttest scores on a HIV knowledge test. **Qualitative measures** are "data collected with the use of narrative and observational approaches to understand individuals' knowledge, perceptions, attitudes and behaviors" (Harris, 2010 p. 208). Qualitative data are usually represented as words that are organized into codes and themes. Examples of qualitative data could include notes generated from observational studies, transcripts from focus groups, and taped recordings of in-depth interviews with key informants. Quantitative and qualitative measures both have their individual strengths and weaknesses, yet their greatest utility may occur when both are used together in the measurement process. While quantitative data are generally associated with better representations of entire populations,

Table 5.1   Comparison of Quantitative and Qualitative Measures

Quantitative Measures	Qualitative Measures
Measures level of occurrence	Provides depth of understanding
Asks how often? and how many?	Asks why?
Studies actions	Studies motivations
Is objective	Is subjective
Provides proof	Enables discovery
Is definitive	Is exploratory
Measures levels of actions and trends, etc.	Allows insights into behavior and trends, etc.
Describes	Interprets

Source: Cottrell & McKenzie (2011, p. 228) from Debus (1988).

qualitative data can provide rich contextual understanding of those same populations. **Table 5.1** provides a comparison of many of the qualities and characteristics of quantitative and qualitative measures.

The Importance of Measurement in Program Planning and Evaluation

As noted earlier in the chapter (see Box 5.1), health education specialists are expected to have the knowledge and skills (NCHEC, SOPHE, & AAHE, 2010) to plan and carry out the processes associated with measurement; for example, (1) when reviewing literature in order to justify a program, health education specialists need to be able to understand the data generated by measurement in order to determine if they have adequate and appropriate evidence for a proposed program; (2) when conducting a needs assessment, health education specialists must understand the basic principles of measurement in order to select and use appropriate data collection instruments; (3) when health education specialists are planning an evaluation to measure whether program objectives have been met, they need to be able to measure related program outcomes; (4) when a funding agency wants evidence that a program it funds is making a difference in a community, health education specialists must apply appropriate measurement techniques to generate the needed evidence; or (5) when health education specialists are asked to interpret the results of a program evaluation to a group of stakeholders, they need to be competent in determining and communicating whether program components actually produced the identified results. Each of these examples demonstrates the need for a sound understanding of the processes associated with measurement. In other words, measurement is an integral part of program planning, implementation, and evaluation.

Levels of Measurement

A fundamental question of measurement is deciding *how* something should be measured (McDermott & Sarvela, 1999). For example, consider a scenario in which planners/evaluators need data on the income levels of program participants to control for differences in socioeconomic status. They could ask about the participants' income level in any of the following three ways:

1. Which of the following categories most closely corresponds with your household income: poor, lower middle class, upper middle class, or wealthy?

2. What income category best describes your household income? $0 to 10,000; $10,001 to 25,000; $25,001 to 40,000; $40,001 to $55,000; 55,001 to 70,000; $70,001+

3. What is your household income? _____

Although these questions all pertain to household income, each question generates a different type and level of data which in turn dictates the type of analysis that can be used. Thus, when planners/evaluators begin to think about data collection, they need to consider both the wording of their questions and how that wording will impact the nature of their analysis.

Nearly 70 years ago, Stevens (1946) proposed that four **levels of measurement**— nominal, ordinal, interval, and ratio—were the basis for all scientific measurement. In fact, these four levels of measurement are widely accepted in social and behavioral research and are necessary to classify the type of data used and to identify the appropriate type of statistical test or analysis that can be applied to the data.

The four levels of measurement proposed originally by Stevens (1946) are considered "hierarchical" in nature. In other words, they progress from more simple or basic to more complex. As mentioned, this hierarchy also relates to an increasing complexity of statistical analysis.

1. Nominal level measures constitute the lowest level in the measurement hierarchy and use names or labels to categorize people, places, or things. While nominal data represent different categories, they do not represent any particular value or order (i.e., they are simply grouped by name). "The two requirements for nominal measures are that the categories have to be mutually exclusive so that each case fits into one of the categories, and the categories have to be exhaustive so that there is a place for every case" (Weiss, 1998, p. 116). For example, a question that would generate nominal data is, "What is your sex?" The possible answers include the categories of "female" and "male." These answers are exhaustive (contain all possible answers) and mutually exclusive (the respondent has to be one or the other, but not both). We can then assign numbers to these categories according to a particular rule we create (e.g., 1 = female, 2 = male).

2. Ordinal level measures like nominal level measures, allow planners to put data into categories that are mutually exclusive and exhaustive, but also permit them to rank-order the categories. The different categories represent relatively more or less of something. However, the distance between categories cannot be measured. For example, the question "How would you describe your level of satisfaction with your health care? (select one) very satisfied—satisfied—not satisfied" creates categories (very satisfied— satisfied—not satisfied) that are mutually exclusive (the respondent cannot select two categories) and exhaustive (there is a category for all levels of satisfaction), and the categories represent more or less of something (amount of satisfaction), thus there is a rank order. We cannot, however, measure the distance (or difference) between the levels of satisfaction (e.g., what the difference is between very satisfied and satisfied). Is the distance between very satisfied and satisfied the same distance between satisfied and not satisfied? Ordinal data categories are not necessarily an equal distance apart. Another example is when a patient is asked how much pain he/she is experiencing on a scale from 1 to 10. While 7 is more severe than 5, this difference may not be the same as the difference between 3 and 1.

3. **Interval level measures** enable planners to put data into categories that are mutually exclusive and exhaustive, and rank-orders the categories. Furthermore, the widths or differences between categories must all be the same (Hurlburt, 2003), which allows for the distance between the categories to be measured. There is, however, no absolute zero value. For example, a question that generates interval data is, "What was the high temperature today?" We know that a temperature of 70°F is different than a temperature of 80°F, that 80° is warmer than 70°, that there is 10°F difference between the two, and if the temperature drops to 0° F there is still some heat in the air (though not much) because 0°F is warmer than –10°F. Similarly, whereas a score of zero on an IQ test may indicate certain things, it does not mean a person is devoid of any intelligence.

4. **Ratio level measures**, the highest level in the measurement hierarchy, enable planners to do everything with data that can be done with the other three levels of measures; however, those tasks are accomplished using a scale with an absolute zero. Example questions that generate interval data include: "What was your score on the test?" "How tall are you in inches?" "How much do you weigh?" and "During an average week, how many minutes do you exercise aerobically?" An absolute zero "point means that the thing being measured actually vanishes when the scale reads zero" (Hurlburt, 2003, p. 17). For example, when a person has a blood pressure reading of zero over zero, there is in fact no blood pressure.

Because interval and ratio data are continuous and rank-ordered values with equal distance between them, and because most statistical procedures are the same for both types of data (Valente, 2002), some have combined them into a single level of measurement and refer to the resulting data as *numerical data.*

When planners/evaluators make decisions about the type of statistical tests and analyses to perform, they need to examine the level of measurement that was produced by their questionnaire or other instrumentation. Generally speaking, nominal and ordinal measures are associated with nonparametric tests (less likely to assume a normal distribution of data, (i.e., bell shaped curve) while interval and ratio data are more often associated with parametric tests (more likely to assume a normal distribution of data).

Types of Measures

Many different types of measures are used to conduct needs assessments or evaluate programs and it is important to match the methods of measurement with the focus of the task. Typically, health promotion programs focus on one or more of the following types of measures (also called variables) related to: demographics, awareness, knowledge, psychosocial characteristics, skills, behaviors, environmental attributes, health outcomes,

Table 5.2   Types of Measures, Data Generated, and Methods of Obtaining the Data

Measure	Example Data	Commonly Used Methods of Data Collection
Demographics	Social and economic characteristics of a population; e.g., sex, age, race, income	Self-report questionnaires, census records
Awareness	Conscious of, for example, location of services, significance of risk factors related to disease	Self-report questionnaires, polls
Knowledge	Bloom's taxonomy* • knowledge (remembering) • comprehension (lowest level of understanding) • application (using learned material) • analysis (ability to analyze learned material) • synthesis (creating from learned material) • evaluation (ability to judge the value)	Written or oral tests
Psychosocial characteristics	Attitudes, beliefs, motivation, and personality traits, e.g., fears, sympathy, belonging, cohesiveness	Self-report validated scales
Skills	Ability to perform a task (i.e., giving an insulin shot or performing CPR)	Observation (skills testing)
Behaviors	Smoking, exercise, alcohol consumption	Self-report questionnaires
Environmental attributes	Factors or conditions outside a person, e.g., social support, access to care, clean air	Self-report questionnaires, observation, checklists, laboratory tests
Health outcomes	Biological and clinical health, e.g., prevalence of HIV or breast cancer in a community	Self-report questionnaires, health screenings
Quality of life (QoL)	Satisfaction, happiness, and fulfillment, health-related quality of life	Self-report validated scales

*Source: Taxonomy of Educational Objectives: The Classification of Educational Goals. Handbook I: Cognitive Domain. L. W. Anderson, D. R. Krathwohl, P. W. Airasian, K. A. Cruikshank, R. E. Mayer, P. R. Pintrich, J. Raths, M. C. Wittrock. Copyright © 2000 by Pearson Education. Reprinted with permission.

and quality of life indicators. **Table 5.2** provides examples of how data can be generated for each of these different types of measures.

Desirable Characteristics of Data

The results of a needs assessment or program evaluation are only as good as the data that are collected and analyzed. If a questionnaire is filled with ambiguous questions and the respondents are not sure how to answer, it is highly unlikely that the data will reflect the true knowledge, attitudes, and so on, of those responding. Therefore, it is of vital importance that planners and evaluators make sure that the data they collect are reliable, valid, fair, and unbiased. Collectively, these three characteristics—reliability, validity, and fairness—are referred to as an instrument's **psychometric qualities** (Cottrell & McKenzie, 2011).

Reliability

Reliability refers to consistency in the measurement process. That is, **reliability** "is an empirical estimate of the extent to which an instrument produces the same result (measure or score), applied once or two or more times" (Windsor et al., 2004, p. 93). However, no instrument will ever provide perfect accuracy in measurement. Green and Lewis (1986) illustrated the theory of reliability with an equation, where total score (obtained score) equals the true score (unobservable) plus an error score. The total score represents the individual's score obtained on a measuring instrument. The true score represents the score for the same individual if all conditions and the measuring instrument were perfect. The error score represents the portion of the total score that is generated from the "imprecision in measurement due to human error, uncontrollable environment occurrences, inappropriateness of measurement instruments, and other unanticipated things" (Dignan, 1995, p. 40). For example, suppose the total score of an individual on a knowledge test was 85 out of a possible 100 points. The question then becomes whether the 85% is a true indication of the person's knowledge. If the conditions under which the score was generated were perfect and the measurement instrument had perfect reliability, the error score would be zero and we could say the 85% score is a true indication of the person's knowledge. However, if the conditions under which the score was generated were *not* perfect (e.g., the person did not have enough time to take the test) and the measurement instrument *did not* have perfect reliability (e.g., it included several poorly worded questions), the error score would *not* be zero and we would conclude that the score of 85% was *not* a true indication of the person's knowledge. The subject may really know more, or maybe less, than was indicated by the score. "Reliability coefficients are highest if no error exists ($r = 1.0$) and lowest when there is only error or no association ($r = 0.0$) between two measures" (Windsor et al., 2004, p. 95).

Planners need to strive to collect data under the best conditions with the most reliable measurement instruments possible (Cottrell & McKenzie, 2011). Several methods of determining reliability are available.

Internal consistency is one of the most commonly used methods of estimating reliability (Windsor et al., 2004). It refers to the intercorrelations among the individual items on the instrument, that is, whether items on the instrument are measuring the same research domain. This can be done by examining the instrument to ensure that the items reflect what is to be measured and that the level of difficulty of all items is consistent. Statistical methods can also be used to determine internal consistency by correlating the items on the test with the total score. A Chronbach's alpha reliability coefficient measures internal consistency and ranges from 0 to 1 with scores of greater than 0.70 typically classified as acceptable and scores of 0.80 classified as good (George & Mallery, 2003). While alpha coefficients of 0.90 or greater are generally considered to be excellent, scores this high can also indicate there is redundancy in the instrumentation (i.e., too many questions may be asking the same thing).

Test–retest reliability, or stability reliability, "is used to generate evidence of stability over a period" (Torabi, 1994, p. 57) of time. To establish this type of reliability, the same instrument is used to measure the same group of people under similar, or the same conditions, at two different points in time, and the two sets of data generated by the measurement are used to calculate a correlation coefficient (Cottrell & McKenzie, 2011). An adequate amount of time should be allowed between the test and retest so that individuals are not responding on the basis of remembering responses they made the first time, but not be so long that other events could occur in the intervening time to influence their responses. To avoid the problems of retesting, parallel forms (equivalent forms) of the test can be administered to the participants and the results can be correlated. While a Cohen's kappa coefficient (Cohen, 1960) equal to or greater to than 0.70 is generally acceptable, a coefficient of 0.80 is ideal and should be documented (Harris 2010; Windsor et al., 2004).

Rater reliability focuses on the consistency between individuals who are observing or rating the same item or when one individual is observing or rating a series of items. If two or more raters are involved, it is referred to as **inter-rater reliability**. If only one individual is observing or rating a series of events, it is referred to as **intra-rater reliability.** There are several different ways to calculate rater reliability. In a research study, most researchers would use Cohen's kappa to calculate rater reliability. However, a quicker and easier method is to calculate it as a percentage of agreement between/among raters or within an individual rater (DiIorio, 2005). An example of inter-rater reliability would be the percent of agreement between two observers who are observing passing drivers in cars for safety belt use. If 10 cars are observed by the raters and they agree 8 out of 10 times on whether the drivers are wearing their safety belts, the inter-rater reliability would be 80%. Intra-rater reliability would be the degree to which one rater agrees with himself or herself on the characteristics of an observation over time. For example, when a rater is evaluating the CPR skills of participants in his or her program, the rater should be consistent while observing and evaluating the skills of the participants.

Parallel forms reliability, or equivalent forms or alternate-forms reliability, focuses on whether different forms of the same measurement instrument when measuring the same subjects will produce similar results (means, standard deviations, and inter-item correlations). The usefulness of having measurement instruments that possess parallel forms reliability is being able to test the same subjects on different occasions (e.g., using a pretest-posttest evaluation design) without concern that the subjects will score better on the second administration (posttest) because they remember questions from the first administration (pretest) of the instrument. A good example of parallel forms reliability is found in the different versions of the standardized college entrance examinations (Cottrell & McKenzie, 2011).

Validity

When designing a data collection instrument, planners/evaluators must ensure that it measures what it is intended to measure. This refers to the **validity** of the measurement—whether it is correctly measuring the concepts under investigation. Using a valid instrument increases the chance that planners/evaluators are measuring what they want to measure, thus ruling out other possible explanations for the results.

Face validity is the lowest level of validity. A measure is said to have face validity if, on the face, it appears to measure what it is supposed to measure (McDermott & Sarvela, 1999). Face validity differs from the other forms of validity in that it lacks some form of systematic logical analysis of the content (Hopkins, Stanley, & Hopkins, 1990). An example of face validity is when a planner/evaluator asks a group of colleagues to look over a series of questions to see whether they seem reasonable to include on a questionnaire about the risk for heart disease. Face validity is a good first step toward creating a valid measurement instrument, but is not a replacement for the other means of establishing validity (Cottrell & McKenzie, 2011).

Content validity refers to "the assessment of the correspondence between the items composing the instrument and the content domain from which the items were selected" (DiIorio, 2005, p. 213). This means that all essential elements of a research domain are included in the instrument. For example, when planning a health promotion program to prevent heart disease, the program planner can conduct a review of the literature in the area of cardiovascular risk reduction in order to ensure that all major risk factors, such as smoking, exercise, and diet, are included in the questionnaire. If some, but not all risk factors are measured, the instrument will not demonstrate content validity.

Content validity is usually established by using a group (jury or panel) of experts to review the instrument. After such a group is identified, they would be asked to review each element of the instrument for appropriateness. The collective opinion of the experts is then used to determine the content of the instrument. McKenzie and colleagues (1999) present a method of establishing content validity that includes both qualitative and quantitative steps.

Criterion-related validity refers to "the extent to which data generated from a measurement instrument are correlated with data generated from a measure (criterion) of the phenomenon being studied, usually an individual's behavior or performance" (Cottrell & McKenzie, 2011, p. 150). Criterion-related validity can be divided into two subtypes: predictive and concurrent validity (DiIorio, 2005).

If the measurement used will be correlated with another measurement of the same phenomenon at another time, as with the use of standardized test scores to predict future college success, the criterion validity is known as **predictive validity**. **Concurrent validity** occurs when a new instrument and an established valid instrument that measure the same characteristics are administered to the same subjects, and the results of the new instrument are compared to the results of the valid instrument. For example, if a planner/evaluator wanted to establish the validity of a new test for breast cancer, he or she would administer both the new instrument with an already valid breast cancer instrument to the same subjects and then compare the results. The new instrument would be valid if the results compared favorably with the established instrument. In both subtypes of criterion-related validity, the aim is to legitimize the inferences that can be made by establishing their predictive ability for a related criterion.

Construct validity "is the degree to which a measure correlates with other measures it is theoretically expected to correlate with. Construct validity tests the theoretical framework within which the instrument is expected to perform" (Valente, 2002, p. 161). Because there are times when there is no existing criterion with which to compare, as in criterion-related validity, or the phenomenon that planners want to measure is more abstract than concrete, validity can be established via construct validity (Cottrell & McKenzie, 2011). An instrument that has construct validity will possess both convergent validity and discriminant validity. **Convergent validity** "is the extent to which two measures which purport to be measuring the same topic correlate (that is, converge)" (Bowling, 2005, p. 12). For example, an instrument that purports to measure a person's self-efficacy for regular exercise should positively correlate with that person's exercise behavior. That is, a person who is self-efficacious with regard to exercise would exercise regularly regardless of the circumstances (e.g., normal day, busy day, inclement weather, while on vacation, etc.). **Discriminant validity** "(also known as divergent validity) requires that the construct should not correlate with dissimilar (discriminant) variables" (Bowling, 2005, p. 12). Thus in the exercise example above, the self-efficacy instrument would not be expected to correlate positively with a person's inactivity.

Sensitivity and Specificity   When speaking about validity, planners should also be familiar with the terms *sensitivity* and *specificity*. These terms are used in health care settings as well as epidemiology to express the validity of screening and diagnostic tests (Cottrell & McKenzie, 2011). **Sensitivity** is defined as the ability of the test to identify correctly those who actually have the disease (Friis & Sellers, 2009). It is recorded as the proportion of true positive cases correctly identified as positive on the test (Timmreck, 1997). The better the sensitivity, the fewer the false positives. **Specificity** is defined as "the ability of the test to identify only non-diseased individuals who actually do not have the disease" (Friis & Sellers, 2009, p. 24). It is recorded as the proportion of true negative cases correctly identified as negative on the test (Timmreck, 1997). And the better the specificity, the fewer the number of false negatives. "An ideal screening test would demonstrate 100% sensitivity and 100% specificity. In practice this does not occur; sensitivity and specificity are usually inversely related" (Mausner & Kramer, 1985, p. 217).

The validity of an instrument is thought to be more important than its reliability. If an instrument does not measure what it is supposed to, then it does not matter if it is reliable (Windsor et al., 2004). **Table 5.3** summarizes the different types of reliability and validity.

Fairness

Fairness deals with the question of whether a measure "is appropriate for the individuals of various ethnic groups with different backgrounds, gender, educational levels, etc." (Torabi, 1994, p. 56). Because planners/evaluators often work with members of priority populations with distinct beliefs, cultures, and needs, they need to be concerned about fairness. Unlike the other psychometric qualities of validity and reliability, there are no quantitative procedures for determining the fairness of a measure (Cottrell & McKenzie, 2011). Instead it becomes the responsibility of the planners/evaluators to seek fairness. A foundation for fairness is the planners/evaluators having an understanding of the culture of those in the priority population. **Culture** is defined as "the patterned ways of thought and behavior that characterize a social group, which are learned through socialization processes and persist through time" (Coreil, Bryant, & Henderson, 2001, p. 29). Therefore, people from different cultures are likely to possess different values, beliefs, traditions, and perceptions. These cultural values, beliefs, traditions, and perceptions affect nearly all activities of individuals, including their health-related behavior (Kline & Huff, 1999) and their response to questions related to health. Thus, culture influences program participants' ability to

Table 5.3 Types of Reliability and Validity

Reliability—"an empirical estimate of the extent to which an instrument produces the same result (measure or score), applied once or two or more times" (Windsor et al., 2004, p. 93).

Internal consistency—the intercorrelations among individual items on the instrument, that is, whether all items on the instrument are measuring part of the total area.

Test-retest (or stability)—"used to generate evidence of stability over time" (Torabi, 1994, p. 57).

Rater (or observer)—associated with the consistent measurement (or rating) of an observed event by the same or different individuals (or judges or raters) (McDermott & Sarvela, 1999).

Parallel (or equivalent or alternate) **forms**—focus on whether different forms of the same instrument when measuring the same participants will produce similar results.

Validity—whether an instrument correctly measures what it is intended to measure.

Face—if, on the face, the measure appears to measure what it is supposed to measure (McDermott & Sarvela, 1999).

Content—"the assessment of the correspondence between the items composing the instrument and the content domain from which the items were selected" (DiIorio, 2005, p. 213).

Criterion-related—"the extent to which data generated from a measurement instrument are correlated with the data generated from a measure (criterion) of the phenomenon being studied, usually an individual's behavior or performance" (Cottrell & McKenzie, 2011, p. 322); two types: concurrent and predictive.

Construct—"the degree to which a measure correlates with other measures it is theoretically expected to correlate with. Construct validity tests the theoretical framework within which the instrument is expected to perform" (Valente, 2002, p. 161); an instrument with construct validity possesses both convergent and discriminant validity.

understand, internalize, and exercise positive health practices that will enhance the quality of life. For example, if we examine the diet of individuals from different cultures (e.g., religion, race), it is easy to see the impact of culture on what people eat. Some cultures see some foods as an important part of their diet while others see the same foods as inappropriate for consumption. Thus, when collecting data from diverse populations, planners/evaluators need to respond appropriately to cultural differences. In other words, planners/evaluators need to work toward being culturally competent. **Cultural competence** is a developmental process defined as a set of values, principles, behaviors, attitudes, and policies that enable health professionals to work effectively across racial, ethnic and linguistically diverse populations (Joint Committee on Terminology, 2012).

Bias Free

Biased data are those data that have been distorted because of the way they have been collected. More specifically, **bias** can be introduced in the selection or sampling process of study participants, in the study's design or measurement process, or in the intervention phase which includes how participants were exposed to the treatment (Hartman, Forsen, Wallace, & Neely, 2002). In order to effectively plan and evaluate health promotion programs, planners/evaluators must work to eliminate bias. Windsor and colleagues (2004) describe ways in which bias can occur in data collection—for example, when participants do not feel comfortable answering a sensitive question, when participants act differently because they know they are being watched, when certain characteristics of the interviewer influence a response, when participants answer questions in a particular way regardless of the questions being asked, or when a biased sample has been selected from the priority population (see information later in this chapter on sampling).

There are a number of steps planners/evaluators can take to limit bias. For example, if data are being collected via observation, the observation should be as unobtrusive as possible. If sensitive questions are being asked of respondents, then those collecting such data need to ensure that the data are being collected in a confidential way (the identity of the respondent can be determined but not released), and consider collecting the data via an anonymous means (there is no way of identifying the respondent). No matter how data are collected, the use of techniques to reduce bias will increase the accuracy of the results.

Measurement Instruments

As presented earlier, many different methods can be used to collect both primary and secondary data (see Chapter 4). The focus here is not to repeat that information but rather to present information on measurement instruments. By **measurement instrument,** we mean the item used to measure the variables (e.g., demographic, psychosocial, behavioral) of interest. Measurement instruments are also sometimes referred to as tools or data collection instruments. The term **instrumentation** is "a collective term that describes all measurement instruments used" (Cottrell & McKenzie, 2011, p. 146).

Measurement instruments can take many different forms and sizes. They can range from the very simple, like a ruler or yardstick, to a questionnaire, to a very complicated piece of machinery that performs DNA sequencing. Although at times health education specialists may use machines or equipment as instruments (e.g., to check blood cholesterol), more commonly they employ a sequence of questions to measure variables of interest (Windsor et al., 2004). These sequences of questions most often take the form of *tests*, *questionnaires*, and *scales*. The term *test* is most often used in the context of educational measurement (DiIorio, 2005), such as an HIV/AIDS knowledge test. Questionnaires (sometimes called *survey instruments*) are instruments that gather information about a variety of factors (e.g., awareness, skills, behaviors, health status) related to one or more specific topics. For example, a questionnaire may be developed about sleep habits and include questions about the average number of hours slept per night, what time a person typically goes to sleep, use of sleep aids, and techniques used to fall asleep. Further, questionnaires can be administered orally via an interview or by telephone, or people can be asked to respond in writing either electronically or on paper. While questionnaires can involve several scales and multiple concepts, a scale is used to measure only one concept (DiIorio, 2005), often dealing with a psychosocial variable like attitudes, beliefs, or opinions. For example, health education specialists may be interested in collecting data about attitudes related to water fluoridation in the priority population. In scales, often the response choice for every question is the same (e.g., always, sometimes, never). Although sometimes the word *scale* is used in a general sense to refer to an entire questionnaire, which is not a technically correct use of the term.

Depending on the nature of the test, questionnaire, or scale, the instrument can also vary in length. Some can be as short as a single question, rating, or item to measure the variable, while others may be multipage instruments. There are advantages and disadvantages to various instrument lengths. Obvious advantages of a shorter instrument are the time for the participants to complete it and for the planners/evaluators to organize and analyze the data. However, longer instruments may do a better job of measuring less stable (i.e., change over time) variables like attitudes (DiIorio, 2005), and longer instruments may be more suitable for statistical calculations (Bowling, 2005).

Using an Existing Measurement Instrument

Even before planners/evaluators create their own measurement instrument, they should search for an existing instrument that is both valid and reliable and that meets their needs. As you will discover in the next section, it takes a great deal of time, effort, and resources to create a measurement instrument with good psychometric qualities. The main advantages of using an existing valid and reliable instrument include less planning time and thus lower costs. The major disadvantage—one that prevents the use of many existing instruments—is that the items on the existing instrument may not be relevant or appropriate for the program being planned or evaluated. Cottrell and McKenzie (2011) offer four steps for identifying, obtaining, and evaluating existing measurement instruments.

Step 1: Identifying measurement instruments. Start by searching the literature to see what others have used. You may not find an actual copy of the measurement instruments in the literature, but you may find a reference to the original source. As you are aware by now, the U.S. government has created many health-related data collection instruments. Conducting a search of applicable Websites (e.g., National Center for Health Statistics, CDC WONDER) can be useful. Remember, government publications are in the **public domain** (available for anyone to use) and thus free of charge and need no permission to use. Also, be aware that a number of commercial companies sell measurement instruments (e.g., Psychological Assessment Resources, Inc. [PAR]). In addition, you may not find a measurement instrument that you can use in whole, but you may find specific questions or a scale that may work for you.

Step 2: Getting your hands on the instrument. Once you have identified potential measurement instruments, you then have to obtain a hard copy. Unless an instrument is copyrighted, or there are plans to do so in the future, most sources are willing to share their measurement instruments. A phone call, letter, or sometimes a "formal" email requesting a copy of an instrument is usually all that it takes to get a copy. Once the source of the measurement instrument is known, be aware that you may have to pay for an instrument, and have to meet certain criteria (e.g., being a licensed psychologist, or agree to certain terms) to be able to obtain and use some measurement instruments.

Step 3: Is it the right instrument? Here are some questions to ask to determine whether an instrument is the right one for your purposes:

(1) Is there sufficient evidence of the psychometric qualities (validity, reliability, and fairness) of the instrument? (2) Has it been used with participants similar to yours? (3) Are standard or normative scores available for various participants? (4) Is the

instrument culturally appropriate for your participants? (5) Has the reading level of the instrument been determined? (6) Is there a cost to administer or have the instrument scored? Can you afford it? (Cottrell & McKenzie, 2011, p. 164)

Step 4: Final steps before proceeding. If you think you have found the right instrument, before proceeding make sure you have done everything necessary to be able to use it. Remember, for instruments that are not in the public domain, "you need the permission of the author for any use of the instrument, usually in writing, and particularly if you need to make any changes" (Dignan, 1995, p. 67). You also may need to fulfill other conditions placed on the use of the instrument by the owner of the copyright before you use it.

Creating a Measurement Instrument

Only when planners/evaluators are unable to use or adapt another instrument for their use should they undertake the process of developing their own (Janz, Champion, & Strecher, 2002). **Box 5.2** provides a list of steps to follow in creating a measurement instrument. Though the list was created to facilitate data collection for research projects, it illustrates the complexity in creating an instrument with good psychometric qualities. For a more detailed discussion of steps in this process, see Cottrell and McKenzie (2011). Next we will present a more general discussion about the presentation, wording, and sequencing of questions in a measurement instrument.

The measurement instrument should begin with an introduction that includes a brief statement of purpose and directions for completing the instrument (see **Box 5.3**). This introduction can be followed by general questions to put the respondent at ease in the case of a written or electronic self-report instrument, or to develop a rapport between the interviewer and the respondent when data are collected via a face-to-face or telephone interview.

General questions are followed by the actual questions of interest. Any questions that deal with sensitive topics should be posed at the end of the questionnaire or interview. Answers to questions about drug use, sexuality, or even demographic information, such as income level, are more readily answered when the respondents understand the need for the information, are assured of confidentiality or anonymity, and feel comfortable with the interviewer or the questionnaire. If the respondent ends the interview or does not complete the instrument when asked sensitive questions, the other information collected can still be used.

The way in which questions are worded is extremely important in gaining the needed information. The result of a poorly worded question was evident to one health promotion planner who was planning a smoking cessation program for employees. When asked "Do you feel we need a smoking cessation program?" most employees said yes. The planner realized later that he should have also asked the question, "If offered, would you attend a smoking cessation program?" since very few employees participated. In general, always try to avoid questions that can be answered with a simple yes or no.

Questions should always be clear and bias free. It is important to avoid leading questions ("How have you enjoyed the class?") that guide the respondent's answer. Two-part questions should also be avoided ("Do you brush and floss your teeth?"). Another

Box 5.2 STEPS FOR CREATING A MEASUREMENT INSTRUMENT

Step 0: Be familiar with the related literature.

Step 1: Determine the specific purpose (or goal) and the objectives of the proposed instrument.

Step 2: Who are the individuals who are to be measured?

Step 3: Identify the conceptual theory/model that will provide the foundation for the instrument.

Step 4: Create a table of specifications for the instrument.

Step 5: Identify items from other existing instruments that could be used.

Step 6: Create new instrument items.

Step 7: Create directions for completing the instrument, and directions and instructions for administering the instrument.

Step 8: Establish procedures for scoring the instrument.

Step 9: Assemble an initial draft of the instrument.

Step 10: Establish face validity for the instrument.

Step 11: Check the readability of the instrument.

Step 12: Establish content validity for the instrument.

Step 13: Pilot-test the instrument.

Step 14: Conduct item analysis, factor analysis, and checks of psychometric qualities.

Step 15: Review, revise, and reassess.

Step 16: Conduct a second pilot-test, if necessary.

Step 17: Determine a cut score.

Step 18: Refine as needed and create the final version.

Source: Health Promotion and Education Research Methods: Using the Five-Chapter Thesis/Dissertation Model. R. R. Cottrell and J. F. McKenzie. Copyright © 2011 by Jones & Bartlett Learning. Reprinted with permission.

problem with question design occurs when the question assumes knowledge that individuals may not have or includes terminology that they may not understand ("What cardiovascular benefits do you feel are gained from aerobic exercise?").

Many different types of questions can be used to create measurement instruments. Consideration must be given to whether the type of question will generate the needed data. For example, assume planners/evaluators were interested in identifying the ages of those in the priority population. A question like "How old are you?" could generate the best data (i.e., ratio level data), but some may not want to share their actual age and thus planners/evaluators may not collect enough data to describe the priority population. In this case, a question that generates ordinal level data such as "I am: 15–24 years old; 25–44 years old; 45–64 years old; 65+ years old" may be a better choice.

Box 5.3	APPLICATION—INTRODUCTION FOR A DATA COLLECTION INSTRUMENT

Health Questionnaire

Purpose: The Health Department is conducting a survey of those living in Delaware County in order to find out more about their health. Obtaining this information is important because it will provide us with a better understanding of the needs of our citizens so that we may in turn provide the programs to improve the health of those in our county.

Directions for completing the questionnaire: You are not required to complete this questionnaire, but your voluntary participation is requested. This is an anonymous survey so do not write your name on this instrument. Please read each of the questions carefully and respond to them by circling the response that best represents your feelings. There are no right or wrong answers. We recognize that some of the questions, by necessity, are quite personal. Be assured that your individual responses will not be shared with anyone and that only summarized group information will be reported. When you have completed the questionnaire, place it in the postage-paid business reply envelope and drop it in the mail. Thank you for your help with this survey.

Another consideration in creating questions is to determine how much freedom you want respondents to have in answering questions. Those with the least freedom are structured or closed questions. Examples include true-false or multiple-choice questions and are most often used to assess knowledge. These types of responses are the easiest to tabulate but do not allow the individual to elaborate on the answers. They may also force a person into a choice because of the limited number of responses to each question. An "other" category, with space to list the exact nature of the response, may serve to give the respondent another option. However, giving the respondents an opportunity to provide their own answers on multiple-choice questions makes it more difficult to categorize responses when the data are analyzed, thus reducing one of the main benefits of such questions. One way to ensure that the most common responses to questions are included in the possible choices is to involve several individuals (especially those in the priority population) in the formation of the instrument.

Attitude questions generally use less structured forms. Scales, such as Likert or semantic differentials, are often used, with respondents choosing a response along a continuum, generally ranging from a 5- to a 7-point scale. For example, responses to the statement "I feel that it is important to limit my use of salt" might be rated on a 5-point scale ranging from "strongly agree" to "strongly disagree."

Unstructured or open-ended questions—such as essay questions, short-answer questions, journals, or logs—may be used to gain descriptive information, but are generally not used when collecting quantitative data. Such responses are often difficult to summarize or to code for analysis. **Box 5.4** provides examples of structured and unstructured types of questions.

Box 5.4	EXAMPLES OF SELF-REPORT QUESTIONS

Structured (Closed)

I. Dichotomous

   1. What is your sex?
     a. Female   b. Male

   2. A risk factor for heart disease is sedentary lifestyle.
     a. True   b. False

II. Multiple Choice

   1. The leading cause of death in the United States for adults is:
     a. cancer   b. heart disease
     c. injuries   d. AIDS

   2. What type of computer do you use?
     a. IBM   b. Apple
     c. Dell   d. Other (please specify): _____

III. Matching

Vitamin deficiencies

   1. Vitamin A   a. Frequent infection
   2. Vitamin C   b. Slow blood clotting
   3. Vitamin D   c. Night blindness
   4. Vitamin K   d. Bone softening

Grams of saturated fats

   1. Butter, 1 tbsp.   a. 9
   2. Ice cream, 4 oz.   b. 7.1
   3. Chicken, 3 oz.   c. 5
   4. One hot dog   d. 1.2

Less Structured (But Still Closed)

I. Likert

   1. Women should be able to have an abortion if they choose to do so.

	Strongly agree	Agree	Neutral	Disagree	Strongly disagree

   2. I feel I can exercise regardless of weather conditions.

	Strongly agree	Agree	Neutral	Disagree	Strongly disagree

II. Semantic Differentials

   1. Smokeless tobacco is   Good ____ ____ ____ ____ ____ Bad

   2. When taking a test, I feel   Nervous ____ ____ ____ ____ ____ Calm

III. Rank Order

   1. Put the following values in order, from most important in your life to least important:
     a. health   _____   d. emotional security _____
     b. love   _____   e. financial security   _____
     c. friendship _____

| **Box 5.4** | (CONTINUED) |

2. Rank-order the following servings of foods from highest to lowest sources of protein:

a. tuna _____   d. cottage cheese _____
b. rice _____   e. bread _____
c. sirloin steak _____   f. broccoli _____

Unstructured (Open)

I. Completions

   1. I like to exercise because _____

   2. The types of foods I generally eat are _____

II. Short-Answer
   1. List five advantages to conducting a worksite health promotion program.

   2. Describe the correct way to lift a heavy object to avoid straining your back.

III. Essay

   1. Explain the difference between aerobic and anaerobic exercise. Include examples of each type of exercise, and discuss the importance of each in total fitness.

   2. Discuss the incidence of tuberculosis in the world today, including who is at risk and the public health measures to reduce the problem.

Sampling

The need to select participants from whom data will be collected can occur at several times during the process of program planning or evaluation. Depending on the size of the priority population, planners/evaluators may want to collect data from all participants, a **census**, or from only some of the participants, a **sample**. Each of the participants is referred to as a sampling unit. A **sampling unit** is the element or set of elements considered for selection as part of a sample (Babbie, 1992). A sampling unit "may be an individual, an organization, or a geographical area" (Bowling, 2005, p. 166).

Figure 5.1 illustrates the relationship between groups of individuals. All individuals, unspecified by time or place, constitute the **universe**—for example, all U.S. citizens, regardless of where they reside in the world. Within the universe is a **population** of individuals specified by time or place, such as all U.S. residents in the 50 states on January 1, 2012. Within this population is a **survey population**, composed of all individuals who are accessible to the researchers. The key term here is *accessible*. For example, all U.S. citizens who are accessible and can be reached by telephone would be a survey population. Obviously, this would not include those without telephones, such as those who chose not to own them, those institutionalized, and the homeless.

A survey population may still be too large to include in its entirety. For this reason, a sample is chosen from the survey population, a process called **sampling**. Those in the sample are the individuals who will be included in the data collection process. Using a sample

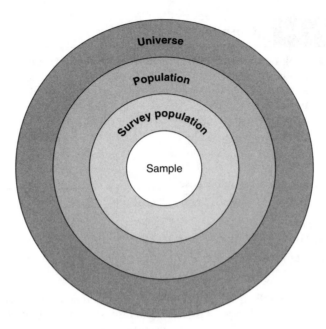

Figure 5.1 Relationship of Study Populations

rather than an entire survey population helps contain costs. For example, using a sample reduces the amount of staff time needed to conduct interviews, the cost of postage for written questionnaires, and the time and cost of travel to conduct observations.

How the sample is chosen is critical to the result of the needs assessment or evaluation: Does the information gained from the sample reflect the knowledge, attitudes, and behaviors of the survey population? According to Green and Lewis (1986), the sampling bias is the difference between the sampling estimate and the actual population value. Sampling bias can be reduced by controlling the sampling procedure—that is, how the sample is chosen. Furthermore, the ability to generalize the results to the survey population is greater when the sampling bias is reduced.

Probability Sample

Increasing the likelihood that the sample is representative of the survey population is achieved by **random selection**. "Randomness minimizes the likelihood that a systematic source of selection bias will occur among the sample, thereby influencing the degree of representativeness of the population" (Windsor et al., 2004, p. 110). When random selection is used, each person in the survey population has an equal chance or probability of being selected, thus creating a **probability sample**.

There are a number of different methods for selecting a probability sample. The most basic of the probability sampling methods is selecting a **simple random sample (SRS)**.

In order to select an SRS, or for that matter any probability sample, the planner must have a list or "quasi-list" (Babbie, 1992) of all sampling units in the survey population. This list is referred to as the **sampling frame**. Oftentimes, sampling frames have the names and contact information for everyone in the survey population such as with membership lists, patients of a clinic, and parents of children enrolled in a certain school or program. Other times the frame may simply be the title of an individual or organization, such as the director of environmental services in the 92 local health departments in Indiana, or a list of all the voluntary health agencies in the county (Cottrell & McKenzie, 2011).

Once the sampling frame has been identified, the planner can proceed with the process of selecting an SRS. It begins with assigning a number with an equal number of digits to each sampling unit in the frame. Suppose, for example, we have a frame of 200 individuals. The first person in the frame would be given the number 000. The rest of the individuals in the frame would be assigned consecutive numbers and the last person in the frame would be assigned the number 199. Once it is decided how large the sample should be, the sample can be selected. For the purpose of this example let's suppose a sample size of 20 is desired. To select these 20 individuals, a computer could be used to randomly select 20 numbers between 000 and 199, or it could be done manually by using a table of random numbers (Cottrell & McKenzie, 2011) (see **Table 5.4**).

In order to use a table of random numbers, the manner in which the table will be used needs to be set forth. Since these tables are generated randomly (by computer), it really does not matter which way one moves through the table as long as it is done in a consistent manner. For example, the process set forth could be to (1) use the first three digits in the columns of numbers (because all individuals in the example frame have a three-digit number, that is, 000 to 199); (2) proceed down the columns (as opposed to up or across the rows); (3) at the bottom of the column proceed to the top of the next column to the right; and (4) proceed in this same manner until the 20 individuals are selected. To ensure that this process is indeed random, the process must begin with a random start. That is, the planner cannot just pick the first number at the top of column

Table 5.4 Abbreviated Table of Random Numbers

Row/Column	A	B	C	D	E
1	75 51	02 17	71 04	33 93	36 60
2	42 75	76 22	23 87	56 54	84 68
3	00 47	37 59	08 56	23 81	22 42
4	74 01	23 19	55 59	79 09	69 82
5	66 22	42 40	15 96	74 90	75 89
6	09 24	34 42	00 68	72 10	71 37
7	89 22	10 23	62 65	78 77	47 33
8	51 27	23 02	13 92	44 13	96 51
9	17 18	01 34	10 98	37 48	93 86
10	02 28	54 60	01 11	28 35	54 32

one and proceed down through the column because every individual in the survey population would not have an equal chance of being selected. The planner can accomplish the random start by closing his or her eyes and pointing to a place on the table of random numbers then proceeding through the table in the way that was set forth above (Cottrell & McKenzie, 2011).

A **systematic sample** also uses a frame and takes every Nth person (determined by dividing the survey population size by the sample size, N/n), beginning with a randomly selected individual. For example, suppose that we want to choose a sample of 10 people from a survey population of 100. We start by randomly choosing a number between 001 and 100, such as 026, using a table of random numbers. We then choose every tenth ($N/n = 100/10 = 10$) person (036, 046, 056, 076, 086, 096, 006, 016) until we have the 10 subjects for the sample. In this way, everyone in the survey population has an equal chance of being selected. A simple random sample or systematic sample can also be used to select "naturally occurring groups or clusters, such as schools, clinics, worksites, or census tracks" (Gilmore, 2012, p. 74). When this occurs, it is called **cluster sampling**.

If it is important that certain groups be represented in a sample, a **stratified random sample** can be selected. Such a method would be used if the planners felt that a certain variable (e.g., size, income, or age, etc.) might have an influence on the data collected from the participants. A stratified random sample might also be used if it is believed that due to small numbers of a certain group in the survey population, representatives from that group may not be selected using a simple random sample. That is, you may have a survey population of 100 participants and in that 100 there are only 8 of one group. If you were to select a sample of 10 from the 100, there is a good chance that none of the 8 from the small group might be selected (Cottrell & McKenzie, 2011).

Here is an example of the use of a stratified random sample. To begin, the planner first must divide the survey population into subgroups, or **strata**, then select a simple random sample from each stratum. Suppose we were interested in collecting data from companies within a particular state concerning the number of health education programs offered for employees. Based on past experience, we suspect the size of the business (i.e., number of employees) would affect the data we want to collect. That is, small companies might have fewer health education programs in general than large companies. Also, we know that relatively few companies in the state have a large number of employees. We could then divide the companies into strata by size, for example small (1–100 employees), medium (101–1,000), and large (1,001+). Once the planners decide how many to select from each stratum, they next decide whether to conduct a proportional stratified random sample or nonproportional stratified random sample. A **proportional stratified random sample** would be used if the planners wanted the sample to mirror, in proportion, the survey population. That is, draw out the companies in the same proportions that they are represented in the survey population. Say our example has 600 small companies, 350 medium companies, and 50 large companies, and the desired sample size is 100. Planners would then select simple random samples of 60 small, 35 medium, and 5 large companies (Cottrell & McKenzie, 2011).

A **nonproportional stratified random sample** may be used if the planners want equal representation from the different strata within the survey population. For example, suppose we want to collect information about the opinions of college students on

Table 5.5   Summary of Probability Sampling Procedures

Sample	Primary Descriptive Elements
Simple Random	Each subject has an equal chance of being selected if table of random numbers and random start are used.
"Fishbowl" (or "Out of a Hat")	Approximates simple random sampling, but not as precise. Can be done with or without replacement.
Systematic	Using a list (e.g., membership list or telephone book), subjects are selected at a constant interval (N/n) after a random start.
Nonproportional Stratified	The population is divided into subgroups based on key characteristics (strata), and subjects are selected from the subgroups at random to ensure representation of the characteristic.
Proportional Stratified	Like the nonproportional stratified random sample, but subjects are selected in proportion to the numerical strength of strata in the population.
Cluster or Area	Random sampling of groups (e.g., teachers' classes) or areas (e.g., city blocks) instead of individuals.
Matrix	The responses of several randomly selected subjects to different items are combined to form the response of one.

Source: Adapted from E. R. Babbie, *The Practice of Social Research*, 6th ed. (Belmont, CA: Wadsworth, 1992); P. C. Cozby, *Methods in Behavioral Research*, 3rd ed. (Palo Alto, CA: Mayfield, 1985); P. D. Leedy, *Practical Research: Planning and Design*, 5th ed. (New York: Macmillan, 1993); and R. J. McDermott and P. D. Sarvela, *Health Education Evaluation and Measurement: A Practitioner's Perspective*, 2nd ed. (New York: McGraw-Hill, 1999).

a medium-size regional campus (the survey population) about a new alcohol use policy that was put in place by the administration and we want to hear equally from the different levels of students (freshmen [$n=4,000$], sophomores [$n=3,000$], juniors [$n=2,000$], and seniors [$n=1,000$]) because it is thought that the policy will affect each class differently. If a sample size of 200 is desired, we would randomly select (using a simple random sample method) 50 students from each of the classes (Cottrell & McKenzie, 2011). (See **Table 5.5** for a summary of probability sampling procedures.)

Nonprobability Sample

There are times when a probability sample cannot be obtained or is not needed. In such cases, planners/evaluators can take **nonprobability samples** in which all individuals in the survey population do not have an equal chance or probability of being selected to participate in the needs assessment or evaluation. Participants can be included on the basis of convenience (because they have volunteered, are available, or can be easily contacted) or because they possess a certain characteristic.

Nonprobability samples have limitations in the extent to which the results can be generalized to the total survey population. Bias may also occur because those who are not included in the sample may differ in some way from those who are included. For example, including only the individuals who complete a health promotion program may bias the results; the findings might be different if all participants, including those who attended but did not complete the program, were surveyed.

Table 5.6   Summary of Nonprobability Sampling Procedures

Sample	Primary Descriptive Elements
Convenience	Includes any available subject meeting some minimum criterion usually being part of an accessible intact group.
Volunteer	Includes any subject motivated enough to self-select for a study.
Grab	Includes whomever investigators can access through direct contact, usually for interviews.
Homogeneous	Includes individuals chosen because of a unique trait or factor they possess.
Judgmental	Includes subjects whom the investigator judges to be "typical" of individuals possessing a given trait.
Snowball	Includes subjects identified by investigators, and any other persons referred by initial subjects.
Quota	Includes subjects chosen in approximate proportion to the population traits they are to "represent."

Source: Health Education Evaluation and Measurement: A Practitioner's Perspective. R. J. McDermott and P. D. Sarveld. Copyright © 1999 by McGraw Hill Companies. Reprinted with permission.

Nonprobability samples can be used when planners/evaluators are unable to identify or contact all those in the survey population. These samples can also be used when resources are limited and a probability sample is too costly or time consuming. It is important that planners/evaluators understand the limitations of this type of sample when reporting the results. (See **Table 5.6** for a summary of nonprobability sampling procedures.)

Sample Size

An often-asked question associated with sampling involves how many individuals are needed for planners/evaluators to feel confident that sampling error is within an acceptable range so that reasonable conclusions can be drawn from the data collected. There is no easy answer to this question. Appropriate sample size is determined by both practical and statistical considerations. From a practical standpoint, often the resources (e.g., personnel, financial) available to collect data are the determining factor on how large the sample will be. Asked another way, is the desired sample size affordable?

When analyzing sample size from a statistical standpoint, three major theoretical considerations are used: central limit theorem (CLT), precision and reliability, and power analysis (Norwood, 2000). The CLT can provide the quickest answer to the sample size question. Mathematically, it has been shown that when a sample size approaches 30 in number, characteristics of that group approach the normal distribution of the group from which it was drawn. Thus, while a sample size of 30 may not properly estimate a research parameter or distinguish research results between groups, a general rule for comparison purposes is, no group should be smaller than 30.

Determining sample size using precision and reliability, or power analysis, is much more complicated (and is not within the scope of this book). **Table 5.7** and **Table 5.8**

Table 5.7 Sample Sizes for Studies Describing Population Proportions When the Population Size Is Known

Population Size	95% Confidence Interval Sample Size for Precision of		
	±1	±3	±5
500	*	*	222
1,000	*	*	286
5,000	*	909	370
10,000	5,000	1,000	385
100,000	9,091	1,099	398
$S\infty$	10,000	1,111	400

* = In these cases the assumption of normal approximation is poor, and the formula used to derive them does not apply.
Source: *Statistics: An Introductory Analysis.* Taro Yamane. Copyright © 1973 by Pearson Education. Adapted with permission.

are offered as examples of the application of these considerations. Detailed explanations of these concepts are presented in many statistics textbooks.

Pilot Testing

Pilot testing (sometimes referred to as *piloting* or a *pilot study*) is a set of procedures used by planners/evaluators to try out the program on a small group of participants prior to actual implementation. In other words, pilot testing can be thought of as a

Table 5.8 Sample Sizes for the One-Sample Case for the Mean

Directional ("One-Tailed") Test for Numerical (Interval or Ratio) Data				
	Alpha = 0.05		Alpha = 0.01	
Effect Size/Power	0.80	0.90	0.80	0.90
.20	155	215	251	326
.50	27	37	43	55
.80	12	17	19	23

Nondirectional ("Two-Tailed") Test for Numerical (Interval or Ratio) Data				
	Alpha = 0.05		Alpha = 0.01	
Effect Size/Power	0.80	0.90	0.80	0.90
.20	197	263	292	372
.50	34	44	50	63
.80	15	19	22	27

Source: *Educational and Psychological Measurement.* D. E. Hinkle, J. D. Oliver, and C. A. Hinkle. Copyright © 1985 by Sage Publications, Inc. Reprinted with permission.

dress rehearsal for planners/evaluators (McDermott & Sarvela, 1999). The purpose of using pilot testing is to identify and, if necessary, correct any problems prior to implementation with the priority population. Thus, pilot testing permits a thorough check of all planned processes to help increase the chances of having a successful program. Throughout the program planning process, planners/evaluators may use pilot testing to detect any problems with sampling, data collection instruments, data collection procedures, data analysis procedures, interventions, curricula, and program evaluation (McDermott & Sarvela, 1999). Because this chapter has focused on measurement and measures, the remaining portions of this discussion will focus on the pilot testing of data collection. Pilot testing will be discussed in later chapters, as it relates to the implementation of a program as well as its role in formative evaluation (see Chapter 12 and Chapter 14).

Once the data collection method has been determined and the instrument has been selected or created, a trial run of the instrument, data collection procedures, and analyses should be conducted. During the piloting process, it would not be uncommon for the planners/evaluators to find problems, such as ambiguous questions, difficulty with coding sheets, and misunderstood directions. Further, the data collected during pilot testing should be statistically analyzed or compiled to make sure there is no difficulty with this step in the data collection process. Revising the data collection process using the information gained from the pilot testing helps ensure that the actual data collection will proceed smoothly.

Several authors have suggested processes for pilot testing (Borg & Gall, 1989; McDermott & Sarvela, 1999; Parkinson & Associates, 1982; Stacy, 1987). They have been combined here into a single process. Several of the preceding authors have presented hierarchies for pilot testing: preliminary review, pre-pilot, pilot tests, and field tests. The first and lowest level in the pilot testing hierarchy is a preliminary review. A **preliminary review** is conducted when those responsible for the data collection process ask colleagues, not people from the priority population, to review the data collection instrument. At a minimum, all data collection instruments should be subjected to this type of review. Specifically, in a preliminary review, colleagues would be asked to complete the instrument as if they were participants in hopes of identifying problems, and also respond to several other questions about the instrument, such as the appropriateness of (1) the instrument's title, (2) the introductory statement explaining the purpose of the data collection, (3) the directions, (4) the order or grouping of the questions, (5) the questions (e.g., unclear or too personal), (6) the length of the instrument, and (7) the method of returning the instrument, to name a few. **Pre-pilots** (or mini-pilots) are used by planners/evaluators with five or six members of the priority population to assess the quality of materials, instruments, and data collection techniques. Methods used to collect this information include observations, interviews, and focus groups. The **pilot test** requires the actual implementation of the instrument. A representative sample of the priority population is used to determine the quality of the instrument. A **field study** is a final pilot test, combining all materials previously tested separately (e.g., instrument, curriculum materials) into a complete program. If enough subjects are used during the field study, it may be possible to check the validity and reliability of the instrument. If at all possible, the use of this sequence of pilot testing techniques is desirable, but planners/evaluators are often limited by time and resources, and so not all the steps may be reasonable to complete.

Ethical Issues Associated with Measurement

Whenever people are being measured as part of a needs assessment or an evaluation, planners/evaluators need to be aware that many of their decisions made and actions taken throughout these processes could have ethical ramifications. Further, planners/evaluators are obligated by law—via the Health Insurance Portability and Accountability Act of 1996—to guard against the misuse of individual identifiable health information.

Ethical issues associated with measurement begin with getting people to voluntarily participate in the process. Before people get involved they should be well informed about the nature of the process and what is expected when they do participate. Further, potential participants should not be coerced or deceived to participate. And, once participation has begun, planners/evaluators should make it clear that participants have the right to discontinue participation at any time without penalty. A second issue is that of private and/or sensitive data. If planners/evaluators need to ask questions that reveal private and sensitive data, they need to ensure anonymity or confidentiality. During data collection, planners/evaluators may hear about illegal acts, such as drug use or other crimes, or they may be provided with access to confidential data. The planners/evaluators must consider the ethical issues and the legal ramifications of such issues.

Once the data have been collected, several ethical issues could arise when the data are analyzed and reported. Inappropriate data analyses can lead to personal harm to participants, the continuation of inappropriate programs, policies or procedures, and the waste of time, effort, and resources (Cottrell & McKenzie, 2011). Regardless of the purposes for which the analyzed data are used, planners/evaluators have an ethical obligation to ensure they do not mislead anyone who relies on them (Dane, 1990). Finally, when the results of a needs assessment or an evaluation are reported, planners/evaluators must ensure not to reveal the identity of those who participated, or individual results of participants, without their permission.

SUMMARY

This chapter focused on helping you understand the terms *measurement, measures, measurement instruments, sampling,* and *pilot testing.* A brief overview of measurement and measures was provided, along with the four levels of measurement: nominal, ordinal, interval, and ratio. Several different examples of questions used at each of the levels were also presented. Next, four desirable characteristics of data were discussed, including reliability, validity, fairness, and the importance of being bias free. Background information was provided to assist you with processes to identify existing measurement instruments and create new ones. Information was also presented on writing measurement instrument questions. This was followed by a discussion of techniques used to draw the various probability and nonprobability samples, and when the various sampling techniques might be most useful. The chapter concluded with short presentations on the importance of using pilot testing and the ethical issues associated with measurement.

REVIEW QUESTIONS

1. What is meant by *measurement,* and *qualitative* and *quantitative measures?*

2. Why is measurement such an important process when it comes to program planning and evaluation?

3. Name and give an example of each of the four levels of measurement.

4. What are the most common types of measures (variables) used in needs assessments and evaluations? Give an example of each type of variable.

5. What is validity? What is reliability? Why are they so important?

6. What is bias in data collection? Name three ways in which it can be reduced.

7. Why must measurement instruments be fair?

8. What are the steps one can follow when identifying, obtaining, and evaluating existing measurement instruments?

9. What are the advantages and disadvantages of using an existing measurement instrument?

10. What are the steps for creating a data collection instrument?

11. Define *census, sample, sampling,* and *sampling frame.*

12. Using a table of random numbers, explain how a simple random sample is selected.

13. Describe three types of probability samples.

14. When, if ever, should nonprobability samples be used?

15. What is the purpose of a preliminary review, a pre-pilot (or mini-pilot), a pilot test, and a field study? How is each conducted?

16. What ethical issues are associated with measurement?

ACTIVITIES

1. Construct a three-page written questionnaire on a health promotion topic of your choice that could be administered to a group of college students.

2. Conduct a pre-pilot test on your written questionnaire developed in activity number 1 on five or six of your friends, colleagues, or classmates. After pilot testing, identify any flaws you see in the questionnaire or data collection process.

3. Assume that your college or university has hired you to conduct a needs assessment on the student body for a new health promotion program. Because there are few secondary data on this group of people, other than national data on college students, you have decided to survey a random sample of students using a written instrument. Your task now is to develop the instrument. Create a draft of an instrument that includes questions that will collect data about the students' health behavior and demographic characteristics. After completing the instrument, pilot test it on 10 students and then tally the data collected.

4. Assume that you are charged with the responsibility of collecting data from all the students on your campus who have enrolled in a fitness course. Assume also that this group of students is too large to collect data from everyone. Explain how you would obtain a representative sample from this population.

5. Review a needs assessment or evaluation instrument. Identify the level of measurement for the questions, types of measurement, and types of questions.

6. Photocopy a page from a local telephone book. Assume that this page represents a sampling frame for your priority population. Go through the frame and divide it into groups of 10 by using the first 10 numbers as group 1, the second 10 as group 2, and so on, until all the numbers are used. Be sure you do not use fax or business numbers. If you have an odd number of telephone numbers (not an even 10), do not use that group. With this information, explain how you would select a simple random sample of 20 numbers, a systematic sample of 10 numbers, a proportional stratified sample of 40 numbers stratified on the first 3 numbers of the telephone numbers, and a cluster sample of 10 groups, assuming that the groups of 10s you formed are your clusters.

WEBLINKS

1. **http://ctb.ku.edu/tools/en/sub_main_1044.htm**

   Community Toolbox

   This page from the Community Toolbox Website, created and maintained by the Work Group on Health Promotion and Community Development at the University of Kansas, defines and describes the process of developing baseline measures.

2. **http://www.welcoa.org/freeresources/pdf/data_dashboard.pdf**

   Wellness Councils of America (WELCOA)

   Visit the WELCOA Website to view the article titled "Developing a Data Dashboard: The Art and Science of Making Sense." For those health education specialists interested in worksite wellness, this article presents a nice overview of the measures (metrics) with which those in the work setting are interested.

3. http://www.cdc.gov/nchs/default.htm

   National Center for Health Statistics (NCHS)

   The NCHS Website is a rich source of measurement instruments used to collect the data about America's health.

4. http://www.surveysystem.com/resource.htm

   Creative Research Systems

   The Creative Research Systems Website includes a lot of information about survey instrument development data collection and includes a calculator for determining appropriate sample size.

CHAPTER 6

Mission Statement, Goals, and Objectives

CHAPTER OBJECTIVES

After reading this chapter and answering the questions at the end, you should be able to:

- Explain what is meant by the terms *mission statement* and *vision statement*.
- Define *goals* and *objectives,* and distinguish between the two.
- Identify the different levels of objectives as presented in the chapter.
- Describe a SMART objective.
- State the necessary elements of an objective as presented in the chapter.
- Specify an appropriate criterion for objectives.
- Write program goals and objectives.
- Describe the use for *Healthy People 2020.*

KEY TERMS

attitude objectives	goal	outcome
awareness objectives	impact objectives	outcome objectives
behavioral objectives	knowledge objectives	process objectives
condition	learning objectives	skill development objectives
criterion	mission statement	SMART objectives
environmental objectives	objectives	vision statement

To plan, implement, and evaluate effective health promotion programs, planners must have a solid foundation in place to guide them through their work. The mission statement, goals, and objectives of a program can provide such a foundation. If prepared properly, a mission statement, goals, and objectives should not only give the necessary direction to a program but also provide the groundwork for the eventual program evaluation (**Box 6.1**). There are two old sayings that help express the need for

Box 6.1   RESPONSIBILITIES AND COMPETENCIES FOR HEALTH
EDUCATION SPECIALISTS

The content of this chapter focuses on the mission, goals, and objectives of a
program. Because the mission, goals, and objectives provide the foundation on
which programs are developed and the criteria used to evaluate the programs, the
information presented in this chapter is applicable to three areas of responsibility:

Responsibility II: Plan Health Education

Competency 2.2: Develop Goals and Objectives

Competency 2.3: Select or Design Strategies and Interventions

Competency 2.4: Develop a Scope and Sequence for the
Delivery of Health Education

Responsibility III: Implement Health Education

Competency 3.2: Monitor Implementation of Health Education

Competency 3.3: Train Individuals Involved in Implementation
of Health Education

Responsibility IV: Conduct Evaluation and Research Related to Health Education

Competency 4.1: Develop Evaluation/Research Plan

Source: NCHEC, SOPHE, & AAHE (2010).

a mission statement, goals, and objectives. The first is: If you do not know where you are
going, then any road will do—and you may end up someplace where you do not want to
be, or you may eventually end up where you want to be, but after wasted time and effort.
The second is: If you do not know where you are going, how will you know when you
have arrived? Without a mission statement, goals, and objectives, a program may lack
direction, and at best it will be difficult to evaluate. **Figure 6.1** shows the relationship
between a mission statement, goals, and objectives. The size of the rectangles presented
in Figure 6.1 has special meaning. The rectangle that represents the mission statement is
the largest, while the rectangle representing the objectives is the smallest, meaning that
ideas presented go from broad to narrow in scope.

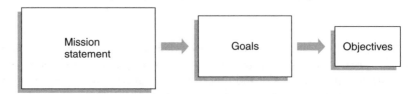

Figure 6.1 Relationship of Mission Statement, Goals, and Objectives

Mission Statement

Sometimes referred to as a program overview or program aim, a **mission statement** is a short narrative that describes the general focus or purpose of the program. The statement not only describes the current focus of a program but also may reflect the philosophy behind it. The mission statement also helps to guide planners in the development of program goals and objectives. **Box 6.2** presents examples of mission statements for several different settings.

Some people mistake a vision statement for a mission statement. They are different. Whereas a mission statement provides a description of the current efforts of a program, a **vision statement** is more of a brief description of where the program will be in the future; typically, in three or more years. A vision statement answers the questions, "What do we want to be?" and "What will we look like in three plus years?" Vision statements are often part of a strategic planning process in which organizations define a strategy or direction for the future. Items that are considered when creating a vision statement are future products (i.e., information, ideas, goods, services, events, and behavior), markets, customers, location, and staffing. Most programs do not include a vision statement. However, if a vision statement were added to Figure 6.1, it would be found in a larger rectangle to the left of the mission statement rectangle.

Box 6.2	EXAMPLES OF MISSION STATEMENTS
Setting	**Mission Statement**
Community Setting	The mission of the Walkup Health Promotion Program is to provide a wide variety of primary prevention activities for residents of the community.
Heath Care Setting	This program is aimed at helping patients and their families to understand and cope with physical and emotional changes associated with recovery following cancer surgery.
School Setting	School District #77 wants happy and healthy students. To that end, the district's personnel strive, through a coordinated school health program, to provide students with experiences that are designed to motivate and enable them to maintain and improve their health.
Worksite Setting	The purpose of the employee health promotion program is to develop high employee morale. This is to be accomplished by providing employees with a working environment that is conducive to good health and by providing an opportunity for employees and their families to engage in behavior that will improve and maintain good health.

Program Goals

Although some individuals use the terms *goals* and *objectives* interchangeably, they are not the same: There are important differences between them. "Goals are broad statements of direction written in nontechnical language" (Cottrell & McKenzie, 2011, p. 217). They are less specific than objectives and are used to explain the general intent of a program to those not directly involved in the program (Cottrell & McKenzie, 2011; Neiger & Thackeray, 1998). "Goals set the fundamental, long-range direction" (CDC, 2008a, p. 1). "Objectives break the goal down into smaller parts that provide specific, measurable actions by which the goal can be accomplished" (CDC, 2008a, p. 1). In comparison to objectives, a **goal** is an expectation that:

1. Is much more encompassing, or global

2. Is written to include all aspects or components of a program

3. Provides overall direction for a program

4. Is more general in nature

5. Usually takes longer to complete

6. Does not have a deadline (CDC, 2003)

7. Usually is not observed, but rather must be inferred because it includes words like *evaluate, know, improve,* and *understand* (Jacobsen, Eggen, & Kauchak, 1989)

8. Is often not measurable in exact terms

Program goals are not difficult to write and need not be written as complete sentences. They should, however, be simple and concise, and should include two basic components: who will be affected, and what will change as a result of the program. Goals typically include verbs such as *improve, increase, promote, protect, minimize, prevent,* and *reduce* (CDC, 2003). A program need not have a set number of stated goals. It is not uncommon for some programs to have a single goal while others have several. **Box 6.3** presents some examples of goals for health promotion programs.

Box 6.3 EXAMPLES OF PROGRAM GOALS

- To reduce the incidence of cardiovascular disease in the employees of the Smith Company.
- All cases of measles in the City of Kenzington will be eliminated.
- To prevent the spread of HIV in the youth of Indiana.
- To reduce the cases of lung cancer caused by exposure to secondhand smoke in Elizabethtown, PA.
- To reduce the incidence of influenza in the residents of the Delaware County Home.
- The survival rate of breast cancer patients will be increased through the optimal use of community resources.

Objectives

As Ross and Mico (1980) have indicated, **objectives** are more precise and represent smaller steps than program goals—steps that, if completed, will lead to reaching the program goal(s). Stated another way, objectives specify intermediate accomplishments or benchmarks that represent progress toward a goal (CDC, 2003). Objectives outline in measurable terms the specific changes that will occur in the priority population at a given point in time as a result of exposure to the program. "Objectives are crucial. They form a fulcrum, converting diagnostic data into program direction and resource allocation over time" (Green & Kreuter, 2005, p. 100). Objectives can be thought of as the bridge between needs assessment and a planned intervention. Knowing how to construct objectives for a program is a most important skill for planners.

Different Levels of Objectives

Several different levels of objectives are associated with program planning. The different levels are sequenced or placed in a hierarchical order to allow for more effective planning (Cleary & Neiger, 1998; Deeds, 1992; Parkinson & Associates, 1982). Objectives are created at each level in order to help attain the program goal. The "objectives should also be *coherent* across levels, with objectives becoming successively more refined and more explicit, and usually multiplied from one level to the next" (Green & Kreuter, 2005, p. 102). Achievement of the lower-level objectives will contribute to the achievement of the higher-level objectives and goals. **Table 6.1** presents the hierarchy of objectives and indicates their relationship to program outcomes and evaluation. Because the hierarchy of objectives was created from the work of several, the labels (names) given to the different levels of objectives have not been consistent. Thus, as we present the description of each type of objective, we identify various labels that have been used.

Process Objectives   The **process objectives** are the daily tasks, activities, and work plans that lead to the accomplishment of all other levels of objectives (Deeds, 1992). They help shape or form the program and thus focus on all program inputs (all that are needed to carry out a program), implementation activities (actual presentation of the program), and stakeholder reactions. More specifically, these objectives focus on such things as program resources (materials, funds, space); appropriateness of intervention activities; priority population exposure, attendance, participation, and feedback; feedback from other stakeholders such as the funding and sponsoring agencies; and data collection techniques, to name a few.

Impact Objectives   The second level of objectives in the hierarchy is **impact objectives**. This level of objectives comprises three different types of objectives: learning objectives, behavioral objectives, and environmental objectives. They are called impact objectives because they describe the immediate observable effects of a program (e.g., changes in awareness, knowledge, attitudes, skills, behaviors, or the environment) and they form the groundwork for impact evaluation (see the last column in Table 6.1).

Table 6.1   Hierarchy of Objectives and Their Relation to Evaluation

Type of Objective	Program Outcomes	Possible Evaluation Measures	Type of Evaluation
Process objectives	Activities presented and tasks completed	Number of sessions held, exposure, attendance, participation, staff performance, appropriate materials, adequacy of resources, tasks on schedule	Process (form of formative)
Impact objectives			
Learning objectives	Change in awareness, knowledge, attitudes, or skills	Increase in awareness, knowledge, attitudes, or skill development/ acquisition	Impact (form of summative)
Behavioral objectives	Change in behavior	Current behavior modified or discontinued, or new behavior adopted	Impact (form of summative)
Environmental objectives	Change in the environment	Measures associated with economic, service, physical, social psychological, or political environments, e.g., protection added to, or hazards or barriers removed from, the environment	Impact (form of summative)
Outcome objectives	Change in quality of life (QOL), health status, or risk, and social benefits	QOL measures, morbidity data, mortality data, measures of risk (e.g., HRA)	Outcome (form of summative)

Source: Adapted from Deeds (1992), Cleary & Neiger (1998), and Parkinson & Associates (1982).

Learning Objectives   **Learning objectives** are the educational or learning tools needed in order to achieve the desired behavior change. They are based upon the analysis of educational and ecological assessment of the PRECEDE-PROCEED model.

Within this category of objectives, there is another hierarchy (Parkinson & Associates, 1982). This hierarchy includes four types of objectives, beginning with the least complex and moving toward the most complex. Complexity is defined in terms of the time, effort, and resources necessary to accomplish the objective. The learning objectives hierarchy begins with **awareness objectives** and moves through **knowledge, attitude, and skill development objectives.** This hierarchy indicates that if those in the priority population are going to adopt and maintain a health-enhancing behavior to alleviate a health concern or problem, they must first be aware of the health concern. Second, they must expand their knowledge and understanding of the concern. Third, they must attain and maintain an attitude that enables them to deal with the concern. And fourth, they need to possess the necessary skills to engage in the health-enhancing behavior.

Behavioral Objectives   **Behavioral objectives** describe the behaviors or actions in which the priority population will engage that will resolve the health problem and move you toward achieving the program goal (Deeds, 1992). Behavioral objectives are commonly written about adherence (e.g., regular exercise), compliance (e.g., taking medication as prescribed), consumption patterns (e.g., diet), coping (e.g., stress-reduction activities), preventive actions (e.g., brushing and flossing teeth), self-care (e.g., first aid), and utilization (e.g., appropriate use of the emergency room).

Environmental Objectives   **Environmental objectives** outline the nonbehavioral causes of a health problem that are present in the social, physical, psychological economic, service, and/ or political environments. Environmental objectives are written about such things as the state of the physical environment (e.g., clean air or water, proximity to facilities, removal of physical barriers), the social environment (e.g., social support, peer pressure), the psychological environment (e.g., the emotional learning climate), the economic environment (e.g., affordability, incentives, disincentives), the service environment (e.g., access to health care, equity in health care), and/or the political environment (e.g., health policy).

Outcome Objectives   Outcome objectives are the ultimate objectives of a program and are aimed at changes in health status, social benefits, risk factors, or quality of life. "They are outcome or future oriented" (Deeds, 1992, p. 36). If these objectives are achieved, then the program goal will be achieved. These objectives are commonly written in terms of reduction of risk, physiologic indicators, signs and symptoms, morbidity, disability, mortality, or quality of life measures.

Developing Objectives

Does every program require objectives from each of the levels just described? The answer is no! However, too often, health promotion programs have too few objectives, all of which fall into one or two levels. Many planners have developed programs hoping solely to change the health behavior of a priority population. For example, a smoking cessation program may have an objective of getting 30% of the participants to stop smoking. Perhaps this program is offered, and only 10% of the participants quit smoking. Is the program a failure? If the program has a single objective of changing behavior, its sponsors would have a good case for saying that the program was not effective. However, it is quite possible that as a result of participating in the smoking cessation program, the participants increased their awareness of the dangers of smoking. They probably also increased their knowledge, maybe changed their attitudes, and developed skills for quitting or cutting back on the number of cigarettes they smoke each day. These are all very positive outcomes—and they could be overlooked when the program is evaluated, if the planner did not write objectives that cover a variety of levels.

Criteria for Developing Objectives

In addition to making sure that the objectives are written in an appropriate manner, planners also need to be realistic with regard to the other parameters of the program. These are some of the questions that planners should consider when writing objectives:

1. Can the objective be realized during the life of the program or within a reasonable time thereafter? It would be quite realistic to assume that a certain number of people

will not be smoking one year after they have completed a smoking cessation program, but it would not be realistic to assume that a group of elementary school students could be followed for life to determine how many of them die prematurely due to inactivity.

2. Can the objective realistically be achieved? It is probably realistic to assume that 30% of any smoking cessation class will stop smoking within one year after the program has ended, but it is not realistic to assume that 100% of the employees of a company will participate in its fitness program.

3. Does the program have enough resources (personnel, money, and space) to obtain a specific objective? It would be ideal to be able to reach all individuals in the priority population, but generally there are not sufficient resources to do so.

4. Are the objectives consistent with the policies and procedures of the sponsoring agency? It may not be realistic to expect to incorporate a no-smoking policy in a tobacco company.

5. Do the objectives violate any of the rights of those who are involved (participants or planners)? Right-to-know laws make it illegal to withhold information that could cause harm to a priority population.

6. If a program is planned for a particular ethnic/cultural population, do the objectives reflect the relationship between the cultural characteristics of the priority group and the changes sought? It would not be realistic to have an objective that eliminates the use of tobacco in a priority population that is comprised of Native Americans because of the ceremonial pipe use in the Native American culture.

Program objectives that meet the six criteria noted above are referred to as **SMART objectives.** SMART stands for specific, measurable, achievable, realistic, and time phased (CDC, 2003). Every objective planners write for their programs should be SMART!

Elements of an Objective

For an objective to provide direction and be useful in the evaluation process, it must be written in such a way that it can be clearly understood, states what is to be accomplished, and is measurable. To ensure that an objective is indeed useful, it should include the following elements:

1. The *outcome* to be achieved, or what will change

2. The *conditions* under which the outcome will be observed, or when the change will occur

3. The *criterion* for deciding whether the outcome has been achieved, or how much change

4. The *priority population,* or who will change

The first element, the **outcome**, is defined as the action, behavior, or something else that will change as a result of the program. In a written objective, the outcome is usually identified as the verb of the sentence. Thus words such as *apply, argue, build, compare, demonstrate, evaluate, exhibit, judge, perform, reduce, spend, state,* and *test* would be considered outcomes (see **Box 6.4** for a more comprehensive listing of appropriate outcome words). It should be noted that not all verbs would be considered appropriate outcomes for an objective; the verb must refer to something measurable and observable. Words such as *appreciate, know, internalize, and understand* by themselves do not refer to something measurable and observable, and therefore are not good choices for outcomes. Some verbs work better than others for specific types of objectives. For example, the verb *list* is an

---

Box 6.4   OUTCOME VERBS FOR OBJECTIVES

abstract	copy	gather	offer	round
accept	count	(information)	order	score
adjust	create	generalize	organize	seek
adopt	criticize	generate	pair	select
advocate	deduce	group	participate	separate
analyze	defend	guess	partition	share
annotate	define	hypothesize	perform	show
apply	delay (response)	identify	persist	simplicity
approximate	demonstrate	illustrate	plan	simulate
argue	derive	imitate	practice	solve
(a position)	describe	improve	praise	sort
ask	design	infer	predict	spend
associate	determine	initiate	prepare	(money)
attempt	develop	inquire	preserve	state
balance	differentiate	integrate	produce	structure
build	discover	interpolate	propose	submit
calculate	discriminate	interpret	prove	subscribe
categorize	dispute	invent	qualify	substitute
cause	distinguish	investigate	query	suggest
challenge	effect	join	question	summarize
change	eliminate	judge	recall	supply
choose	enumerate	justify	recite	support
clarify	estimate	keep	recognize	symbolize
classify	evaluate	label	recommend	synthesize
collect	examine	list	record	tabulate
combine	exemplify	locate	reduce	tally
compare	exhibit	manipulate	regulate	test
complete	experiment	map	reject	theorize
compute	explain	match	relate	translate
conceptualize	express	measure	reorganize	try
connect	extend	name	repeat	unite
construct	extract	obey	replace	visit
consult	extrapolate	object	represent	volunteer
contrast	find	(to an idea)	reproduce	weigh
convert	form	observe	restructure	write

appropriate verb for an awareness-level objective, but not for a knowledge-level objective. The verb *explain* would be much better suited for a knowledge-level objective.

The second element of an objective is the **condition** under which the outcome will be observed, or when it will be observed. "Typical" conditions found in objectives might be "upon completion of the exercise class," "as a result of participation," "by the year 2020," "after reading the pamphlets and brochures," "orally in class," "when asked to respond by the facilitator," "one year after the program," "by May 15th," or "during the class session."

The third element of an objective is the **criterion** for determining when the outcome has been achieved, or how much change will occur. The purpose of this element is to provide a standard by which the planners/evaluators can determine if an outcome has been performed in an appropriate and/or successful manner. Examples might include "to no more than 105 per 1,000," "by 10% over the baseline," "300 pamphlets," "33% of the county residents," "75% of the motor vehicle occupants," "at least half of the participants," "according to CDC guidelines," or "all people who preregistered." One of the most difficult parts of creating appropriate objects for a program is to determine what would be the appropriate criterion for an objective. Should program planners expect a 10% increase over baseline? Should they anticipate half of the employees to participate? What should be expected? There is no hard-and-fast rule for determining the criterion, but remember SMART objectives should be realistic and based on evidence whenever possible. Several different criterion-(target)-setting methods have been used in writing the objectives for the *Healthy People* initiative over the past three plus decades. **Box 6.5** provides a brief description of the target-setting methods used.

The last element that needs to be included in an objective is mention of the priority population, or who will change. Examples are "1,000 teachers," "25% of employees of the company," and "those residing in the Muncie and Provo areas." **Figure 6.2** summarizes the key elements of a well-written objective. There is one exception to the priority population always being the *who* of an objective. That exception applies to process-level objectives. Because some of these objectives guide the work of the program planners and/or implementers. In those cases, the *who* is the staff or group entrusted with instituting the program instead of the priority population (Cottrell & McKenzie, 2011). (See **Box 6.6** for examples of objectives that would include the four primary elements.)

In summary, well-written objectives will always answer the question "WHO is going to do WHAT, WHEN, and TO WHAT EXTENT?" (CDC, 2008a, p. 2). Although it is easy to describe the components of well-written objectives, it is not always easy to write them. **Box 6.7** provides a template to help program planners write objectives.

Goals and Objectives for the Nation

A chapter on goals and objectives would not be complete without at least a short discussion of the health goals and objectives of the nation. These goals and objectives have been most helpful to planners throughout the United States.

The goals and objectives of the nation, which have been referred to as the *health agenda* or the *blueprint of public health planning* for the United States, are the primary

| **Box 6.5** | TARGET SETTING METHODS FOR THE OBJECTIVES OF THE *HEALTHY PEOPLE* INITIATIVE |

- Better than best—When no baseline data were available, target was set based on a comparison to racial/ethnic group with best, or most favorable rate.
- Consistent with another program—Target was set based on the results of an already completed program.
- Consistent with national strategy—Target was set based on the national strategy to improve health.
- Consistent with regulations/policies/laws—Target was set based on data included in the regulations/policies/laws.
- Evidence-based approach—Target set based on results of completed research.
- Expert opinion—If no other data were available, the target was set based on the opinion of experts.
- Minimal statistical significance—Target was set using the smallest improvement that results in a statistically significant difference when tested against the baseline value.
- Modeling/projection of trend (or trend analysis)—Target was set using a model or based on trend data.
- No increase from baseline (maintain baseline)—Target was set based on the belief there would be no change from baseline.
- One state per year—Target was set based on getting one state (or the District of Columbia) to meet a criterion each year.
- Percent improvement—Target was based on a reasonable expected percent change in the priority population compared to previous improvement.
- Retain previous set of objectives target—Target was retained if the previous target was not reached and was still appropriate.
- Threshold analysis—Target was set after analyzing at what point change would begin to produce an effect.
- Total coverage or elimination—Target was set based on the belief that a criterion of 100% could be achieved.

Sources: Gurley (2007, April), USDHHS (2007b), USDHHS (2010a).

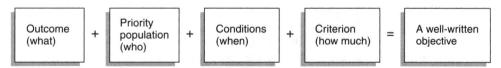

Figure 6.2 Elements of a Well-Written Objective

Box 6.6 EXAMPLES OF OBJECTIVES TO SUPPORT THE PROGRAM GOAL "TO REDUCE THE PREVALENCE OF HEART DISEASE IN THE RESIDENTS OF FRANKLIN COUNTY"

Process Objectives

A. By 2015, the program planners will increase the number of heart healthy educational sessions offered to the county residents from the baseline of 15 to 25 per year.

Outcome (what): Increase the number of heart healthy educational sessions
Priority Population (who): Program planners
Conditions (when): By 2015
Criterion (how much): From the baseline of 15 to 25 per year

B. By August 4, the volunteers will distribute the informational brochure to 33% of the county residents.

Outcome (what): Will distribute the informational brochure.
Priority Population (who): Volunteers.
Conditions (when): By August 4.
Criterion (how much): 33% of the county residents.

C. During the pilot testing, the program facilitators will receive a "good" rating from at least half of the participants.

Outcome (what): Will receive a "good" rating.
Priority Population (who): Program facilitators.
Conditions (when): During the pilot testing.
Criterion (how much): At least half of the participants.

D. Prior to the start of the program, the program staff will deliver the program notebooks to all people who preregistered for the program.

Outcome (what): Will deliver the program notebooks.
Priority Population (who): Program staff.
Conditions (when): Prior to the start of the program.
Criterion (how much): All people who preregistered.

Impact – Learning Objectives

A. Awareness level: After the American Heart Association's pamphlet on cardio-vascular health risk factors has been placed in grocery bags, at least 20% of the shoppers will be able to identify two of their own risks.

Outcome (what): Identify their own risks.
Priority population (who): Shoppers.
Conditions (when): After distribution of the pamphlet.
Criterion (how much): 20%.

B. Knowledge level: When asked over the telephone, one out of three viewers of the heart special television show will be able to explain the four principles of cardiovascular conditioning.

Outcome (what): Able to explain the four principles of cardiovascular conditioning.
Priority population (who): Television viewers.
Conditions (when): When asked over the telephone.
Criterion (how much): One out of three.

Box 6.6 (CONTINUED)

C. Attitude level: During one of the class sessions, 50% of the participants will defend their reason for regular exercise.

Outcome (what): Defend their reason for regular exercise.
Priority population (who): Class participants.
Conditions (when): During one of the class sessions.
Criterion (how much): 50%.

D. Skill development level: After viewing the video "How to Exercise," half of those participating will be able to locate their pulse and count it every time they are asked to do it.

Outcome (what): Locate their pulse and count it.
Priority population (who): Those participating.
Conditions (when): After viewing the video.
Criterion (how much): Half of those participating.

Impact—Behavioral Objectives

A. One year after the formal exercise classes have been completed, 40% of those who completed a majority of the classes will still be involved in a regular aerobic exercise program.

Outcome (what): Will still be involved.
Priority population (who): Those who completed a majority of the classes.
Conditions (when): One year after the classes.
Criterion (how much): 40%.

B. During the telephone interview follow-up, 50% of the residents will report having had their blood pressure taken during the previous six months.

Outcome (what): Will report having their blood pressure taken.
Priority population (who): Residents.
Conditions (when): During the telephone interview follow-up.
Criterion (how much): 50%.

Impact—Environmental Objectives

A. By the year 2020, 10% of the clinic patients will have been able to schedule an appointment either after 5 p.m. or on a Saturday.

Outcome (what): Will have been able to schedule.
Priority Population (who): Clinic patients.
Conditions (when): By the year 2020.
Criterion (how much): 10%.

B. By the end of the year, all senior citizens who want it will be provided transportation to the congregate meals.

Outcome (what): Provided transportation.
Priority population (who): Senior citizens who want it.
Conditions (when): By end of year.
Criterion (how much): All.

(Box 6.6 continues)

Box 6.6 (CONTINUED)

Outcome Objectives

  A. By the year 2020, heart disease deaths will be reduced to no more than 100 per 100,000 in the residents of Franklin County.

    Outcome (what): Reduce heart disease deaths.
    Priority population (who): Residents of Franklin County.
    Conditions (when): By the year 2020.
    Criterion (how much): To no more than 100 per 100,000.

  B. By 2020, increase to at least 25% the proportion of men in Franklin County with hypertension whose blood pressure is under control.

    Outcome (what): Blood pressure under control.
    Priority population (who): Men in Franklin County with hypertension.
    Conditions (when): By 2020.
    Criterion (how much): At least 25%.

  C. Half of all those in the county who complete a regular, aerobic, 12-month exercise program will reduce their "risk age" on their follow-up health risk assessment by a minimum of two years compared to their preprogram results.

    Outcome (what): Will reduce their "risk age."
    Priority population (who): Those who complete an exercise program.
    Conditions (when): After the 12-month exercise program.
    Criterion (how much): Half.

  D. Two-thirds of those who participate in a formal exercise program will use 10% fewer sick days during the life of the program than those who do not participate.

    Outcome (what): Use 10% fewer sick days.
    Priority population (who): Those who participate.
    Conditions (when): During the life of the program.
    Criterion (how much): Two-thirds.

---

component of the U.S. *Healthy People* initiative. The *Healthy People* initiative was launched with the publication of *Healthy People: The Surgeon General's Report on Health Promotion and Disease Prevention* (USDHEW, 1979). Shortly thereafter, the first set of goals and objectives, *Promoting Health/Preventing Disease: Objectives for the Nation* (USDHHS, 1980) were published. The goals and objectives were written to cover the 10-year period from 1980 to 1990 and were divided into three main areas: preventive services, health protection, and health promotion. Each of these areas contained 5 focus areas, or 15 in all. From the 15 areas came a total of 226 objectives. Since the creation of the first set of goals and objectives, three additional sets have been developed and published under the titles of *Healthy People 2000: National Health Promotion and Disease Prevention Objectives* (USDHHS, 1990a), *Healthy People 2010* (USDHHS, 2000), and *Healthy People 2020* (USDHHS, 2010a). Formal reviews (i.e., measured progress) of these objectives are conducted both at midcourse (i.e., half way through the

---

Box 6.7   APPLICATION—TEMPLATE FOR WRITING OBJECTIVES FOR HEALTH PROMOTION PROGRAMS

(Insert one *when* from column A here), (insert one *how much* from column B here) of the (insert one *who* from column C here), will (insert one *what* from column D here).

Column A—*When?*

By December 2020

After the program

During a class session

One year after the classes

Column B—*How much?*

10%

half

a majority

at least 25

Column C —*Who?*

participants

people enrolled in the program

employees

university students

Column D—*What?*

be able to demonstrate how to prepare a low-fat meal

be able to explain the difference between exercise and physical activity

have stopped smoking

list the risk factors for skin cancer

10-year period) and again at the end of 10 years. The midcourse review provides an opportunity to update the document based on the events of the first half of the decade for which the objectives are written. For example, in *Healthy People 2010*, a number of objectives were changed, updated, or deleted because of the events 9/11 and Hurricanes Katrina and Rita. Both the results of the midcourse and end reviews along with other available data are used to help create the next set of goals and objectives. Each set of goals and objectives has become more detailed than the previous. "The evolution from the first decade's objectives to each subsequent set of objectives reflected changing societal concerns, evidence-based technologies, theories, and discourses of those decades. Such accommodations changed the contours of the initiative over time in attempts to make it more relevant to specific partners and other stakeholders" (Green & Fielding, 2011, p. 451).

Healthy People 2020, which was released at the end of 2010, will guide U.S. public health practice and health education specialists through 2020. **Table 6.2** presents the vision statement, a mission statement, and four overarching goals for *Healthy People 2020*. In addition, *Healthy People 2020* includes almost 600 science-based objectives (see **Box 6.8**) spread over 42 different topic areas (see **Table 6.3**) (USDHHS, 2010a). On the Healthy People.gov Website each topic has its own Webpage. At a minimum each page contains a concise goal statement, a brief overview of the topic that provides the background and context for the topic, a statement about the importance of the topic backed up by appropriate evidence, and references.

Table 6.2   *Healthy People 2020* Vision, Mission, and Goals

Vision

A society in which all people live long, healthy lives.

Mission

Healthy People 2020 strives to:

- Identify nationwide health improvement priorities.
- Increase public awareness and understanding of the determinants of health, disease, and disability and the opportunities for progress.
- Provide measurable objectives and goals that are applicable at the national, state, and local levels.
- Engage multiple sectors to take actions to strengthen policies and improve practices that are driven by the best available evidence and knowledge.
- Identify critical research, evaluation, and data collection needs.

Overarching *Goals*

- Attain high-quality, longer lives free of preventable disease, disability, injury, and premature death.
- Achieve health equity, eliminate disparities, and improve the health of all groups.
- Create social and physical environments that promote good health for all.
- Promote quality of life, healthy development, and healthy behaviors across all life stages.

Source: USDHHS (2010a).

The developers of the *Healthy People 2020* felt that the best way to achieve the goals would be to implement the national objectives with the framework referred to as MAP-IT (see **Figure 6.3**). MAP-IT stands for **m**obilize, **a**ssess, **p**lan, **i**mplement, and **t**rack. The mobilize step of MAP-IT deals with bringing interested parties together within communities to deal with health issues. The second step, assess, is used to find out who is affected by the health problem and examine what resources are available to deal with the problem. In the plan step, goals and objectives are created and an intervention is planned that has the best chances of dealing with the health problem. The implement step deals with putting the intervention into action. And the final step, track, deals with evaluating the impact of the intervention on the health problem. (USDHHS, 2010a).

The importance of the *Healthy People* initiative serving as a blueprint for the nation's health agenda is evidenced by their widespread use. Since the publication of the first *Healthy People* goals and objectives in 1980, a number of other documents have been created that can help planners develop or adopt appropriate goals and objectives for their

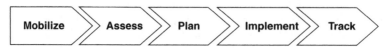

Figure 6.3 MAP-IT: The Action Model to Achieve Healthy People Goals

Source: USDHHS (2010a).

| **Box 6.8** | EXAMPLE GOAL AND OBJECTIVES FROM *HEALTHY PEOPLE 2020* |

Educational and Community-Based Programs (ECBP)

Goal: Increase the quality, availability, and effectiveness of educational and community-based programs designed to prevent disease and injury, improve health, and enhance quality of life.

Objective: ECBP-10 Increase the number of community-based organizations (including local health departments, tribal health services, nongovernmental organizations, and state agencies) providing population-based primary prevention services in the following areas

ECBP 10.8 Nutrition

Target: 94.7 percent.

Baseline: 86.4 percent of community-based organizations (including local health departments, tribal health services, nongovernmental organizations, and state agencies) provided population-based primary prevention services in nutrition in 2008

Target setting method: 10 percent improvement.

Data source: National Profile of Local Health Departments, National Association of County and City Health Officials (NACCHO)

ECBP 10.9 Physical Activity

Target: 88.5 percent.

Baseline: 80.5 percent of community-based organizations (including local health departments, tribal health services, nongovernmental organizations, and state agencies) provided population-based primary prevention services in physical activity in 2008.

Target setting method: 10 percent improvement.

Data source: National Profile of Local Health Departments, National Association of County and City Health Officials (NACCHO)

Source: USDHHS (2010a).

programs. A number of states and U.S. territories have taken the national objectives and created similar documents specific to their own residents. In addition, a number of agencies/organizations have taken similar steps to create documents that could be used by their members and clients in various planning efforts.

The national goals and objectives have been important components in the process of health promotion planning since 1980. It is highly recommended that planners review these objectives before developing goals and objectives for programs. The national objectives may be helpful in providing a rationale for a program and in focusing program goals and objectives toward the areas of greatest need, as planners work toward the year 2020.

Table 6.3   *Healthy People 2020* Topic Areas

1. Access to Health Services
2. Adolescent Health
3. Arthritis, Osteoporosis, and Chronic Back Conditions
4. Blood Disorders and Blood Safety
5. Cancer
6. Chronic Kidney Disease
7. Dementias, Including Alzheimer's Disease
8. Diabetes
9. Disability and Health
10. Early and Middle Childhood
11. Educational and Community-Based Programs
12. Environmental Health
13. Family Planning
14. Food Safety
15. Genomics
16. Global Health
17. Healthcare-Associated Infections
18. Health Communication and Health Information Technology
19. Health-Related Quality of Life and Well-Being
20. Hearing and Other Sensory or Communication Disorders
21. Heart Disease and Stroke
22. HIV
23. Immunization and Infectious Diseases
24. Injury and Violence Prevention
25. Lesbian, Gay, Bisexual, and Transgender Health
26. Maternal, Infant, and Child Health
27. Medical Product Safety
28. Mental Health and Mental Disorders
29. Nutrition and Weight Status
30. Occupational Safety and Health
31. Older Adults
32. Oral Health
33. Physical Activity
34. Preparedness
35. Public Health Infrastructure
36. Respiratory Diseases
37. Sexually Transmitted Diseases
38. Sleep Health
39. Social Determinants of Health
40. Substance Abuse
41. Tobacco Use
42. Vision

Source: USDHHS (2010a).

SUMMARY

The mission statement provides an overview of a program and is most useful in the development of goals and objectives. It should not be confused with a vision statement. The terms *goals* and *objectives* are sometimes used interchangeably, but they are quite different. Together, the two provide a foundation for program planning and evaluation. Goals are more global in nature and often are not measurable in exact terms, whereas objectives are more specific and consist of the steps used to reach the program goals. Objectives can and should be written for several different levels. For objectives to be useful, they should be written so as to be observable and measurable. At a minimum, an objective should include the following elements: a stated outcome (what), conditions under which the outcome will be observed (when), a criterion for considering that the outcome has been achieved (how much), and mention of the priority population (who). As planners develop their goals and objectives for their programs, they should find the *Healthy People 2020* document and other information at its Website very useful.

REVIEW QUESTIONS

1. What is a mission statement? Why is it important? How is it different from a vision statement?

2. What is (are) the difference(s) between a goal and an objective?

3. What is the purpose of program goals and objectives?

4. What are the different levels of objectives?

5. What are the necessary elements of an objective?

6. What are the characteristics of a SMART objective?

7. What are the goals and objectives for the nation? How can they be used by program planners?

8. Briefly explain the *Healthy People* initiative.

9. How can planners use the *Healthy People 2020* goals and objectives in their program planning efforts?

ACTIVITIES

1. Write a mission statement, a goal, and supporting objectives (one at each level) for a program you are planning.

2. Identify which of the following objectives include all four elements necessary for a complete objective; revise those objectives that do not include all the elements:

   a. After the class on objective writing, the students will know the difference between a goal and an objective.

   b. The students know how a skinfold caliper works.

   c. After completing this chapter, the students will be able to write objectives for each of the levels based on the four elements outlined in the chapter.

   d. Given appropriate instruction, the employees will be able to accurately take blood pressure readings of fellow employees.

   e. Program participants will be able to list the reasons why people do not exercise.

3. Using data available from the County Health Rankings (http://www.countyhealthrankings.org/) for the county in which you currently reside, write a goal aimed at improving a health behavior and write one process, three impact (i.e., one each for knowledge, behavior, and environment), and one outcome objective to help reach the goal.

4. Using data available from the Kaiser State Health Facts Website (http://www.statehealthfacts.org) for the state in which you currently reside, write a goal aimed at improving a health status topic and write one process, three impact (i.e., one each for awareness, skill, and environment), and one outcome objective to help reach the goal.

5. Assume that you are a health education specialist working in a primary care clinic. Based on some data provided by personnel at the local hospital regarding birth outcomes for the clinic patients, your supervisor has asked that you create a new program to decrease the percentage of female patients of childbearing age who smoke. After completing a needs assessment you have found that the highest rate of smokers was found among those patients who were 18–24 years of age, covered by a health insurance plan, and have more than one child. In addition, the average number of cigarettes smoked per day by the patients was 22. Write a mission statement, a goal, and at least six objectives to help reach the stated goal.

WEBLINKS

1. http://www.cdc.gov/phin/communities/resourcekit/tools/evaluate/smart_objectives.html

   Communities of Practice for Public Health: Resource Kit

   On this page of the Centers for Disease Control and Prevention Website, you will find more information about SMART objectives and some related resources that provide templates for writing SMART objectives.

2. **http://www.healthypeople.gov/2020/default.aspx**

   Healthy People 2020

   This is the home page for *Healthy People 2020*. At this site you can navigate to background information about *Healthy People 2020*, a listing of the 42 topic areas and the almost 600 objectives, and suggestions for implementing *Healthy People 2020*.

3. **http://ctb.ku.edu/en/default.aspx**

   Community Tool Box

   On the home page of the Community Tool Box (CTB), you can use the "Search the CTB" function to locate information on creating mission statements, goals, and SMART objectives.

CHAPTER 7

Theories and Models Commonly Used for Health Promotion Interventions

After reading this chapter and answering the questions at the end, you should be able to:

- Define *theory, model, constructs, concepts,* and *variables.*
- Explain why health promotion interventions should be planned using theoretical frameworks.
- Describe how the concept of the ecological perspective applies to using theories.
- Explain the difference between a continuum theory and a stage theory.
- Briefly explain the theories and models presented in this chapter.

action stage
attitude toward the behavior
aversive stimulus
behavior change theories
behavioral capability
concepts
construct
contemplation stage
continuum theory
decisional balance
direct reinforcement
efficacy expectations
elaboration
emotional–coping response
expectancies

expectations
intention
lapse
likelihood of taking recommended preventive health action
locus of control
maintenance stage
model
negative punishment
negative reinforcement
outcome expectations
perceived barriers
perceived behavioral control
perceived benefits

perceived seriousness/ severity
perceived susceptibility
perceived threat
planning models
positive punishment
positive reinforcement
precontemplation stage
preparation stage
processes of change
punishment
recidivism
reciprocal determinism
reinforcement
relapse

Key Terms, continued

relapse prevention (RP)	social context	subjective norm
self-control	social network	temptation
self-efficacy	socio-ecological approach	termination
self-regulation	(ecological perspective)	theory
self-reinforcement	stage	variable
social capital	stage theory	vicarious reinforcement

Whenever there is a discussion about the theoretical bases for health education and health promotion, we often find the terms *theory* and *model* used. We begin this chapter with a brief explanation of these terms, to establish a common understanding of their meaning.

One of the most frequently quoted definitions of **theory** is one in which Glanz, Lewis, and Viswanath (2008b) modified an earlier definition written by Kerlinger (1986). It states, "A *theory* is a set of interrelated concepts, definitions, and propositions that presents a *systematic* view of events or situations by specifying relations among variables in order to *explain* and *predict* the events of the situations" (p. 26). In other words, a theory is a systematic arrangement of fundamental principles that provide a basis for explaining certain happenings of life. "The role of theory is to untangle and simplify for human comprehension the complexities of nature" (Green et al., 1994, p. 398). For health education specialists, theories "provide a framework for generating testable hypotheses and integrating empirical evidence and, over time, a road map for the design and implementation of intervention strategies. The structure and perspective afforded by a theory in the behavioral sciences can be reassuring as it helps to make sense of the complex network of beliefs and behaviors that characterize a particular behavioral domain and guides decisions about how to prioritize the distribution of intervention resources" (Rothman, 2009, p. 150S).

Nutbeam and Harris (1999) have stated that a fully developed theory would be characterized by three major elements: "It would explain:

- the major factors that influence the phenomena of interest, for example those factors which explain why some people are regularly active and others are not;

- the relationship between these factors, for example the relationship between knowledge, beliefs, social norms and behaviours [sic] such as physical activity; and

- the conditions under which these relationships do or do not occur: the how, when, and why of hypothesised [sic] relationships, for example, the time, place and circumstances which, predictably lead to a person being active or inactive" (p. 10).

In comparison, a **model** "is a composite, a mixture of ideas or concepts taken from any number of theories and used together" (Hayden, 2009, p. 1). Stated a bit differently: "Models draw on a number of theories to help understand a specific problem in a particular setting or content. They are not always as specific as theory" (Rimer & Glanz, 2005, p. 4). Unlike theories, models do "not attempt to explain the processes underlying learning, but only to represent them" (Chaplin & Krawiec, 1979, p. 68).

Though we just went to some effort to make a distinction between the words *theory* and *model*, when the term *theory-based* is used (such as in *theory-based planning, theory-based practice,* or *theory-based research*), it is commonly understood in our profession that the word *theory* is used in a general way to mean either theory and model. In fact, some of the best-known and often used theories in health education/health promotion use the word *model* in their title (e.g., Health Belief Model). Goodson (2010) provides an explanation for the discrepancy in the use of term *model* for things we refer to as "theory." She has indicated that when some of these models were created they were properly titled as models. They were created using theoretical constructs to explain specific phenomena. They had little empirical testing to prove their worth. Over time, these models have been tested and refined and thus have gained theory status. Goodson (2010) concludes by saying in our work "because we tend to borrow the theories we employ from other disciplines and fields and because our concern usually centers in applying these theories (or models) to practice or research, it seems to matter little to us whether we deal with theories or with models; it seems to matter even less what labels we attach to them" (p. 228). Thus, as we use the terms *theory* and *theory-based* throughout the remainder of this book, we use them to be inclusive of endeavors based on either a theory *or* a model.

Concepts are the primary elements or building blocks of a theory (Glanz et al., 2008b). When a concept has been developed, created, or adopted for use with a specific theory, it is referred to as a **construct** (Kerlinger, 1986). "The key concepts of a theory are its constructs" (Rimer & Glanz, 2005, p. 4). The operational (practical use) form of a construct is known as a **variable**. Variables "specify how a construct is to be measured in a specific situation" (Glanz et al., 2008b, p. 28). Thus, variables need to be matched "to constructs when identifying what needs to be assessed during evaluation of a theory-driven program" (Rimer & Glanz, 2005, p. 4).

> Consider how these terms are used in practical application. A personal belief is a *concept* related to various health behaviors. For example, people are more likely to behave in a healthy way—say exercise regularly—if they feel confident in their ability to actually engage in a healthy form of exercise. Such a concept is captured in a *construct* of the Social Cognitive Theory (SCT) called self-efficacy. If health education specialists develop an intervention to assist people in exercising, being able to measure the peoples' self-efficacy toward exercise would help with the creation of the intervention. The measurement may consist of a few questions that ask people to rate their confidence in their ability to exercise. This measurement, or operational form, of the self-efficacy construct is a *variable*. However, because of the complexity of getting a non-exerciser to become an exerciser, the health education specialist may need to use a *model*, composed of constructs from several theories, to plan the intervention (Cottrell et al., 2012, p. 101).

Based on these descriptions, it seems logical to think of theories as the backbone of the processes used to plan, implement, and evaluate health promotion interventions. They can help by (1) identifying why people are not behaving in healthy ways, (2) identifying information needed before developing an intervention, (3) providing a conceptual framework for selecting constructs to develop the intervention, (4) providing direction and justification for program activities, (5) providing insights into how best to deliver the intervention, and (6) identifying what needs to be measured to evaluate the impact of the intervention (Cowdery et al., 1995; Crosby, Kegler, & DiClemente, 2009; Glanz et al., 2008b).

Theory also "provides a useful reference point to help keep research and implementation activities clearly focused" (Crosby et al., 2009, p. 11), and it infuses ethics and social justice into practice (Goodson, 2010). In addition, "[u]sing theory as a foundation for program planning and development is consistent with the current emphasis on using evidence-based interventions in public health, behavioral medicine, and medicine" (Rimer & Glanz, 2005, p. 5). Getting people to engage in health behavior change is a complicated process that is very difficult under the best of conditions. Without the direction that theories provide, planners can easily waste valuable resources in trying to achieve the desired behavior change. Therefore, program planners should ground their planning process in the theories that have been the foundation of other successful health promotion efforts.

There are many theories that health education specialists can use to plan programs. There is no best theory. "The 'best theory' is a function of how well it serves the objectives that must be met to achieve sustainable protective behaviors among a specified popula- tion. In essence, the range of behavioral and social science theories available for both health promotion practice and research affords the practitioner and researcher an opportunity to select the theories that are the most appropriate, feasible, and practical for a particular setting or population" (Crosby et al., 2009, p. 15). In addition, "No single theory or conceptual framework dominates research or practice in health promotion and

---

Box 7.1 RESPONSIBILITIES AND COMPETENCIES FOR HEALTH EDUCATION SPECIALISTS

The content of this chapter focuses on theories and models used in the practice of health promotion. Specifically, theories and models provide a "road map" for plan- ners to use when creating interventions and evaluating the effectiveness of those interventions. The responsibilities and competencies related to these tasks include:

Responsibility I: Assess Needs, Assets, and Capacity for Health Education
                     Competency 1.1: Plan Assessment Process
                     Competency 1.2: Access Existing Information and Data Related to Health

Responsibility II: Plan Health Education
                     Competency 2.3: Select or Design Strategies and Interventions

Responsibility III: Implement Health Education
                     Competency 3.1: Implement a Plan of Action

Responsibility VI: Serve as a Health Education Resource Person
                     Competency 6.2: Provide Training

Responsibility VII: Communicate and Advocate for Health and Health Education
                     Competency 7.2: Identify and Develop a Variety of Communi- cation Strategies, Methods, and Techniques

Source: NCHEC, SOPHE, & AAHE (2010).

education today" (Glanz et al., 2008b, p. 31). In a review of 10 leading health, medicine, and psychology journals, Painter, Borba, Hynes, Mays, & Glanz (2008) found that "dozens of theories and models" (Glanz, 2008b, p. 31) had been used in the reported literature. We have no intention of introducing all of them. However, approximately 10 theories and models are used regularly to plan programs. The remaining sections of this chapter and in parts of several other chapters we present an overview of the theories that are most often used in creating health promotion interventions. As you read about and study the various theories, you will find that some express the same general ideas, but employ "a unique vocabulary to articulate the specific factors considered to be important" (Glanz et al., 2008b, p. 28). Also, be aware that the presentation of theories that follows is by no means comprehensive in nature. For those readers who would like to examine these and other theories in more depth, we would recommend six books: *Health Behavior and Health Education: Theory, Research and Practice* (Glanz, Rimer, & Viswanath, 2008a); *Introduction to Health Behavior* (Hayden, 2009); *Emerging Theories in Health Promotion Practice and Research: Strategies for Improving Public Health* (DiClemente, Crosby, & Kegler, 2009); *Theory in Health Promotion Research and Practice* (Goodson, 2010); *Behavior Theory in Health Promotion Practice and Research* (Simons-Morton, McLeroy, & Wendel, 2012); and *Health Behavior Theory for Public Health* (DiClemente, Salazar, & Crosby, 2013). **Box 7.1** identifies the responsibilities and competencies for health education specialists that pertain to the material presented in this chapter.

Types of Theories and Models

There are several ways of categorizing the theories and models associated with health education/promotion practice. One way of doing so is to divide them into two groups. The first group includes those theories and models used for planning, implementing, and evaluating health promotion programs. This group has been called **planning models**. The planning models were presented earlier (Chapter 3). The second group is referred to as **behavior change theories**. Behavior change theories "specify the relationships among causal processes operating both within and across levels of analysis" (McLeroy, Steckler, Goodman, & Burdine, 1992, p. 3). In other words, they help explain how change takes place.

Behavior Change Theories

As noted earlier, there are many behavior change theories that health education specialists could use to plan programs. Because of the peculiarities of the theories and multitude of factors that could impact a specific planning situation, some theories work better in some situations than others. Before we present the theories focusing on behavior change, it is important to introduce the concept of socio-ecological approach.

The underlying concept of the **socio-ecological approach** (sometimes referred to as the **socio-ecological perspective**) is that behavior has multiple levels of influences. As related to health behavior, this approach "emphasizes the interaction between, and the interdependence of factors within and across all levels of a health problem" (Rimer & Glanz,

2005, p. 10). That is to say, "[i]ndividuals influence and are influenced by their families, social networks, the organizations in which they participate (workplaces, schools, religious organizations), the communities of which they are a part, and the society in which they live" (IOM, 2001, p. 26). In other words, the health behavior of individuals is shaped in part by the *social context* in which they live. **Social context** has been "defined as the sociocultural forces that shape people's day-to-day experiences and that directly and indirectly affect health and behavior (Burke, Joseph, Pasick, & Barker, 2009, p. 56S). Therefore, a central conclusion of the socio-ecological approach is that interventions must be aimed at multiple levels of influence in order to achieve substantial changes in health behavior (Sallis, Owen, & Fisher, 2008).

McLeroy, Bibeau, Steckler, and Glanz (1988) identified five levels of influence: (1) intrapersonal or individual factors, (2) interpersonal factors, (3) institutional or organizational factors, (4) community factors, and (5) public policy factors. **Table 7.1** presents and defines each of the five levels, while **Box 7.2** provides an example of how the levels can impact health behavior.

Because of the underlying concepts that are captured in the constructs of individual theories, certain theories are more useful in developing programs aimed at specific levels of influence. For example, some theories were developed to help explain behavior change in individuals, while others were developed to help explain change at the community level. Though there are five distinct levels of influence, for the purposes of program planning the five levels are often condensed to three—intrapersonal, interpersonal, and community (Glanz & Rimer, 1995; Rimer & Glanz, 2005). "In practice, addressing the community level requires taking into consideration institutional and public policy factors, as well as social networks and norms" (Rimer & Glanz, 2005, p. 11). To assist program planners with matching theories appropriate to level of influence, we have presented our discussion of the theories according to the level of influence at which they are most useful.

In addition to theories being placed into a level of influence at which they may be most useful, theories can also be categorized by the approach—continuum or stage theories—they

Table 7.1 An Ecological Perspective: Levels of Prevention

Concept	Definition
Intrapersonal Level	Individual characteristics that influence behavior, such as knowledge, attitudes, beliefs, and personality traits
Interpersonal Level	Interpersonal processes and primary groups, including family, friends, and peers that provide social identity, support, and role definition
Community Level	
Institutional Factors	Rules, regulations, policies, and informal structures that may constrain or promote recommended behaviors
Community Factors	Social networks and norms, or standards, that exist as formal or informal among individuals, groups, and organizations
Public Policy	Local, state, and federal policies and laws that regulate or support healthy actions and practices for disease prevention, early detection, control, and management

Source: Rimer and Glanz (2005, p. 11)

Box 7.2 APPLICATION OF THE SOCIO-ECOLOGICAL APPROACH

A good example of the use of the socio-ecological approach (ecological perspective) is the comprehensive method used to reduce cigarette smoking in the United States. At the *intrapersonal* (or *individual*) *level*, a large majority of smokers know that smoking is bad for them and a slightly smaller majority have indicated they would like to quit. Many have tried—some have tried on many occasions. At the *interpersonal level*, many smokers are encouraged by their physician and/or family and friends to quit. Some smokers may attempt to quit on their own or join a formal smoking cessation group to try to quit. At the *institutional* (or *organizational*) *level*, a number of institutions (e.g., churches and worksites) have developed policies that prohibit smoking in and/or on institution property (i.e., buildings and grounds). At the *community level*, a number of towns, cities, and counties have passed ordinances that prohibit smoking in public places. At the *public policy level*, a number of states have passed clean indoor air acts that limit smoking, and have passed laws increasing the tax on a package of cigarettes. Also at this level, the U.S. government has spent many dollars for public service announcements (PSAs) and other forms of media advertising the dangers of tobacco use. Attacking the smoking problem from all levels has contributed to the decrease in the percentage of smokers in the United States.

---

use to explain behavior. **Continuum theories** are those behavior change theories that identify variables which influence actions (e.g., beliefs, attitudes) and combine them into a single equation that predicts the likelihood of action (Weinstein, Rothman, & Sutton, 1998; Weinstein, Sandman, & Blalock, 2008). "These theories acknowledge *quantitative* differences among people in their positions on different variables" (Weinstein et al., 2008, p. 124) and "thus, each person is placed along a continuum of action likelihood" (Weinstein et al., 1998, p. 291).

A **stage theory** is one that is comprised of an ordered set of categories into which people can be classified, and which identifies factors that could induce movement from one category to the next (Weinstein & Sandman, 2002b). More specifically, stage theories have four principal elements: (1) a category system to define the stages, (2) an ordering of stages, (3) common barriers to change facing people in the same stage, and (4) different barriers to change facing people in different stages (Weinstein et al., 1998; Weinstein & Sandman, 2002a). Advocates of stage theories "claim that there are *qualitative* differences among people and question whether changes in health behaviors can be described by a single prediction equation" (Weinstein et al., 2008, pp. 124–125). **Table 7.2** lists the theories presented in this book by level of influence and theory approach.

Intrapersonal Level Theories

The intrapersonal or "individual level is the most basic one in health promotion practice, so planners must be able to explain and influence the behavior of individuals" (Rimer & Glanz, 2005, p. 12). Intrapersonal theories focus on factors within the individual such as knowledge, attitudes, beliefs, self-concept, feelings, past experiences, motivation, skills, and behavior (Rimer & Glanz, 2005). With much of the work of health education specialists taking place at this level of influence, a number of theories could be used. They are discussed below.

Table 7.2 Theories by Level of Influence and Category

Level of Influence	Chapter Where Found in This Book
• Intrapersonal Level	
Continuum Theory	
Stimulus Response Theory	Chapter 7
Theory of Reasoned Action	Chapter 7
Theory of Planned Behavior	Chapter 7
Health Belief Model	Chapter 7
Protection Motivation Theory	Chapter 7
Elaboration Likelihood Model of Persuasion	Chapter 7
Information-Motivation-Behavioral Skills Model	Chapter 7
Stage Theory	
Transtheoretical Model	Chapter 7
Precaution Adoption Process Model	Chapter 7
• Interpersonal Level	
Continuum Theory	
Social Cognitive Theory	Chapter 7
Social Network Theory	Chapter 7
Social Capital Theory	Chapter 7
• Community Level	
Continuum Theory	
Communication Theory	Chapters 8 & 11
Community Organizing	Chapter 9
Community Building	Chapter 9
Diffusion of Innovations	Chapter 11
Stage Theory	
Community Readiness Model	Chapter 7

Stimulus Response (SR) Theory One of the theories used to explain and modify behavior is the stimulus response, or SR, theory (Thorndike, 1898; Watson, 1925; Hall, 1943). This theory reflects the combination of classical conditioning (Pavlov, 1927) and instrumental conditioning (Thorndike, 1898) theories. These early conditioning theories explain learning based on the associations among stimulus, response, and reinforcement (Parcel & Baranowski, 1981; Parcel, 1983). "In simplest terms, the SR theorists believe that learning results from events (termed 'reinforcements') which reduce physiological drives that activate behavior" (Rosenstock, Strecher, & Becker, 1988, p. 175). The behaviorist B. F. Skinner believed that the frequency of a behavior was determined by the reinforcements that followed that behavior.

In Skinner's view, the mere temporal association between a behavior and an immediately following reward is sufficient to increase the probability that the behavior will be repeated. Such behaviors are called *operants*; they operate on the environment to bring about changes resulting in reward or reinforcement (Rosenstock et al., 1988). Stated another way, operant behaviors are behaviors that act on the environment to produce consequences. These consequences, in turn, either reinforce or do not reinforce the behavior that preceded.

There are two broad categories of environmental consequences: **reinforcement** or **punishment** (McDade-Montez, Cvengros, & Christensen, 2005): Individuals can learn from both. Reinforcement has been defined by Skinner (1953) as any event that follows a behavior, which in turn increases the probability that the same behavior will be repeated in the future. Stated differently, reinforcement has "a *strengthening effect* that occurs when operant behaviors have certain consequences" (Nye, 1992, p. 16). Behavior has a greater probability of occurring in the future: (1) if reinforcement is frequent and (2) if reinforcement is provided soon after the desired behavior. This immediacy clarifies the relationship between the reinforcement and appropriate behavior (Skinner, 1953). Simons-Morton and colleagues (2012) have stated that when a behavior is sufficiently reinforced it tends to recur. If a behavior is complex in nature, smaller steps working toward the desired behavior with appropriate reinforcement will help to shape the desired behavior. This was found to be true in getting pigeons to play Ping-Pong, and it can be useful in trying to change a complex health behavior like smoking or exercise. Whereas reinforcement will increase the frequency of a behavior, punishment will decrease the frequency of a behavior. However, both reinforcement and punishment can be either positive or negative. The terms *positive* and *negative* in this context do not mean good and bad; rather, *positive* means adding something (effects of the stimulus) to a situation, whereas *negative* means taking something away (removal or reduction of the effects of the stimulus) from the situation.

If individuals act in a certain way to produce a consequence that makes them feel good or that is enjoyable, it is labeled **positive reinforcement** (or *reward*). Examples of this would be an individual who is involved in an exercise program and "feels good" at the end of the workout, or one who participates in a weight loss program and receives verbal encouragement from the facilitator, again making that person "feel good." Stimulus response theorists would note that in both of these situations, the pleasant experiences (internal feelings and verbal encouragement, respectively) occur right after the behavior, which in turn increases the chances that the frequency of the behavior will increase.

While positive reinforcement helps individuals learn by shaping behavior, behavior that avoids punishment is also learned because it reduces the tension that precedes the punishment (Rosenstock et al., 1988). "When this happens, we are being conditioned by *negative reinforcement:* A response is strengthened by the *removal* of something from the situation. In such cases, the 'something' that is removed is referred to as a *negative reinforcer* or *aversive stimulus* (these two phrases are synonymous)" (Nye, 1979, p. 33). A good example of **negative reinforcement** is a weight loss program that requires weekly dues. When participants stop paying dues because they have met their goal weight, this removal of an obligation should increase the frequency of the desired behavior (weight maintenance). Or in the case of exercise, "negative reinforcements would include decreased poor self-image and decreased fatigue" (McDade-Montez et al., 2005, p. 64).

Some people think of negative reinforcement as a form of punishment, but it is not. While negative reinforcement increases the likelihood that a behavior will be repeated, punishment typically suppresses behavior. "Skinner suggests two ways in which a response can be punished: by *removing a positive reinforcer* or by *presenting a negative reinforcer*

		Consequences	
		Positive (adding to)	Negative (taking away)
Behavior	Increase in frequency	Positive reinforcement (reward)	Negative reinforcement
	Decrease in frequency	Positive punishment	Negative punishment

Figure 7.1 2 × 2 Table of the Stimulus Response Theory

(aversive stimulus) as a consequence of the response" (Nye, 1979, p. 43). Punishment is usually linked to some uncomfortable (physical, mental, or otherwise) experience and decreases the frequency of a behavior. An aversive smoking cessation program that circulates cigarette smoke around those enrolled in the program as they smoke is an example of **positive punishment**. It decreases the frequency of smoking by presenting (adding) a negative reinforcer or **aversive stimulus** (smoke) as a consequence of the response. Examples of **negative punishment** (removing a positive reinforcer) would include not allowing employees to use the employees' lounge if they continue to smoke while using it, or reducing the health insurance benefits of employees who continue to participate in health-harming behavior such as not wearing a safety belt. Stimulus response theorists would note that taking away the privilege of using the employees' lounge or reducing health insurance benefits would decrease the frequency of smoking among the employees and increase the wearing of safety belts, respectively. **Figure 7.1** illustrates the relationship between reinforcement and punishment.

Finally, if reinforcement is withheld—or, stating it another way, if the behavior is ignored—the behavior will become less frequent and eventually will not be repeated. Skinner (1953) refers to this as extinction. Teachers frequently use this technique with disruptive children in the classroom. If a child is acting up in class, the teacher may choose to ignore the behavior in hopes that the nonreinforced behavior will go away.

Theory of Reasoned Action (TRA)   Another theory that has received considerable attention in the literature of health behavior change is Fishbein's (1967) *theory of reasoned action (TRA)*. This theory was developed to explain not just health behavior but all volitional behaviors "that is, behaviors that can be performed at will" (Luszczynska & Sutton, 2005, p. 73). While the stimulus response theory discussed earlier in this chapter was concerned with behavior, this one provides a framework to study attitudes toward behaviors.

Fishbein and Ajzen (1975) distinguish among *attitude, belief, intention,* and *behavior,* and they present a conceptual framework for the study of the relationship among these four constructs. **Intention** "is an indication of a person's readiness to perform a given behavior, and it is considered to be an immediate antecedent of behavior" (Ajzen, 2006). According to this theory, individuals' intention to perform given behaviors are functions of their *attitudes* toward the behavior and their *subjective norms* associated with the behaviors.

Attitude toward the behavior "is the degree to which performance of the behavior is positively or negatively valued. According to the expectancy-value model, attitude toward a behavior is determined by the total set of accessible behavioral beliefs linking the behavior to various outcomes and other attributes" (Ajzen, 2006). Thus a person who has strong beliefs about positive attributes or outcomes from performing the behavior will have a positive attitude toward behavior (Montaño & Kasprzyk, 2008). For example, if a person feels strongly about exercise being able to help control weight, then that person will have a positive attitude toward exercise. The converse is true as well. Weak beliefs about the outcomes or attributes of exercise will produce a negative attitude toward it.

Subjective norm "is the perceived social pressure to engage or not engage in a behavior" (Ajzen, 2006). For many health behaviors, the social pressure comes from a person's peers, parents, partner, close friends, teachers, role models, boss, and co-workers, as well as experts or professionals like physicians or lawyers. Thus individuals who believe that certain people think they should perform a behavior and are motivated to meet the people's expectations will hold a positive subjective norm (Montaño & Kasprzyk, 2008). Similar to behavioral beliefs, the converse is also true. An example of a positive subjective norm are employees who see their co-workers as important people in their lives and believe that these people approve of them participating in a company exercise program.

Theory of Planned Behavior (TPB)   The theory of reasoned action has proved to be most successful when dealing with purely volitional behaviors, but complications are encountered when the theory is applied to behaviors that are not fully under volitional control. A good example of this is a smoker who intends to quit but fails to do so. Even though intent is high, nonmotivational factors—such as lack of requisite opportunities, skills, and resources—could prevent success (Ajzen, 1988).

The *theory of planned behavior (TPB)* (see **Figure 7.2**) is an extension of the theory of reasoned action that addresses the problem of incomplete volitional control. The major difference between TPB and TRA is the addition of a third, conceptually independent determinant of intention. Like TRA, TPB includes attitude toward the behavior and subjective norm, but it has added the concept of perceived behavioral control. Perceived behavioral control is similar to the Social Cognitive Theory's concept of self-efficacy. **Perceived behavioral control** "refers to people's perceptions of their ability to perform a given behavior" (Ajzen, 2006). Stated differently, perceived behavioral control refers to the perceived ease or difficulty of performing the behavior and is assumed to reflect past experience as well as anticipated impediments and obstacles. As a general rule, the more favorable the attitude and subjective norm with respect to a behavior, and the greater the perceived behavioral control, the stronger should be the individual's intentions to perform the behavior under consideration (Ajzen, 1988).

Figure 7.2 illustrates two important features of this theory. First, perceived behavioral control has motivational implications for intentions. That is, without perceived control, intentions could be minimal even if attitudes toward the behavior and subjective norm were strong. Second, there may be a direct link between perceived behavioral control and behavior. Behavior depends not only on motivation but also on actual control. *Actual behavioral control* "refers to the extent to which a person has the skills, resources, and other prerequisites needed to perform a given behavior. Successful performance of

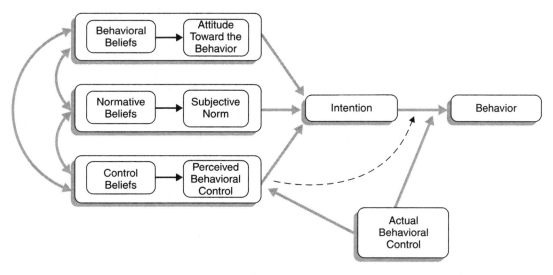

Figure 7.2 Theory of Planned Behavior Diagram

Source: Theory of Planned Behavior Diagram. Icek Ajzen. Copyright © 2006 by Icek Ajzen. Reprinted with permission.

the behavior depends not only on a favorable intention but also on a sufficient level of behavioral control. To the extent that perceived behavioral control is accurate, it can serve as a proxy of actual control and can be used for the prediction of behavior" (Ajzen, 2006). To use the example of smoking once again as a behavior not fully under volitional control, TPB predicts that individuals will give up smoking if they:

- Have a positive attitude toward quitting
- Think others whom they value believe it would be good for them to quit
- Perceive that they have control over whether they quit

Health Belief Model (HBM)   The *health belief model* (HBM), which is the one most frequently used in health behavior applications, is also a value-expectancy theory. "According to this class of theory, the tendency to perform a particular act is a function of the expectancy that the act will be followed by certain consequences (e.g., 'How vulnerable am I to the danger?') and the value of those consequences (e.g., 'How severe is the danger?')" (Prentice-Dunn & Rogers, 1986, p. 157). It was developed in the 1950s by a group of psychologists to help explain why people would or would not use health services (Rosenstock, 1966). The HBM is based on Lewin's decision-making model (Lewin, 1935, 1936; Lewin et al., 1944). Since its creation, the HBM has been used to help explain a variety of health behaviors (Becker, 1974; Janz & Becker, 1984).

The HBM hypothesizes that health-related action depends on the simultaneous occurrence of three classes of factors:

1. The existence of sufficient motivation (or health concern) to make health issues salient or relevant.

2. The belief that one is susceptible (vulnerable) to a serious health problem or to the sequelae of that illness or condition. This is often termed **perceived threat**.

3. The belief that following a particular health recommendation would be beneficial in reducing the perceived threat, and at a subjectively acceptable cost. Cost refers to the **perceived barriers** that must be overcome in order to follow the health recommendation; it includes, but is not restricted to, financial outlays (Rosenstock et al., 1988, p. 177). In fact, the lack of self-efficacy is also seen as a perceived barrier to taking a recommended health action (Strecher & Rosenstock, 1997).

Figure 7.3 provides a diagram of the HBM as presented by Becker, Drachman, and Kirscht (1974).

In recent years, self-efficacy has become a more meaningful concept in the perceived barriers construct of the HBM. When the HBM was first conceived, self-efficacy was not explicitly a part of it. "The original model was developed in the context of circumscribed

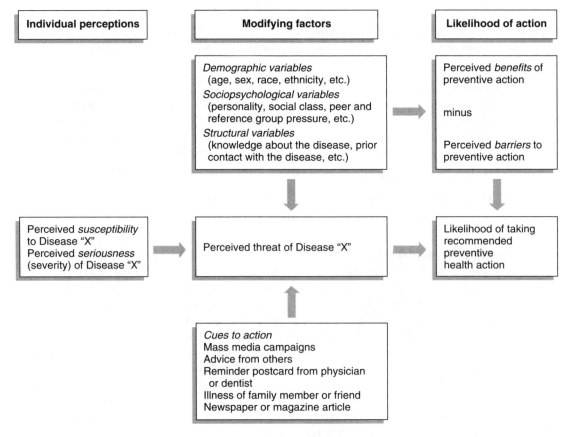

Figure 7.3 The HBM as a Predictor of Preventive Health Behavior

Source: "A New Approach to Explaining Sick-Role Behavior in Low Income Populations." M. H. Becker et al, from *American Journal of Public Health*, *Vol. 64*, No. 3, pp. 205–216. Copyright © 1974 by the American Public Health Association. Reprinted with permission.

preventive health actions (accepting a screening test or an immunization) that were not perceived to involve complex behaviors" (Champion & Skinner, 2008, p. 49). However, when program planners want to use the HBM to plan health promotion interventions for priority populations in need of lifestyle behaviors requiring long-term changes, self-efficacy must be included in the model. Therefore, "[f]or behavior change to succeed, people must (as the original HBM theorizes) feel threatened by their current behavioral patterns (perceived susceptibility and severity) and believe that change of a specific kind will result in a valued outcome at acceptable cost. They must also feel themselves competent (self-efficacious) to overcome perceived barriers to taking action" (Champion & Skinner, 2008, p. 50).

Here is an example of the HBM applied to exercise. Someone watching television sees an advertisement about exercise. This is a cue to action that starts her thinking about her own need to exercise. There may be some variables (demographic, sociopsychological, and structural) that cause her to think about it a bit more. She remembers her college health course that included information about heart disease and the importance of staying active. She knows she has a higher than normal risk for heart disease because of family history, poor diet, and slightly elevated blood pressure. Therefore, she comes to the conclusion that she is susceptible to heart disease (**perceived susceptibility**). She also knows that if she develops heart disease, it can be very serious (**perceived seriousness/severity**). Based on these factors, the individual thinks that there is reason to be concerned about heart disease (perceived threat). She knows that exercise can help delay the onset of heart disease and can increase the chances of surviving a heart attack if one should occur (**perceived benefits**). But exercise takes time from an already busy day, and it is not easy to exercise in the variety of settings in which she typically finds herself, especially during bad weather (perceived barriers). Her confidence in being able to exercise regularly will also be important. She must now weigh the threat of the disease against the difference between benefits and barriers. This decision will then result in a likelihood of exercising or not exercising (**likelihood of taking recommended preventive health action**).

Protection Motivation Theory (PMT) The *protection motivation theory* (PMT), a value-expectancy theory, was originally (Rogers, 1975) "proposed to provide explanations of the effects of fear appeals on health attitudes and behavior" (Floyd, Prentice-Dunn, & Rogers, 2000, p. 409). The PMT was later revised and extended (Rogers, R., 1983) to a more general theory of persuasive communication that included reward and self-efficacy components. The PMT has some similarities to the HBM. Both are premised on expectancy-value theory, both contain a cost-benefit analysis in which the individual weighs the costs of taking a precautionary action against the expected benefits of taking action, and both share an emphasis on cognitive processes mediating attitudinal and behavioral change (Floyd et al., 2000; Prentice-Dunn & Rogers, 1986).

As explained by the PMT, inputs come from environmental sources of information such as verbal persuasion and observational learning, and from intrapersonal sources such as one's personality and feedback from personal experiences associated with the targeted maladaptive and adaptive responses (Floyd et al., 2000) (see **Figure 7.4**). Based on these inputs people make a cognitive assessment of whether there is a threat to their health.

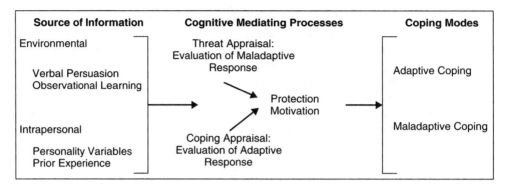

Figure 7.4 Overall Model of Protection Motivation Theory

Source: "A Meta-Analysis of Research on Protection Motivation Theory." Donna L. Floyd, Steven Prentice-Dunn, Ronald W. Rogers, from *Journal of Applied Social Psychology, Volume 30.* Copyright © 2000 by John Wiley & Sons, Inc. Reprinted with permission.

Information about a threat to one's health arouses two cognitive mediating processes: threat appraisal and coping appraisal (Floyd et al., 2000; McClendon & Prentice-Dunn, 2001) (see **Figure 7.5**).

The threat appraisal process is addressed first because a threat to one's health must be perceived or identified before there can be an assessment of the coping options (Floyd et al., 2000). Threat appraisal assesses maladaptive behaviors (e.g., physical inactivity, smoking, overeating, binge drinking). The assessment includes: (1) a review of intrinsic (e.g., physical and psychological pleasure such as feeling "good") and extrinsic (e.g., peer approval such as receiving attention) rewards; and (2) a review of the perceived severity of and the perceived vulnerability to the threat. "Rewards increase the probability of selecting the maladaptive response (not to protect self or others), whereas threat will

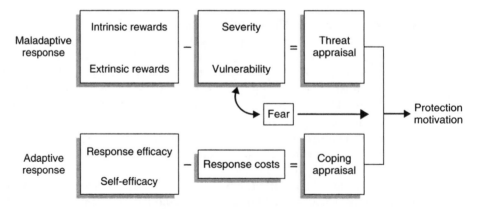

Figure 7.5 The Cognitive Mediating Processes of Protection Motivation Theory

Source: "Protection motivation theory." R. W. Rogers and S. Prentice-Dunn, from *Handbook of Health Behavior Research*, D. Gochman (Ed.). Copyright © 1997 by Plenum Press. Reproduced with permission.

decrease the probability of selecting the maladaptive response" (Floyd et al., 2000, p. 410). "Thus the rewards minus the sum of severity and vulnerability indicate the amount of threat experienced by the individual" (McClendon & Prentice-Dunn, 2001, p. 322).

Coping appraisal assesses adaptive behaviors (e.g., health enhancing behaviors). This type of assessment includes: (1) a review of response efficacy (e.g., belief that the coping action will avert the threat) and self-efficacy (i.e., belief that the person is capable of completing the coping action); and (2) a review of the response costs (e.g., "inconvenience, expense, unpleasantness, difficulty, complexity, side effects, disruption of daily life, and overcoming habit strength" [Rogers, 1984, p. 104]). "Response efficacy and self-efficacy will increase the probability of selecting the adaptive response, whereas response costs will decrease the probability of selecting the adaptive response" (Floyd et al., 2000, p. 411). In sum, the amount of coping appraisal experienced is indicated by the sum of response efficacy and self-efficacy minus the response costs" (McClendon & Prentice-Dunn, 2001, p. 322).

When the results of the threat appraisal and coping appraisal processes are combined it is the protective motivation that an individual possesses. Stated a bit differently, "The output of these appraisal-mediating processes is the decision (or intention) to initiate, continue, or inhibit the applicable adaptive responses (or coping modes)" (Floyd et al., 2000, p. 411). When using the PMT to design an intervention protection motivation has been measured using behavioral intentions (Floyd et al., 2000).

Prentice-Dunn and Rogers (1986, p. 156) offered the following summary of the PMT:

> PMT assumes that protection motivation is maximized when: (i) the threat to health is severe; (ii) the individual feels vulnerable; (iii) the adaptive response is believed to be an effective means for averting the threat; (iv) the person is confident in his or her abilities to complete successfully the adaptive response; (v) the rewards associated with the maladaptive behavior are small; and (vi) the costs associated with the adaptive response are small. Such factors produce protection motivation and, subsequently, the enactment of the adaptive, or coping, response.

Since its development, the *protection motivation theory* has been successfully used to create program interventions for a number of different health behaviors (Floyd et al., 2000). Some applications of the theory have included: breast self-examination (Fry & Prentice-Dunn, 2006), living wills (Allen, Phillips, Whitehead, Crowther, & Prentice-Dunn, 2009), sun protection behavior/skin cancer (McMath & Prentice-Dunn, 2005; Prentice-Dunn, McMath, & Cramer, 2009), and weight loss and bariatric surgery (Boeka, Prentice-Dunn, & Lokken, 2010).

Elaboration Likelihood Model of Persuasion (ELM) *The Elaboration Likelihood Model of Persuasion*, or the *Elaboration Likelihood Model* (ELM) for short, was initially developed to help explain inconsistencies in the results from research dealing with the study of attitudes (Petty, Barden, & Wheeler, 2009). Specifically, the model was designed to help explain how persuasion messages (communication) aimed at changing attitudes were received and processed by people. Though not created specifically for health communication, since its development the ELM has been used to help interpret and predict the impact of health messages (see **Figure 7.6**).

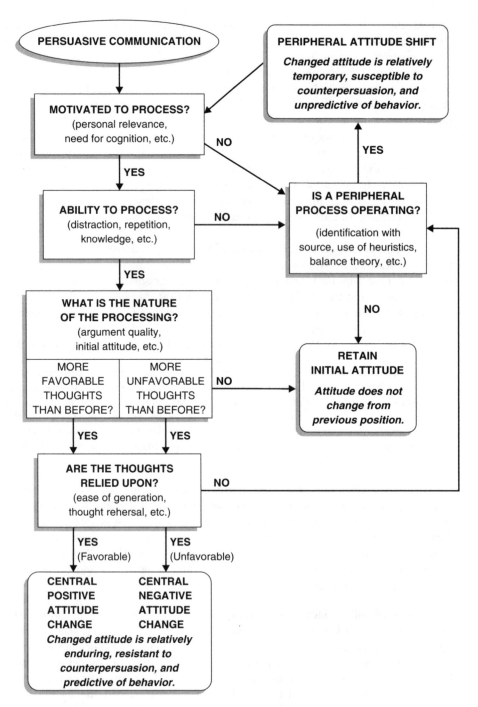

Figure 7.6 The Elaboration Likelihood Model of Persuasion (ELM)

Source: "The Elaboration Likelihood Model of Persuasion" by R. E. Petty, J. Barden, and G. R. Alexander, from *Emerging Theories in Health Promotion Practice and Research: Strategies for Improving Public Health, 2e,* Ed. J. R. DiClemente, R. A. Crosby, and M. C. Kegler. Copyright © 2009 by Jossey-Bass. Reprinted with permission.

The utility of the ELM is that it does three things. First, the ELM proposes that attitudes can be formed as a result of two different types of routes to persuasion—peripheral and central processing routes (Petty et al., 2009). The distinction between the two routes is the amount of elaboration. **Elaboration** refers to the amount of cognitive processing (i.e., thought) that a person puts into receiving messages. The peripheral route processes involve minimal thought and rely on superficial cues or mental shortcuts (called *heuristics*) about issue-relevant information as primary means for attitude change (Petty et al., 2009). For example, people may form an attitude after hearing a persuasive message simply because the person delivering the message is someone that they admire. On the other hand, central route processes involve thoughtful consideration (or effortful cognitive elaboration) of issue-relevant information and one's own cognitive responses as the primary bases for attitude change (Petty et al., 2009). "Two conditions are necessary for effortful processing to occur—the recipient of the message must be both *motivated* and *able* to think carefully" (Petty et al., 2009, p. 188). An example of central route processing would be a motorcyclist's formation of an attitude about wearing a helmet based on thoughtful consideration of a message about the pros and cons of helmet use along with recalling knowledge gained in a motorcycle safety class and possibly the results of a motorcycle crash in which his or her cousin was involved.

It should be clear that the distinction between the peripheral and central routes is the amount of consideration given to the issue-relevant information and how the information is processed, not the type of information itself (Petty, Wheeler, & Bizer, 1999). Yet not all messages fall neatly into either peripheral or central categories of processing. People really receive messages along an elaboration likelihood continuum. The continuum stretches from one end and is anchored with processes requiring no thinking, like classical conditioning (see discussion on stimulus response theory earlier in the chapter), to processes requiring some effortful thinking such as inferences based on one's experiences, to processes requiring careful consideration (Petty et al., 2009).

Second, when comparing the consequences of the two routes there are times when the result is similar. However, the two routes usually lead to attitudes with different consequences. "High effort central route processes are more likely to lead to attitudes that are persistent over time, resistant to counterattack, and influential in guiding thought and behavior than are peripheral process" (Petty et al., 2009, pp. 207–208).

Third, "the model specifies how variables have an impact on persuasion" (Petty et al., 2009, p. 197). The variable can have an influence on people's motivation to think or ability to think, as well as the valence of people's thought or the confidence in the thoughts generated (Petty et al., 2009). For example, variables that have an impact on how a message is processed are the source of the message (e.g., friend, expert), the message itself (e.g., funny, serious), the context (e.g., delivered person-to-person, on the Internet), and various characteristics of the recipient (e.g., intelligence, age, attentiveness).

The ELM has been used to develop a variety of interventions for health promotion programs. The one area where the ELM has been most useful in health promotion has been with message tailoring. *Tailored messages* are those that are "crafted for and delivered to each individual based on individual needs, interests, and circumstances" (NCI, 2002, p. 251). In other words, tailored messages are matched to the needs, interests, and circumstances of the intended recipient. It has been found that the more tailored the persuasive communication, the more relevant it is to the recipient, and the more likely the message will be processed through the central route. And, if a message is processed through the central route the more likely it will impact attitude and behavior change.

Information-Motivation-Behavioral (IMB) Skills Model   The *information-motivation-behavioral skills model* (IMB) (see **Figure 7.7**) was initially created to address the critical need for a strong theoretical basis for HIV/AIDS prevention efforts (Fisher & Fisher, 1992). There is empirical evidence to support that it has been useful in these efforts (Fisher, Fisher, & Shuper, 2009). Since its development, and because of it success in dealing with HIV/AIDS prevention behavior, it has been applied to a number of other risk-reduction behaviors (Fisher et al., 2009). According to the IMB model, the constructs of information, motivation, and behavioral skills are the fundamental determinants of preventive behavior. The information provided needs to be relevant, easily enacted based on the specific circumstances, and serve as a guide to personal preventive behavior. "In addition to facts that are easy to translate into behavior, the IMB model recognizes additional cognitive processes and content categories that significantly influence performance of preventive behavior" (Fisher et al., 2009, p. 27). Such as the simple decision rules a person may hold, like "if my best friend is willing to ride a motorcycle without a helmet, it must be okay."

Even though people are well informed about a particular health issue, they may not be motivated to act. According to the IMB model, prevention motivation includes both personal motivation to act (i.e., one's attitude toward a specific behavior) and social motivation to act (is there social support for the preventive behavior?) (Fisher et al., 2009). Both types of motivation are necessary for action to occur.

In addition to people being well informed and motivated to act, the IMB model also asserts that people must possess behavioral skills to engage in the preventive behavior. The behavioral skills component of the IMB model includes an individual's objective ability and his or her perceived self-efficacy to perform the preventive behavior.

In applying the IMB model, health education specialists cannot simply use their own judgment to determine what information to provide, how best to motivate, and what behavioral skills to teach to a given population. The process should begin by

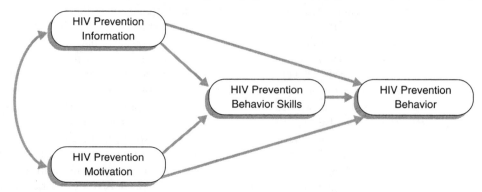

Figure 7.7 The Information-Motivation-Behavioral Skills Model of HIV Prevention

Source: "Changing AIDS-Risk Behavior." J. D. and W. A. Fisher from *Psychological Bulletin 111*(3). Copyright © 1992 by the American Psychological Association. Adapted with permission.

eliciting information from a subsample of the priority population to identify deficits in their health-relevant information, motivation, and behavior skills. Next health education specialists need to design and implement "*conceptually-based, empirically-targeted, population-specific*" (p. 29) interventions, constructed on the bases of the elicited findings (Fisher et al., 2009). Then, after the implementation of the intervention, health education specialists must evaluate the intervention to determine if it had significant and sustained effects on the information, motivation, and behavioral skill determinants of the preventive behavior and on the preventive behavior itself (Fisher et al., 2009).

The Transtheoretical Model (TTM) "The Transtheoretical Model is an integrative framework for understanding how individuals and populations progress toward adopting and maintaining health behavior change for optimal health. The Transtheoretical Model uses stages of change to integrate processes and principles of change from across major theories of intervention, hence the name 'Transtheoretical'" (Prochaska, Johnson, & Lee, 1998, p. 59). The model has its roots in psychotherapy and was developed by Prochaska (1979) after he completed a comparative analysis of 18 therapy systems and a critical review of 300 therapy outcome studies. From the analysis and review, Prochaska found that some common processes were involved in change.

As this model has evolved, researchers have applied it to many different types of health behavior change, including but not limited to alcohol and substance abuse, anxiety and panic disorders, delinquency, eating disorders and obesity, exercise, high-fat diets, HIV/AIDS prevention, mammography screening, medication compliance, unplanned pregnancy prevention, pregnancy and smoking, sedentary lifestyles, weight control, sun exposure, and physicians practicing preventive medicine (Prochaska, Redding, & Evers, 2008; Spencer, Adams, Malone, Roy, & Yost, 2006).

The core constructs of the *transtheoretical model* include the stages of change, the processes of change, the pros and cons of changing, self-efficacy, and temptation. (see **Table 7.3**). In addition, this model is "based on critical assumptions about the nature of behavior change and interventions that can best facilitate change" (Prochaska et al., 1998, p. 60). These constructs and assumptions will be discussed next.

Behavioral change does not occur overnight. A person does not go to bed at night as a nonexerciser and wake up the next morning as an exerciser. Behavior change occurs over time. Thus, the **stage** construct is an important part of the transtheoretical model because it represents the temporal dimension of change (Prochaska et al., 2008). The model suggests that "people move from *precontemplation,* not intending to change, to *contemplation,* intending to change within 6 months, to *preparation,* actively planning change, to *action,* overtly making changes, and into *maintenance,* taking steps to sustain change and resist temptation to relapse" (Prochaska, Redding, Harlow, Rossi, & Velicer, 1994). The **precontemplation stage** is defined as a time in which "people do not intend to take action in the near term, usually measured as the next six months. The outcome interval may vary, depending on behavior. People may be in this stage because they are uninformed or under-informed about the consequences of their behavior. Or they may have tried to change a number of times and become demoralized about their abilities to change" (Prochaska et al., 2008, p. 100). People in this stage "tend to avoid reading, talking, or thinking about their high-risk behaviors" (Prochaska et al., 1998).

Table 7.3   Transtheoretical Model Constructs

Constructs	Description
Stages of Change	
Precontemplation	No intention to take action within the next 6 months
Contemplation	Intends to take action within the next 6 months
Preparation	Intends to take action within the next 30 days and has taken some behavioral steps in this direction
Action	Has changed overt behavior for less than 6 months
Maintenance	Has changed overt behavior for more than 6 months
Decisional Balance	
Pros	The benefits of changing
Cons	The costs of changing
Self-Efficacy	
Confidence	Confidence that one can engage in the healthy behavior across different challenging situations
Temptation	Temptation to engage in the unhealthy behavior across different challenging situations
Processes of Change	
Consciousness Raising	Finding and learning new facts, ideas, and tips that support the healthy behavior change
Dramatic Relief	Experiencing the negative emotions (fear, anxiety, worry) that go with unhealthy behavioral risks
Self-Reevaluation	Realizing that the behavior change is an important part of one's identity as a person
Environmental Reevaluation	Realizing the negative impact of the unhealthy behavior, or the positive impact of the healthy behavior, on one's proximal social and/or physical environment
Self-Liberation	Making a firm commitment to change
Helping Relationships	Seeking and using social support for the healthy behavior change
Counterconditioning	Substitution of healthier alternative behaviors and/or cognitions for the unhealthy behavior
Reinforcement Management	Increasing the rewards for the positive behavior change and/or decreasing the rewards of the unhealthy behavior
Stimulus Control	Removing reminders or cues to engage in the unhealthy behavior and/or adding cues to reminders to engage in the healthy behavior
Social Liberation	Realizing that social norms are changing in the direction of supporting the healthy behavior change

Source: SPM Handbook for Health Assessment Tools. Colleen A. Redding, Joseph S. Rossi, S. R. Rossi, W. F. Velicer, and J. O. Prochaska. Copyright © 1999 by the Society of Prospective Medicine. Reprinted with permission from the authors.

The second stage, **contemplation** is the stage in which "people intend to change their behaviors in the next six months" (Prochaska et al., 2008, p. 100). It occurs when people are aware that a problem exists and are seriously thinking about a behavior change but have not yet made a commitment to take action. They are more open to feedback and information about the problem behavior than those in the precontemplation stage

(Redding et al., 1999). For example, most smokers know that smoking is bad for them and consider quitting, but are not quite ready to do so. The third stage is called **preparation** and combines intention and behavioral criteria. In this stage, "people intend to take action soon, usually measured as the next month. Typically, they have already taken some significant step toward the behavior in the past year. They have a plan of action, such as joining a health education class, consulting a counselor, talking to their physician, buying a self-help book, or relying on a self-change approach" (Prochaska et al., 2008, p. 100). "These are the people we should recruit for such action-oriented programs as smoking cessation, weight loss, or exercise" (Prochaska et al., 1998, p. 61).

People are in the fourth stage, the **action stage**, when they have made overt changes in their behavior, experiences, or environment in order to overcome their problems within the past six months. This stage of change reflects a consistent behavior pattern, is usually the most visible, and receives the greatest external recognition (Prochaska, DiClemente, & Norcross, 1992). Since the behavior change is very new in this stage and the chance of relapse is high, considerable attention still must be given to relapse prevention (Redding et al., 1999). Also, "not all modifications of behavior count as action in this model. People must attain a criterion that scientists and professionals agree is sufficient to reduce risks of disease" (Prochaska et al., 2008, p. 102). For example, in smoking, reduction in the number of cigarettes smoked does not count, only total abstinence (Prochaska et al., 1998). If those making changes continue with their new pattern of behavior, they will move into the fifth stage, maintenance.

Working to prevent relapse is the focus of the **maintenance stage**. People in this stage have made specific, overt modifications in then lifestyles for at least six months and are increasingly more confident that they can continue their changes (Prochaska et al., 2008; Prochaska et al., 1998; Redding et al., 1999). The person's change has become more of a habit and the chance of relapse is lower, but it still requires some attention (Redding et al., 1999).

The final stage is **termination**. This stage is defined as the time when individuals who have changed have zero temptation to return to their old behavior and they have 100% self-efficacy—that is, a lifetime of maintenance. No matter what their mood, they will not return to their old behavior (Prochaska et al., 2008). This is a stage that few people reach with certain behaviors (e.g., drinking for alcoholics). Since this may not be a practical goal for the majority of people, it has been given less attention in the research (Prochaska et al., 2008). **Figure 7.8** provides a summary of the stages of change.

The second major construct of the transtheoretical model is the **processes of change** (see Table 7.3 for an explanation of the 10 processes). "These are the covert and overt activities that people use to progress through the stages" (Prochaska et al., 2008, p. 101). Studies over the years have indicated that some of the processes are more useful at specific stages of change. The experimental set of processes (consciousness raising, dramatic relief, self-reevaluation, environmental reevaluation, and social liberation) are most often emphasized in earlier stages (precontemplation, contemplation, and preparation) to increase intention and motivation, whereas the behavioral set of processes (helping relationships, counterconditioning, reinforcement management, stimulus control, and self-liberation) are most often utilized in the later stages (preparation, action, maintenance) as observable behavior change efforts get underway and need to be maintained (Redding et al., 1999) (see **Table 7.4**).

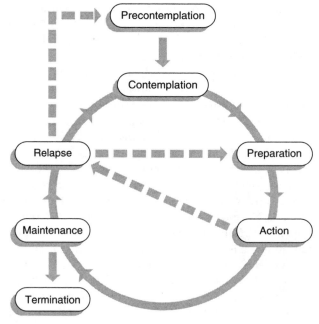

Figure 7.8 The Stages of Change

Source: "Models for Provider-Patient Interaction: Applications to Health Behavior Change." M. G. Goldstein from *The Handbook of Health Behavior Change*. Sally Shumaker (ed.). Copyright © 1998 by Sally Shumaker. Reprinted with permission.

The construct of **decisional balance** refers to the pros and cons of the behavioral change. That is, individuals' decisions to move from one stage to the next are based on the relative importance (pro), or the lack thereof (con), of the behavior change for the individuals. "Characteristically, the pros of healthy behavior are low in the early stages and increase across the stages of change, and the cons of the healthy behavior

Table 7.4 Processes of Change That Mediate Progression Between the Stages of Change

	Precontemplation	**Contemplation**	**Preparation**	**Action**	**Maintenance**
Processes	Consciousness raising				
	Dramatic relief				
	Environmental reevaluation				
		Self-reevaluation	Self-liberation		
				Counter conditioning	
				Helping relationships	
				Reinforcement management	
				Stimulus control	

Source: "The Transtheoretical Model and Stages of Change." J. O. Prochaska, C. A. Redding, K. E. Evers, in *Health Behavior and Health Education: Theory, Research, and Practice*. K. Glanz, B. K. Rimer, and K. Viswanath (eds.). Copyright © 2008 by Jossey-Bass. Reprinted with permission.

are high in the early stages and decrease across the stages of change" (Redding et al., 1999, p. 90).

The fourth construct of the *transtheoretical model* is **self-efficacy**. The developers of this model see self-efficacy as it was defined by Bandura (1977b), as people's confidence in their ability to perform a certain behavior or task. The final construct of the transtheoretical model is temptation. **Temptation** "reflects the converse of self-efficacy—the intensity of urges to engage in a specific behavior when in difficult situations. Typically, three factors reflect the most common types of temptations: negative affect or emotional distress, positive social situations, and craving" (Prochaska et al., 2008, p. 102). As one might guess, temptation decreases as one moves through the stages; however, even in the maintenance stage temptation is still present.

As noted at the beginning of this discussion, the *transtheoretical model* not only includes the five core constructs but it is also based on five critical assumptions (Prochaska et al., 2008):

1. No single theory can account for all the complexities of behavior change. A more comprehensive model will most likely emerge from an integration across major theories.

2. Behavior change is a process that unfolds over time through a sequence of stages.

3. Stages are both stable and open to change just as chronic behavioral risk factors are stable and open to change.

4. The majority of at-risk populations are not prepared for action and will not be served by traditional action-oriented behavior change programs.

5. Specific processes and principles of change should be emphasized at specific stages to maximize efficacy (p. 103).

Since its development, the *transtheoretical model* has been useful in several different ways. The first is that it makes program planners aware that not everyone is ready for change "right now," even though there is a program that can help them modify their behavior. People proceed through behavior change at different paces. Second, if individuals are not ready for action right now, then other programs can be developed to help them become ready for action. **Box 7.3** provides an example how to "stage" a person with a series of transtheoretical model type questions. With such information, planners can match a person's stage to a specific intervention, which in turn can increase the chances that the intervention will have an effect.

Precaution Adoption Process Model (PAPM) The *precaution adoption process model* (PAPM) is more recent than the *transtheoretical model* (TTM) (Weinstein, 1988; Weinstein & Sandman, 1992). Its goal "is to explain how a person comes to the decision to take action, and how he or she translates that decision into action" (Weinstein et al., 2008, p. 126). Though the TTM and PAPM are both stage models and appear similar, "it is mainly the names that have been given to the stages that are similar. The number of stages is not the same in the two theories, and those with similar names are defined quite differently" (Weinstein & Sandman, 2002a, p. 125). The PAPM is most applicable for use with the adoption of a new precaution, or the abandonment of a

> **Box 7.3** APPLICATION—AN EXAMPLE OF USING QUESTIONS BASED ON THE *TRANSTHEORETICAL MODEL* TO "STAGE" A PERSON
>
> **1.** Do you eat at least five servings of fruits and vegetables each day?
>
> Yes—Move to question #2
>
> No—Skip to question #3
>
> **2.** Have you been doing so for more than six months?
>
> Yes—Maintenance stage
>
> No—Action stage
>
> **3.** Do you intend to in the next 30 days?
>
> Yes—Preparation stage
>
> No—Move to question #4
>
> **4.** Do you intend to in the next six months?
>
> Yes—Contemplation stage
>
> No—Precontemplation stage

risky behavior that requires a deliberate action. It can also be used to explain why and how people make deliberate changes in habitual patterns. It is not applicable for actions that require the gradual development of habitual patterns of behavior such as exercise and diet (Weinstein et al., 2008).

The PAPM includes seven stages along the full path from ignorance to action (see **Figure 7.9**).

At some initial point in time, people are unaware of the health issue (Stage 1) [Unaware]. When they first learn something about the issue, they are no longer unaware, but they are not yet engaged by it either (Stage 2) [Unengaged]. People who reach the decision-making stage (Stage 3) [Deciding about acting] have become engaged by the issue and are considering their response. This decision-making process can result in one of three outcomes: they may suspend judgment, remaining in Stage 3 for the moment; they may decide to take no action, moving to Stage 4 [Decide not to act] and halting the precaution

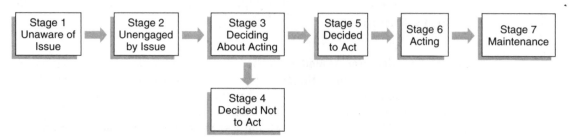

Figure 7.9 Stages of the Precaution Adoption Process Model

Source: Health Behavior and Health Education: Theory, Research, and Practice, by Karen Glanz, Barbara K. Rimer, and K. Viswanath. Copyright © 2008 by John Wiley & Sons, Inc. Reproduced with permission.

Box 7.4	APPLICATION—AN EXAMPLE OF USING A QUESTION BASED ON THE *PRECAUTION ADOPTION PROCESS MODEL* TO "STAGE" A PERSON

What are your intentions for receiving the new vaccine for shingles?
- I have already gotten it. (Stage 6)
- I have decided to get it. (Stage 5)
- I have thought about it and decided not to get it. (Stage 4)
- I am not sure. I am still trying to decide whether to get it or not. (Stage 3)
- I heard there was a vaccine, but I really haven't thought much about it. (Stage 2)
- I was not aware there was a vaccine for shingles. (Stage 1)

adoption process, at least for the time being; or they may decide to adopt the precaution, moving to Stage 5 [Decide to act]. For those who decide to adopt the precaution, the next step is to initiate the behavior (Stage 6) [Acting]. A seventh stage, if relevant, indicates that the behavior has been maintained over time (Stage 7) [Maintenance]. (Weinstein et al., 2008, p. 126; note: names of the stages were inserted by McKenzie, Neiger, & Thackeray.)

As with the TTM, the usefulness of this model is its ability to identify various stages of the behavior change process (see **Box 7.4**). Once it is known what stage the program participants are in, then the program planners can develop a stage-specific intervention to move the participants toward action. **Table 7.5** presents the important issues that need to be addressed to move participants from one stage to the next.

Table 7.5 Examples of Factors Likely to Determine Progress Between Stages

Stage Transition	Important Issues
Stage 1 to Stage 2	• Media messages about the hazard and precaution
Stage 2 to Stage 3	• Media messages about the hazard and precaution
	• Communication from significant other
	• Personal experience with hazard
Stage 3 to Stage 4 or Stage 5	• Beliefs about hazard likelihood and severity
	• Beliefs about personal susceptibility
	• Beliefs about precaution effectiveness and difficulty
	• Behaviors and recommendations of others
	• Perceived social norms
	• Fear and worry
Stage 5 to Stage 6	• Time, effort, and resources needed to act
	• Detailed "how-to" information
	• Reminders and other cues to action
	• Assistance in carrying out action

Source: Health Behavior and Health Education: Theory, Research, and Practice, by Karen Glanz, Barbara K. Rimer, and K. Viswanath. Copyright © 2008 by John Wiley & Sons, Inc. Reproduced with permission.

Interpersonal Level Theories

"At the interpersonal level, theories of health behavior assume individuals exist within, and are influenced by, a social environment. The opinions, thoughts, behavior, advice, and support of the people surrounding an individual influence his or her feelings and behavior, and the individual has a reciprocal effect on those people" (Rimer & Glanz, 2005, p. 19). Those individuals who have the greatest influence on others include spouse/partner, other family members, friends, peers (i.e., fellow students and coworkers), fellow members of social groups, health care providers, religious leaders, and others (Rimer & Glanz, 2005).

Though social relationships can have an impact on many different human behaviors, research has shown that they can be a powerful influence on health and health behaviors (Heaney & Israel, 2008). Therefore a number of theories have been created to explain concepts such as *social learning* (learning that occurs in a social context), *social power* (ability to influence others or resist activities of others), *social integration* (structure and quality of relationships), *social networks* ("web of social relationships that surround individuals") (Heaney & Israel, 2008, p. 190), *social support* ("aid and assistance exchanged through social relationships and interpersonal transactions") (Heaney & Israel, 2008, p. 191), *social capital* ("relationships between community members including trust, reciprocity, and civic engagement") (Minkler, Wallerstein, & Wilson, 2008, p. 294), and *interpersonal communication*. In the sections that follow, we present a detailed description of a well-established interpersonal theory—the social cognitive theory, and we present brief overviews of two newer theories—the social network theory and the social capital theory. These latter two theories may be theories in name only. Earlier in this chapter we made a distinction between theories and models. You may remember we said that there are some theories that have the term "model" in their title because that is the way they were initially identified and now that there is empirical evidence to call them theories the "model title" has remained because that is what we have gotten used to calling them. Well we believe that the social network and the social capital theories may have been prematurely called theories and are probably more in the model stage. But again as Goodson (2010) stated, ". . . it seems to matter little to us whether we deal with theories or with models; it seems to matter even less what labels we attach to them" (p. 228). Therefore, the important point of presenting the social network and social capital theories (or models) is to make you aware of the important concepts contained in each.

Social Cognitive Theory (SCT)   The social learning theories (SLT) of Rotter (1954) and Bandura (1977b)—or, as Bandura (1986) relabeled them, the *social cognitive theory (SCT)*—combine SR theory and cognitive theories. Stimulus response theorists emphasize the role of reinforcement in shaping behavior and believe that no "thinking" or "reasoning" is needed to explain behavior. However, Bandura (2001) stated, "If actions were performed only on behalf of anticipated external rewards and punishments, people would behave like weather vanes, constantly shifting directions to conform to whatever influence happened to impinge upon them at the moment" (p. 7). Cognitive theorists believe that reinforcement is an integral part of learning, but emphasize the role of subjective hypotheses or expectations held by the individual (Rosenstock et al., 1988). In other words, reinforcement contributes to learning, but reinforcement along with an individual's expectations of the consequences of behavior determine the behavior. "Behavior, in this perspective, is a function of the subjective value of an outcome and the subjective probability (or 'expectation') that a particular action will achieve that outcome. Such formulations are generally termed 'value-expectancy' theories" (Rosenstock et al., 1988, p. 176). In brief, SCT explains human functioning in terms of triadic reciprocal causation (Bandura, 1986). "In this model of reciprocal causality, internal personal factors in the form of cognitive, affective, and biological events, behavioral patterns, and environmental influences all operate as interacting determinants that influence one another bidirectionally" (Bandura, 2001, pp. 14–15). The constructs of the SCT that have been most often used in designing health promotion interventions will be presented here.

As already noted, reinforcement is an important component of SCT. According to SCT, reinforcement can be accomplished in one of three ways: directly, vicariously, or through self-reinforcement (Baranowski, Perry, & Parcel, 2002). An example of **direct reinforcement** is a group facilitator who provides verbal feedback to participants for a job well done. **Vicarious reinforcement** is having the participants observe someone else being reinforced for behaving in an appropriate manner. This has been referred to as *observational learning* (Baranowski et al., 2002) or *social modeling*. In a system of reinforcement by **self-reinforcement**, the participants would keep records of their own behavior, and when the behavior was performed in an appropriate manner, they would reinforce or reward themselves.

If individuals are to perform specific behaviors, they must know first what the behaviors are and then how to perform them. This is referred to as **behavioral capability**. For example, if people are to exercise aerobically, first they must know that aerobic exercise exists, and second they need to know how to do it properly. Many people begin exercise programs, only to quit within the first six months (Dishman, Sallis, & Orenstein, 1985), and some of those people quit because they do not know how to exercise properly. They know they should exercise, so they decide to run a few miles, have sore muscles the next day, and quit. Skill mastery is very important. The construct of **expectations** refers to the ability of human beings to think, and thus to anticipate certain things to happen in certain situations. For example, if people are enrolled in a weight loss program and follow the directions of the group facilitator, they will expect to lose weight. **Expectancies**, not to be confused with expectations, are the values that individuals place on an expected outcome. "Expectancies influence behavior according to the hedonic principle: if all other things are equal, a person will choose to perform an activity that maximizes a positive outcome or minimizes a negative outcome" (Baranowski et al., 2002, p. 173). Someone who enjoys the feeling of not smoking more than that of smoking is more likely to try to do the things necessary to stop. The construct of **self-control** or **self-regulation** states that individuals may gain control of their own behavior through monitoring and adjusting it (Clark et al., 1992). When helping individuals to change their behavior, it is a common practice to have them monitor their behavior over a period of time, through 24-hour diet or smoking records or exercise diaries, and then to have them reward (reinforce) themselves based on their monitored performance.

One construct of SCT that has received special attention in health promotion programs is self-efficacy (Strecher et al., 1986), which refers to the internal state that individuals experience as "competence" to perform certain desired tasks or behavior, "including confidence in overcoming the barriers to performing that behavior" (Baranowski et al., 2002, p. 173). "Unless people believe they can produce desired results and forestall detrimental ones by their actions, they have little incentive to act or to persevere in the face of difficulties" (Bandura, 2001, p. 10). Self-efficacy is situation specific; that is, individuals may be self-efficacious when it comes to aerobic exercise but not so when faced with reducing the amount of fat in their diet. People's competency feelings have been referred to as **efficacy expectations**. Thus, people who think they can exercise on a regular basis no matter what the circumstances have efficacy expectations. Even though people have efficacy expectations, they still may not want to engage in a behavior because they may not think the outcomes of that behavior would be beneficial to them. Stated another way, they may not feel that the reward (reinforcement) of performing the behavior is great enough for them. These beliefs are called **outcome expectations**. For example, in order for individuals to quit smoking for health reasons (behavior), they must believe both that they are capable of quitting (efficacy expectation) and that cessation will benefit their health (outcome expectation) (I. M. Rosenstock, personal communication, April 1986).

Individuals become self-efficacious in four main ways:

1. Through performance attainments (personal mastery of a task)

2. Through vicarious experience (observing the performance of others)

3. As a result of verbal persuasion (receiving suggestions from others)

4. Through emotional arousal (interpreting one's emotional state)

The construct of **emotional–coping response** states that for people to learn, they must be able to deal with the sources of anxiety that may surround a behavior. For example, fear is an emotion that can be involved in learning; according to this construct, participants would have to deal with the fear before they could learn the behavior.

The construct of **reciprocal determinism** states, unlike SR theory, that there is an interaction among the person, the behavior, and the environment, and that the person can shape the environment as well as the environment shape the person. All these relationships are dynamic. Glanz and Rimer (1995) provide a good example of this construct:

> A man with high cholesterol might have a hard time following his prescribed low-fat diet because his company cafeteria doesn't offer low-fat food choices that he likes. He can try to change the environment by talking with the cafeteria manager or the company medical or health department staff, and asking that healthy food choices be added to the menu. Or, if employees start to dine elsewhere in order to eat low-fat lunches, the cafeteria may change its menu to maintain its lunch business. (p. 15)

Finally, there is one other construct that grew out of the social learning theory of Rotter (1954) that needs to be mentioned because of its association with health behavior. "Rotter posited that a person's history of positive or negative reinforcement across a variety of situations shapes a belief as to whether or not a person's own actions lead to those reinforcements" (Wallston, 1994, p. 187). Rotter referred to this construct as **locus of control**. He felt that people with internal locus of control perceived that reinforcement was under their control, whereas those with external locus of control perceived rein-forcement to be under the control of some external force. In the 1970s, Wallston and his colleagues at Vanderbilt University began testing the usefulness of this construct in predicting health behavior (Wallston, 1994). They explored the concept of whether indi-viduals with internal locus of control were more likely to participate in health-enhancing behavior than those with external locus of control. They began their work by examining locus of control as a two-dimensional construct (internal versus external), then moved to a multidimensional construct when they split the external dimension into "powerful others" and "chance" (Wallston, Wallston, & DeVellis, 1978). After a number of years of work by many different researchers, Wallston has come to the conclusion that locus of control accounts for only a small amount of the variability in health behavior (Wallston, 1992). The internal locus of control belief about one's own health status is a necessary but not sufficient determinate of health-enhancing behavior (Wallston, 1994). Since the rise of the construct of self-efficacy, Wallston (1994) feels that self-efficacy is a better pre-dictor of health-promoting behavior than locus of control. This is not to say that locus of control is not a useful construct in developing health promotion programs. Knowing the locus of control orientation of those in the priority population can provide planners with valuable information when considering social support as part of a planned intervention. **Table 7.6** provides a summary of the constructs of the SCT and an example of how each construct might be operationalized.

Social Network Theory (SNT)   The term **social network** ("web of social relationships that surround people") (Heaney & Israel, 2008, p. 190) arose in the 1950s from the work of a sociologist who studied Norwegian villages. Barnes (1954) created the term to describe social relationships and characteristics of the villagers that could not be de-scribed through traditional social units such as families (Edberg, 2007; Heaney & Israel, 2009). Since that time, the concept has continued to be used and studied by sociolo-gists and professionals in various other disciplines including health education/health promotion. To support the work of health education specialists there is now evidence from social epidemiological observational studies that have clearly documented the beneficial effects of supportive networks on health status (Heaney & Israel, 2008). But is there enough evidence to suggest there is such a thing as a *social network the-ory* (SNT)? Heaney and Israel (2008) feel that the social network, and the closely related concept of social support, "do not connote theories per se. Rather, they are concepts that describe the structure, processes, and functions of social relationships" (p. 193). They feel that intervention studies are "needed to identify the most potent causal agents and critical time periods for social network enhancement" (p. 197). For example, it is not known how much social networking is enough to enhance health or how much is too much. It is also not known what are the characteristics of "good networks" that result in positive health behavior (e.g., regular exercise) versus "bad networks" that lead to negative health behavior (e.g., smoking). But what is known is that people who are part of social networks are as a whole healthier than those who are not involved in networks.

Table 7.6   Often-used Constructs of the Social Cognitive Theory and Examples
of Their Application

Construct	Definition	Example
Behavioral capability	Knowledge and skills necessary to perform a bahavior.	If people are going to exercise aerobically, they need to know what it is and how to do it.
Expectations	Beliefs about the likely outcomes of certain bahaviors.	If people enroll in a weight-loss program, they expect to lose weight.
Expectancies	Values people place on expected outcomes.	How important is it to people that they become physically fit?
Locus of control	Perception of the center of control over reinforcement.	Those who feel they have control over reinforcement are said to have internal locus of control.
		Those who perceive reinforcement under the control of an external force are said to have external locus of control.
Reciprocal determinism	"Environmental factors influence individuals and groups, but individuals and groups can also influence their environments and regulate their own behavior" (McAlister, Perry, & Parcel, 2008, p. 171).	Lack of use of vending machines could be result of the choices within the machine. Notes about the selections from the nonusing consumers to the machine's owners could change the selections and change the selections and change the behavior of the nonusing consumers to that of users.
Reinforcement (directly, vicariously, self-management)	Responses to behaviors that increase the chances of recurrence.	Giving verbal encouragement to those who have acted in a healthy manner.
Self-control, or **self regulation**	Gaining control over one's own behavior through monitoring and adjusting it.	If clients want to change their eating habits, have them monitor their current habits for seven days.
Self-efficacy	People's confidence in their ability to perform a certain desired task or function	If people are going to engage in a regular exercise program, they must feel they can do it.
Collective efficacy	Beliefs about the ability of the group to perform concerted actions that bring desired outcomes (McAlister et al., 2008, p. 171).	If a group of people is going to work to change a community's culture toward healthy behavior, they must feel that they can do it.
Emotional-coping response	For people to learn, they must be able to deal with the sources of anxiety that surround a behavior.	Fear is an emotion that can be involved in learning, and people would have to deal with it before they could learn a behavior.

Source: Principles and Foundations of Health Promotion and Education. Randall R. Cottrell, James T. Girvan, and James F. McKenzie. Copyright © 2012 by Pearson Education. Reprinted with permission.

One person who has written about SNT is Edberg (2007). He has described different types of social networks (e.g., ego-centered networks and full relational networks) (see **Figure 7.10**) and indicated that the key components to social network theory are the relationships between and among individuals and how the nature of those relationships influences beliefs and behaviors. He further states that those who use the SNT need

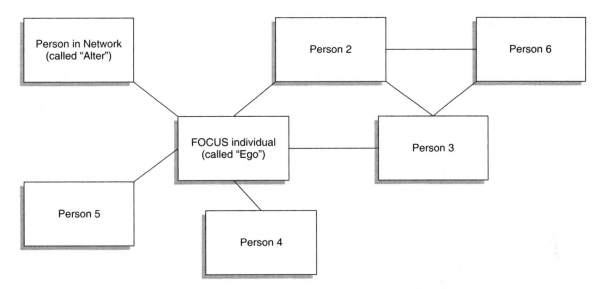

Figure 7.10 A Simple Sociogram, Centered on a "Focus Individual" or "Ego."

Source: Essentials of Health Behavior: Social and Behavioral Theory in Public Health. M Edberg. Copyright © 2007 by Jones & Bartlett Learning. Reprinted with permission.

to consider the items on the following list when assessing the role of a network on the health behavior of individuals who are part of the network (Edberg, 2007):

- Centrality versus marginality of individuals in the network—how much involvement does the person have in the network?

- Reciprocity of relationships—are relationships one-way or two-way?

- Complexity or intensity of relationships in the network—are the relationships between two people or are they multiplexed?

- Homogeneity or diversity of people in the network—do all members of the network have similar characteristics or are they different?

- Subgroups, cliques, and linkages—are there concentrations of interactions among some members and do they interact or are they isolated from others?

- Communication patterns in the network—how does information pass between the members in the network?

In summary, we know that social networks can impact health, but the specifics of who is most impacted and how best to set up and use social networks are unknown. Nevertheless, because of the impact of social networks, health education specialists planning interventions need to consider if social networks should be a part of the strategy they use to bring about change. And finally, with the power of the Internet and social networking, the impact of social networks in the work of health education specialists will to continue to grow.

Social Capital Theory   The often-quoted definition of **social capital** is "the relationships and structures within a community, such as civic participation, networks, norms of reciprocity, and trust, that promote cooperation of mutual benefit" (Putnam, 1995, p. 66). "Social capital is a collective asset, a feature of communities rather than the property of individuals. As such, individuals both contribute to it and use it, but they cannot own it" (Warren, Thompson, & Saegert, 2001, p. 1). The term got its start in political science and has been used in the health education/promotion field since the mid-1990s. The influence of social capital is well documented (Crosby et al., 2009). There are epidemiological studies that show that greater social capital is linked to several different positive outcomes (i.e., reduced mortality). There are also correlational studies that show that lack of social capital is related to poorer health outcomes (e.g., Kawachi, Kennedy, Lochner, & Prothrow, 1997). But as with social networks, a cause-effect relationship has not been established between social capital and better health. "Social capital does not provide theories of change, tools, or time lines for change; nor does it necessarily guarantee improved outcomes if social capital is improved" (Minkler & Wallerstein, 2005, p. 38), but it does seem to have an impact on health.

Figure 7.11 provides a graphic representation of the social capital. This particular figure includes the key concepts of Putman's (1995) definition of social capital and three different types of network resources—bonding, bridging, and linking social capital. These three types are differentiated based on the strength of the relationships between/among those people in the social network (Hayden, 2009). Originally, *bonding social capital* (sometimes referred to as exclusive social capital) was defined as "the type that brings closer

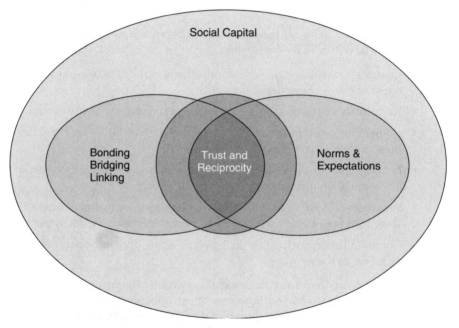

Figure 7.11 Social Capital

Source: Introduction to Health Behavior Theory. J. Hayden. Copyright © 2009 by Jones & Bartlett Learning. Reprinted with permission.

together people who already know each other" (Gittell & Vidal, 1998, p.15), but since then it has been expanded to encompass people who are similar or people who are members of the same group. Bonding social capital would come from those who are members in a service organization (e.g., Lions, Elks, American Legion) or religious community, for example. *Bridging social capital* (sometimes referred to as inclusive social capital), was originally defined as "the type that brings together people or groups who previously did not know each other" (Gittell & Vidal, 1998, p. 15), though now bridging social capital is seen more as the resources that people obtain from their interaction with people from outside their group, oftentimes from people with different demographic characteristics. An example would be people from different parts of a community working to create a community park.

The most recently recognized, and weakest, network resource is *linking social capital* (Hayden, 2009). In this type of network resource social capital comes from relationships between/among "individuals and groups in different social strata in a hierarchy where power, social status, and wealth are accessed by different groups" (UK Office of National Statistics, 2001, p. 11). An example would be when a boss and an employee work together on a project.

Again, as with social networks it is important that health education specialists be aware of the concept of social capital when planning interventions. It is not an intervention in itself, but it is a concept that needs to be considered and monitored.

Community Level Theories

As noted earlier in this chapter, the community level theories include any theory that would apply to the last three levels of the ecological perspective—institutional, community, or public policy. Community level theories "explore how social systems function and change and how to mobilize community members and organizations. They offer strategies that work in a variety of settings such as health care institutions, schools, worksites, community groups, and government agencies" (Rimer & Glanz, 2005, p. 22). Like the other levels already discussed in this chapter, a number of different community-level theories are available for health planners. Several community level theories involve community organizing and developing (see Chapter 9). The following section presents a discussion of a stage model for communities—the community readiness model.

Community Readiness Model (CRM) The community readiness model is a stage theory for communities. The concept of community readiness got its start back in the early 1990s, growing out of the need to understand the problems associated with developing and maintaining community programs. (See Edwards, Jumper-Thurman, Plested, Oetting, & Swanson, 2000, for a description of the origin of the CRM.) What was evident from the beginning is that few communities were alike. They may have had similar problems, but the dynamics in each community did not mean that the starting point for dealing with the problem could be the same. "Communities are fluid—always changing, adapting, growing" (Edwards et al., 2000, p. 291), and like individuals, communities are in various stages of readiness for change. Yet, the stages of change for communities are not the same as for individuals. "The stages of readiness in a community have to deal with group processes and group organization, characteristics that are not relevant to personal readiness" (Edwards et al., 2000, p. 296–297).

Though the model was developed initially to deal with alcohol and drug abuse, it has been useful in helping with a variety of health and nutrition topics (e.g., AIDS awareness, elimination of heart disease, depression awareness, reduction of sexually transmitted diseases), environmentally centered programs (e.g., air quality and recycling), and social programs (e.g., intimate partner violence programs) (Edwards et al., 2000).

The community readiness model defines nine stages:

1. *No Awareness.* The problem is not generally recognized by the community or leaders.

2. *Denial.* There is little or no recognition in the community that there is a problem; if so, the feeling is nothing can be done about it.

3. *Vague Awareness.* Feeling among some in the community there is a problem and something should be done, but no motivation or leadership to do so.

4. *Preplanning.* The clear recognition by some that there is a problem and something should be done. There are leaders, but no focused or detailed planning.

5. *Preparation.* There is planning going on but it is not based on collected data. There is leadership, resources are being sought, and there is modest support for efforts.

6. *Initiation.* Information is available to justify and begin efforts. Staff is in, or has just completed, training. Leaders are enthusiastic and there is usually little resistance and involvement from the community members.

7. *Stabilization.* Program is running, staffed, and supported by community and decision makers. Program is perceived as stable with no need for change. May include routine tracking, but no in-depth evaluation.

8. *Confirmation/Expansion.* Standard efforts are in place and supported by the community and decision makers. Program has been evaluated and modified, and efforts are in place to seek resources for new efforts. Data are collected on an ongoing basis to link risk factors and problems.

Table 7.7   Community Readiness Stages and Goals

Stage	Goal
1. *No Awareness*	Raise awareness of the issue
2. *Denial*	Raise awareness that the problem or issue exists in the community
3. *Vague Awareness*	Raise awareness that the community can do something
4. *Preplanning*	Raise awareness with the concrete ideas to combat condition
5. *Preparation*	Gather existing information to help plan strategies
6. *Initiation*	Provide community-specific information
7. *Stabilization*	Stabilize efforts/programs
8. *Confirmation/Expansion*	Expand and enhance service
9. *Professionalism*	Maintain momentum and continue growth

Source: "Community readiness: Research to practice." Ruth W. Edwards, Pamela Jumper-Thurman, Barbara A. Plested, Eugene R. Oetting, Louis Swanson, in *Journal of Community Psychology* 28(3). Copyright © 2000 by John Wiley & Sons, Inc. Reprinted with permission.

9. *Professionalism.* Much is known about prevalence, risk factors, and cause of problems. Highly trained staff runs effective programs, aimed at general population and appropriate subgroups. Programs have been evaluated and modified. Community is supportive but should hold programs accountable (Edwards et al., 2000).

A community's readiness can be assessed through interviews with key informants. Once the stage of readiness is known, like the other stage theories, there are suggested processes for moving a community from one stage to the next. **Table 7.7** presents the nine stages and the goal for each stage.

Cognitive-Behavioral Model of the Relapse Process

For most people, relapse is a part of change. **Relapse** "refers to the breakdown or failure in a person's attempt to change or modify a particular habit pattern, such as stopping 'bad habits' or developing new, optimal health behaviors" (Marlatt & George, 1998, p. 33). Marlatt and George (1998) differentiate between relapse (an indication of total failure) and a **lapse** (a single slip or mistake). The first drink or cigarette following a period of abstinence would be considered a lapse. It has been said that getting people to change behavior is hard, but having them maintain the behavior is much harder. This is nicely illustrated by the old saying, "Giving up smoking is easy; I've done it a hundred times." At one time, it was enough for program planners just to get people to change their behavior; now they need to do more. Because of the difficulty of maintaining a new behavior, program planners need to give special attention to helping those in the priority population avoid slipping back to their previous behaviors.

Although much of the early research dealing with this concept of slipping back was conducted using addictive behaviors, such as substance abuse and gambling, the concept applies to all behavior change, including preventive health behaviors. Marlatt (1982) indicates that a high percentage of individuals who enter programs for health behavior change relapse to their former behaviors within one year. More specifically, researchers have warned program planners of **recidivism** problems with participants in exercise (Dishman, Sallis, & Orenstein, 1985; Horne, 1975; Simkin & Gross, 1994), oral health care treatment (McCaul et al., 1990), weight loss (Stunkard & Braunwell, 1980), and smoking cessation (Leventhal & Cleary, 1980) programs. Therefore, planners need to make sure that program interventions include the skills necessary for dealing with those difficult times during behavior change.

Marlatt (1982) refers to the process of trying to prevent slipping back as relapse prevention. Relapse prevention, which is based on the social cognitive theory, combines behavioral skill-training procedures, cognitive therapy, and lifestyle rebalancing (Marlatt & George, 1998). **Relapse prevention (RP)** is "a self-control program designed to help individuals to anticipate and cope with the problem of relapse in the habit-changing process" (Marlatt & George, 1998, p. 33). Relapse is triggered by *high-risk situations.* "A high-risk situation is defined broadly as any situation (including emotional reactions to the situation) that poses a threat to the individual's sense of control and increases the risk of potential relapse" (Marlatt & George, 1998, p. 38). Cummings, Gordon, and Marlatt (1980), in a study of clients with a variety of problem behaviors (e.g., drinking, smoking,

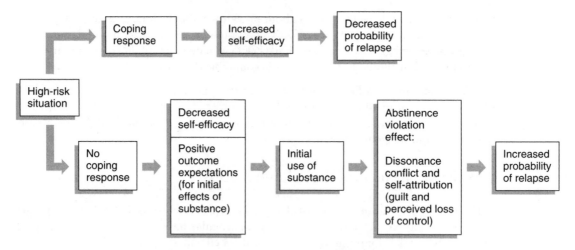

Figure 7.12 Cognitive-Behavioral Model of the Relapse Process

Source: Relapse Prevention: Maintenance Strategies in the Treatment of Addictive Behaviors. G. Alan Marlatt and J. R. Gordon. Copyright © 1985 by Guilford Publications, Inc. Reprinted with permission.

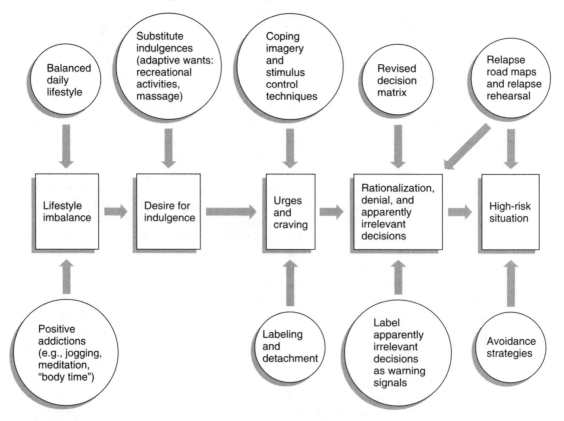

Figure 7.13 Relapse Prevention: Global Self-Control Strategies

Source: Relapse Prevention: Maintenance Strategies in the Treatment of Addictive Behaviors. G. Alan Marlatt and J. R. Gordon. Copyright © 1985 by Guilford Publications, Inc. Reprinted with permission.

heroin addiction, gambling, and overeating), found high-risk situations tend to fall into two major categories: intrapersonal and interpersonal determinants. They found that 56% of the relapse situations were caused by intrapersonal determinants, such as negative emotional states (35%), negative physical states (3%), positive emotional states (4%), testing personal control (5%), and urges and temptations (9%). The 44% of the situations represented by interpersonal determinants included interpersonal conflicts (16%), social pressure (20%), and positive emotional states (8%). These determinants can be referred to as the *covert antecedents* of relapse. That is to say, these high-risk situations do not just happen; instead, they are created by what Marlatt (1982) calls *lifestyle imbalances.*

People who have the coping skills to deal with a high-risk situation have a much greater chance of preventing relapse than those who do not. **Figure 7.12** illustrates the possible paths one may take in a high-risk situation (Marlatt, 1982).

Marlatt has developed both global (see **Figure 7.13**) and specific (see **Figure 7.14**) self-control strategies for relapse intervention. Specific intervention procedures are designed

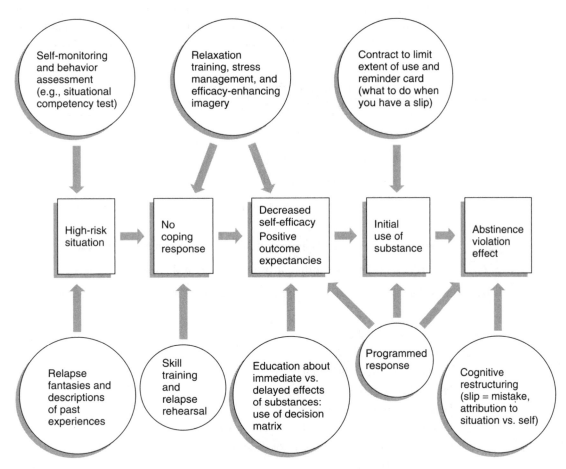

Figure 7.14 Relapse Prevention: Specific Intervention Strategies

Source: Relapse Prevention: Maintenance Strategies in the Treatment of Addictive Behaviors. G. Alan Marlatt and J. R. Gordon. Copyright © 1985 by Guilford Publications, Inc. Reprinted with permission.

to help participants anticipate and cope with the relapse episode itself, whereas the global intervention procedures are designed to modify the early antecedents of relapse, including restructuring of the participant's general style of life. A complete application of the relapse prevention model would include both specific and global interventions (Marlatt, 1982).

SUMMARY

Many theories are available to program planners, and it is important to remember that no one theory is best. This chapter presented an overview of the theories that are most often used in health promotion programs. These theories are important for planners because they provide information about why people are, or are not, engaging in health-enhancing behaviors; how to create interventions; and what factors to look for when evaluating a program. Theories can be categorized in a number of ways. This chapter presents two categories. The first categorizes theories by the level of influence at which it is most effective; the second classifies theories as either the continuum or stage theories. **Table 7.8** summarizes the theories presented in the chapter and the major components of each.

REVIEW QUESTIONS

1. Define *theory,* using your own words.

2. How is a theory different from a model?

3. How do concepts, constructs, and variables relate to theories?

4. Why is it important to use theories when planning and evaluating health promotion programs?

5. How can the socio-ecological approach be used to select a theory for use?

6. What makes stage theories different from continuum theories?

7. What is the underlying concept for each of the following continuum theories?
   a. Stimulus response theory
   b. Social cognitive theory
   c. Theory of reasoned action
   d. Theory of planned behavior
   e. Health belief model
   f. Protection motivation theory
   g. Elaboration likelihood model of persuasion
   h. Information-motivation-behavioral skills model
   i. Social network theory
   j. Social capital theory

Table 7.8   Major Components of the Theories That Underlie Health Promotion Interventions

Stimulus Response Theory	Social Cognitive Theory	Theory of Reasoned Action	Theory of Planned Behavior	Protection Motivation Theory	Motivation-Behavioral Skills Model Information
Operant behavior	Reinforcement 1. Direct 2. Vicarious 3. Self-management	Attitude toward behavior	Attitude toward behavior	Maladaptive response Intrinsic rewards Extrinsic rewards Perceived severity Perceived vulnerability	Information
Consequences	Behavioral capability	Subjective norm	Subjective norm	Adaptive response Response efficacy Self-efficacy Costs	Motivation
Positive reinforcement	Expectations	Intentions	Behavior	Protective motivation	Behavior skills
Negative reinforcement	Expectancies	Behavior	Intentions		
Positive punishment	Self-control		Perceived behavioral control		
Negative punishment	Self-efficacy				
	Emotional-coping response				
	Reciprocal determinism				

Health Belief Model	Transtheoretical Model	Cognitive-Behavior Model of the Relapse Process	Elaboration Likelihood Model of Persuasion	Precaution Adoption Process Model	Community Readiness Model
Perceived susceptibility	Stages of change	High-risk situation	Central route	Stages	Key informant interviews
Perceived seriousness	Decisional balance	Global self-control strategies	Peripheral route	Factors	Stages and goals
Perceived benefits	Processes of change	Specific intervention strategies	Elaboration likelihood continuum		Strategies
Perceived barriers	Self-efficacy		Variables		
Motivation (cues to action)	Temptation				
Self-efficacy					

8. What are the major components of the following stage theories?

    a. Transtheoretical model
    b. Precaution adoption process model
    c. Community readiness model

9. What is the major difference between the transtheoretical model and the precaution adoption process model?

10. How is the community readiness model different from the other stage models?

11. How can program planners help to prepare those in the priority population for relapse prevention?

ACTIVITIES

1. Assume that you have identified a need (health problem) for a given priority population. In a two-page paper:

    a. State who the priority population is and what the need is.
    b. Select a theory to use as a guide in developing an intervention to address the problem.
    c. Explain why you chose the theory that you did.
    d. Defend why you think this is the best theory to use.
    e. Show how the problem "fits into" the theory.

2. In a two-page paper, identify a theory that you plan to use in developing the intervention for the program you are planning. Explain why you chose the theory, and why you think it is a good fit for the problem you are addressing.

3. Write a paragraph on each of the following:

    a. Using the stimulus response theory, explain why a person might smoke.
    b. Using the social cognitive theory (SCT), explain how you could help people change their diets.
    c. Explain how the SCT construct of behavioral capability applies to managing stress.
    d. Explain the differences between, and the relationship of, the SCT constructs of expectations and expectancies.
    e. Explain what would have to take place for individuals to be self-efficacious with regard to taking their insulin.
    f. Use the information-motivation-behavioral skills model to explain how to encourage a person to eat a healthy diet.
    g. Use the theory of planned behavior to explain how a smoker stops smoking.
    h. Use protection motivation theory to explain how you could create a public service announcement to encourage people to exercise.
    i. Apply the health belief model to getting a person to take a flu shot.
    j. Apply the transtheoretical model to get a person to change any health behavior.

    k. Using the precaution adoption process model, explain how a person decides to get screened for blood cholesterol.

    l. Explain how a social network could be used to encourage people to adopt a healthy behavior.

    m. Explain how the community readiness model could be used by planners who are interested in getting a citywide smoking ordinance passed.

    n. Explain how you might increase the social capital of a community.

4. Your supervisor at the local health department has asked you to create a new program to encourage people in your county to get the influenza vaccine. After conducting a needs assessment it was found that the priority population for the program would be senior citizens. Which theory/model do you feel would be the best to use as the foundation for the intervention you will create? Write a brief rationale defending your choice.

5. You have been asked to create a brief education program to prepare outpatients for a screening colonoscopy for the gastroenterology department at the hospital where you work. The request was made because feedback from a significant number of patients who received the screening last year indicated that they wished they would have known what to expect in advance. Which theory/model do you feel would be the best to use to plan the education program around? Write a brief rationale defending your choice.

6. After tallying the results of an employee satisfaction survey, the director of the human resources (HR) department in the company where you work wants to begin an incentive program to encourage more people to participate in the employee health promotion program. The HR director would like you to create the incentive-based intervention for the program. Which theory/model do you feel would be the best to use to create the incentive-based intervention? Write a brief rationale defending your choice.

WEBLINKS

1. http://www.uri.edu/research/cprc/index-old.htm

   Cancer Prevention Resource Center (CPRC), University of Rhode Island

   CPRC is the home of the Transtheoretical Model. At this Website, you can obtain information about the model, as well as measures that can be used to "stage" a person.

2. http://www.cdc.gov/std/program/community/9-PGcommunity.htm

   National Center for HIV/AIDS, Viral Hepatitis, STD, and TB Prevention, Division of Sexually Transmitted Diseases

   This Website provides an overview of the following behavior change theories: health belief model, theory of reasoned action, social (cognitive) learning theory, transtheoretical model (stages of change), diffusion of innovations, and empowerment theory/empowerment.

3. **http://www.cancer.gov/cancertopics/cancerlibrary/theory.pdf**

   National Cancer Institute (NCI)

   This URL will allow you to access *Theory at a Glance: A Guide for Health Promotion Practice*. This volume presents a single, concise summary of health behavior theories that is both easy to read and practical.

4. **http://www.people.umass.edu/aizen/tpb.html**

   Theory of Planned Behavior

   This is part of the Website of Dr. Icek Ajzen, creator of the theory of planned behavior. The site provides great detail about the theory, as well as sample questionnaires to show how data can be collected using this theory.

5. **http://cancercontrol.cancer.gov/brp/constructs/index.html**

   National Cancer Institute (NCI), Behavioral Research

   This page at the NCI's Behavioral Research Website presents definitions, background information, references, published examples, and information about the best measures of a number of theoretical constructs used in health promotion practice and research.

CHAPTER 8

Interventions

After reading this chapter and answering the questions at the end, you should be able to:

- Define the word *intervention* and apply it to a health promotion setting.
- Provide a rationale for selecting an intervention strategy.
- Explain the advantages of using a combination of several intervention strategies rather than a single intervention strategy.
- List and explain the different categories of intervention strategies.
- Explain the terms *curriculum, scope, sequence, units of study, lessons, lesson plans, health advocacy, health literacy,* and *health numeracy*.
- Briefly explain the modified framework for instructional design.
- List some of the documents that provide guidelines or criteria for developing health promotion interventions.
- Discuss the ethical concerns related to intervention development.
- Create an intervention for a health promotion program.
- Describe how to adapt an evidence-based intervention.

KEY TERMS

best experience	contingencies	health literacy
best practices	contract	health numeracy
best processes	cultural audit	incentive
codes of practice	curriculum	intervention
communication channel	disincentives	lessons
community advocacy	dose	lesson plan
community building	GINA	literacy
community organization	health advocacy	multiplicity
contest	health communication	numeracy

Key Terms, continued

penetration rate	sequence	tailoring
scope	social media	treatment
segmenting	strategy	units of study

Once the goals and objectives have been developed, planners need to decide on the most appropriate means of reaching or attaining those goals and objectives. The planners must design an activity or set of activities that would permit the most *effective* (leads to desired outcome) and *efficient* (uses resources in a responsible manner) achievement of the outcomes stated in the goals and objectives. These planned activities make up the intervention, or what some refer to as **treatment.** The **intervention** is the theory-based strategy or experience to which those in the priority population will be exposed or in which they will take part. In the strictest sense, intervention means "to come or occur between two things, events, or points in time; to come in or between so as to hinder or alter an action" (Anderson, Fortson, Kleindler, & Schonthal, 2002, p. 447). When applied to the planning of health promotion programs, it is usually thought of as something that occurs between the beginning and the end of a program or between pre- and post-program measurements. For example, let's say that you want the employees of Company S to increase their use of safety belts while riding in company-owned vehicles. You can measure their safety belt use before doing anything else, by observing them driving out of the motor pool. This would be a pre-program measure. Then you can intervene in a variety of ways. For example, you could provide an incentive by stating that all employees seen wearing their safety belts would receive a $10 bonus in their next paycheck. Or you could put in each employee's pay envelope a pamphlet on the importance of wearing safety belts. You could institute a company policy requiring all employees to wear safety belts while driving company-owned vehicles. Each of these activities for getting employees to increase their use of safety belts would be considered part of an intervention. After the intervention, you would complete a post-program measurement of safety belt use to determine the success of the program.

The term *intervention* is used to describe all the activities that occur between the two measurement points. Thus an intervention may use a single activity, or it may be a combination of two or more activities. In the case of the example just given, you could use an incentive by itself and call it an intervention, or you could use an incentive, pamphlets, and a company policy all at the same time to increase safety belt use and refer to the combination as an intervention.

The above discussion about the number of activities that make up an intervention in part speaks to the *size* of an intervention. Two terms that relate to the size of an intervention are *multiplicity* and *dose.* **Multiplicity** refers to the number of components or activities that make up the intervention. We have known for a number of years (Erfurt et al., 1990; Kline & Huff, 1999; Shea & Basch, 1990) that interventions that include several activities are more likely to have an effect on the priority population than are those that consist of a single activity. What has become more apparent in recent years is that these intervention activities are more likely to be effective if they are aimed at multiple levels of influence that affect individuals' and populations' behaviors and health status (Glanz & Bishop, 2010). In other words, they have a greater chance of being successful if they use a socio-ecological approach. Few people change their behavior based on a single exposure; instead, multiple exposures are generally needed to change most behaviors. It stands to reason that "hitting" the priority population from several angles or through multiple channels should increase the chances of making an impact. Although research has shown that using several activities is better than one, it has not identified an exact number of activities or a specific combination of activities that will ensure the most effective results (Kline & Huff, 1999). The right combination of activities will depend on the needs of those in the priority population and the specific planning situation.

When speaking about the **dose** of an intervention, we are referring to the number of program units delivered. For example, say that it was decided that the intervention for a skin cancer program would consist of multiple activities (*multiplicity*) and those activities would include an educational class for the public, distribution of brochures to those at high risk, and radio and television public service announcements (PSAs). The dose questions related to these activities would be: How many times would the class be offered? How many brochures would be distributed? And, how many times would the PSAs run? Again, like multiplicity, we know that the greater the dose of an intervention, the greater the chance for change. (Chapter 14 includes additional information about multiplicity and dose as they relate to process evaluation.)

Box 8.1 identifies the responsibilities and competencies for health education specialists that pertain to the material presented in this chapter.

Box 8.1   RESPONSIBILITIES AND COMPETENCIES FOR HEALTH EDUCATION SPECIALISTS

The content of this chapter focuses on the creation of the intervention that will be used in the program that is being planned. The intervention is really the heart of a program. It is the component of the program that will cause the change in the priority population. The responsibilities and competencies related to the tasks of creating an intervention include:

Responsibility I: Assess Needs, Assets, and Capacity for Health Education

Competency 1.6: Examine Factors that Enhance or Compromise the Process of Health Education

Responsibility II: Plan Health Education

Competency 2.3: Select or Design Strategies and Interventions

Competency 2.4: Develop a Scope and Sequence for the Delivery of Health Education

Source: NCHEC, SOPHE, & AAHE (2010).

Types of Intervention Strategies

As mentioned earlier, there are many different types of strategies that planners can use as part of an intervention. By **strategy**, we mean "a general plan of action for affecting a health problem. A strategy may encompass several activities" (CDC, 2003, glossary). Here, we present several categories of intervention strategies based on a modification of the Centers for Disease Control and Prevention's (2003) terminology for intervention strategies. These categories cover the more common strategies used by planners, but in actuality the variety of strategies is limited only by the planners' imagination. Note that the categories presented here are not always independent of each other—that is, some of the examples that we use to help explain the strategies could be used in more than one category. Even with this limitation, the strategies have been categorized into the following seven groups:

1. Health communication strategies

2. Health education strategies

3. Health policy/enforcement strategies

4. Environmental change strategies

5. Health-related community service strategies

6. Community mobilization strategies

7. Other strategies

Health Communication Strategies

Health communication has been defined as "the study and use of communication strategies to inform and influence individual and community decisions that affect health" (USDHHS, 2011a, para. 1). It can also be defined by the form it takes in health promotion programs (e.g., mass media, media advocacy, risk communication, public relations, entertainment education, print material, electronic communication). Of the various intervention strategies used in health promotion, we present health communication strategies first for several reasons. First, almost all health promotion interventions include some form of communication ranging from simple, such as speaking and listening, to the more complex communication campaigns delivered through various forms of media. Second, communication strategies are useful in reaching many of the goals and objectives of health promotion programs. They have been shown to create awareness of an issue, change attitudes toward a health behavior, encourage and motivate individuals to follow recommended health behaviors, reinforce attitude and behavior change, increase demand and support for services, and build social norms (Ammary-Risch, Zambon, & Brown 2010; NCI 2004). But be aware that health communication also has its limitations. For example, health communication alone is rarely sufficient to change behavior and reduce the risk of disease. Third, communication strategies probably have the highest **penetration rate** (number in the priority population exposed or reached) of any of the intervention strategies. And fourth, they are much more cost effective and less threatening than most other types of strategies.

In previous editions of this book much of what was presented about health communication strategies dealt with the traditional communication model. In the traditional communication model, a sender relays a message through a channel to receivers (i.e., consumers)—a vertical or top-down process. In such a model, the sender is the gatekeeper of the information, while the consumers play a less active, almost passive, role in receiving the message (Thackeray & Neiger, 2009). An example is when a health department posts information on its Website for public consumption. However, with the enhanced capabilities of the Internet and the development of other emerging communication technologies, the means of delivering health communications have been greatly expanded and blurred the strict roles of the sender and receiver. With the new technology has come a new communication model: the multidirectional communication (MDC) model (Thackeray & Neiger, 2009) (see **Figure 8.1**). In the MDC model, communication occurs through a combination of: (1) sender top-down (vertical) messages, (2) consumer created bottom-up

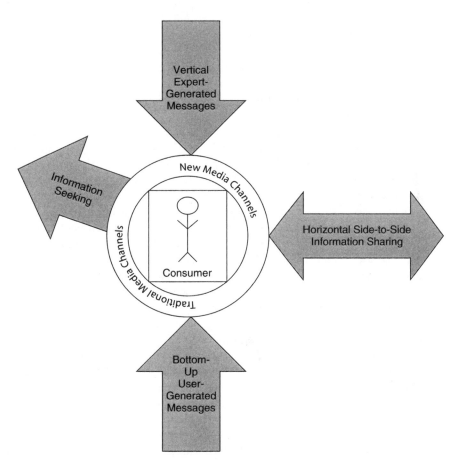

Figure 8.1 A Multidirectional Communication Model

Source: Thackeray, R., & Neiger, B. L. (2009). A multidirectional communication model: Implications for social marketing practice. *Health Promotion Practice, 10*(2), 171–175.

messages, (3) consumer shared horizontal (side-to-side) messages, and (4) consumers seeking information. Thus in the MDC model consumers not only receive information but also actively seek, develop, and share information (Thackeray & Neiger, 2009).

An underlying concept of the MDC model is that the sophistication with which health information is communicated has changed dramatically in recent years due in large part to new technology. To compete for the attention and participation of consumers, those who plan health promotion programs must either develop a working knowledge of these communication technologies or have the foresight to access those who can provide the necessary expertise. Research indicates that effective health communication campaigns adapt audience-centered approaches (USDHHS, 2000). This requires that planners understand consumer tendencies, needs, and preferences before designing campaigns and messages.

There are literally hundreds of communication activities that could be used with a health communication strategy. Communication channels is one way to subdivide these activities. A **communication channel** is the route through which a message is disseminated to the priority population. "Understanding communications channels is imperative to conducting strategic, effective and user-centric health interventions, campaigns and outreach" (CDC, 2009c, para. 1). Selecting appropriate channels for a priority population is often related to, or in some cases limited by, the setting where the communication will be delivered (Kreps, Barnes, Neiger, & Thackeray, 2009). "For example, if the home is identified as the prime setting, appropriate channels could include one-on-one home visits, technology via the telephone, or mass media via television or radio" (Kreps et al., 2009, p. 91). The four traditional communication channels include intrapersonal (one-on-one communication), intrapersonal (small group communication), organization and community, and mass media. These channels are hierarchical in nature with regards to the number of people they reach. The intrapersonal channel typically reaches the fewest number of people, while the mass media channel reaches the largest number of people.

Because of the Internet and the other emerging technologies we are adding *social media* as a fifth communication channel. **Social media**, or *interactive media*, is an overarching term for any type of media that uses the Internet and other technologies to enhance social interaction. Unlike the other four communication channels, social media does not have a set place in the hierarchy because it "cuts across" several different levels. That is, depending on the type and purpose of social media it can be used to generate social interaction at any of the levels of the traditional communication channel hierarchy. After we address each of the four traditional communication channels found in the hierarchy, we will present information on social media.

Over the years, the *intrapersonal channel* has most often been used, but by no means exclusively, in health care settings when the health care provider and patient interact. This is a familiar channel for most people and one they trust. It is typically an effective communication channel, but it is also typically the most time and resource intensive channel for the number of people reached. This is especially true when the health communication is *tailored* for the recipient. **Tailoring** has been defined as "any combination of information or change strategies intended to reach one specific person, based upon characteristics that are unique to that person, related to the outcome of interest, and have been derived from an individual assessment" (Kreuter & Skinner, 2000, p. 1). Tailoring takes more effort than *personalizing* (i.e., placing the recipient's name on/in the communication) or *targeting* (i.e., providing standardized information to a segmented group like Asian American adolescent girls) communication (Kreuter, Farrell, Olevitch, & Brennan, 1999; Suggs & McIntyre, 2009).

In more recent years, the tailoring of intrapersonal communication has been greatly enhanced by the use of technology. Tailoring of messages has been used with electronic mail (i.e., email) messages (Kreuter et al., 1999) and with information delivered through Websites (Suggs & McIntyre, 2009). Another example involves the use of telephones. Though most people no longer think of the telephone as "technology," it too is used for health promotion interventions via the intrapersonal channel. Planners have used it for "gathering information, disseminating information, providing health education and counseling, promoting health education programs, offering cues to action and social support" (Soet & Basch, 1997, p. 760) on a variety of health topics ranging from asthma management to weight loss. Health education delivered by telephone "can be classified into two broad categories: *individual initiated*, whereby the individual must actively seek contact and assistance from a health information hotline; and *outreach*, whereby the individual is called by a health educator or counselor" (Soet & Basch, 1997, p. 760). Individual-initiated health information hotlines or help lines usually provide information, and sometimes education and counseling, whereas outreach activities range from brief, one-time preappointment reminders to long-term interactive professional health counseling (Soet & Basch, 1997) or coaching. Soet and Basch (1997) present a generic process for developing a telephone intervention activity that includes three areas: "designing the intervention protocol, selection and training of the health educator/counselor(s), and developing the documentation and data collection protocol" (p. 763).

Within the intrapersonal channel, one health communication activity in particular has received much attention in recent years—*health coaching*. Health coaching is the process by which a trained health coach, using the results from some type of personal health assessment (e.g., health risk appraisal), assists a client/consumer in identifying health-enhancing goals and uses behavioral psychology principles to help motivate the client to work toward the goals. This confidential communication relationship often takes place via a series of telephone conversations but can be conducted in face-to-face sessions. There are a number of commercial companies that offer health coaching services most often as part of an employee health promotion program to help enhance employee health and reduce health care costs. Most recently, health coaching is also being used by some primary health care providers.

Examples of the *interpersonal channel* are support groups and small classes. This channel has many of the same characteristics of the intrapersonal channel, but reaches larger numbers of people with fewer resources.

Many people receive a lot of information through *organization* and *community channels*. Often health promotion programs have priority populations that are part of or entirely comprise already existing groups (e.g., workers of a particular company, social groups, or members of a religious organization), or who may participate in a community activity. As such, organizational and community channels provide excellent ways to reach priority populations. Thus church bulletins, company or agency newsletters, organizations or community bulletin boards, and community activities are often used as a part of communication activities.

Probably the most visible communication channel to most people is the *mass media channel*. Mass media interventions can seek to influence people either directly or indirectly. When done directly the intervention identifies a problem of concern and targets the people who can change it, while when it is done indirectly the interventions seek to influence people by creating beneficial changes in the places or environments (e.g., homes, schools, worksites, roads, grocery stores, cities) in which people live and work (Abroms & Maibach, 2008). For example, to increase the number of children who are immunized properly a direct mass media intervention would target the parents/guardians of the children. A mass media intervention to counter the advertising of unhealthy foods and drinks in a specific neighborhood would be an example of indirect mass media intervention. The mass media channel includes both print and electronic formats, such as billboards; direct mail; daily papers with national or local circulation; local weekly newspapers; local, public, and network television, including cable television; public and commercial radio stations; and magazines with either a broad readership or a narrow focus. There are many ways to convey a message using the mass media. These include news coverage, public affairs coverage, talk shows, public service roundtables, entertainment, public service announcements (PSAs), paid advertisements, editorials, letters to the editor, comic strips, and columnists' commentaries (Arkin, 1990).

With the growth of and the developments in technology, the *social media* channel has significantly changed the way people communicate both formally and informally. Social media, sometimes referred to as *interactive media* or *Web 2.0*, has several characteristics that set it apart from the other communication channels already discussed. The unique characteristics of social media include: 1) it is user or consumer generated, organized, and distributed; (2) information can be revised or updated almost immediately; (3) it is typically low cost in terms of creation and maintenance; and (4) it is generally entertaining to use. There are many different forms of social media that allow for content management (collaborative writing, e.g., wikis), content sharing (e.g., podcasts, Webinars), social bookmarking (i.e., tagging, saving, searching, and rating Websites, e.g., Digg), social gaming, social journaling (e.g., blogs), social networking (e.g., Facebook, MySpace, LinkedIn, Twitter, text messaging), social news (i.e., tagging, voting for, and commenting on news articles, e.g., Newsvine), social video and photo sharing (e.g., YouTube, Flickr), and syndication (e.g., real simple syndication [RSS] feeds).

Though the use of social media in health promotion interventions may be limited only by planners' creativity, we feel that its greatest potential lies in three uses: (1) the Internet as a platform to deliver behavior change interventions (e.g., weight loss programs; see Bennett & Glasgow, 2009); (2) the Internet to promote health promotion programs (e.g., viral marketing; see Thackeray, Neiger, Hanson, & McKenzie, 2008); and (3) the Internet and mobile devices for community mobilization or advocacy (e.g., organizing youth to get involved in civic affairs; see Thackeray & Hunter, 2010). However, as with other channels of communication, when using social media planners need to think strategically about what they are trying to accomplish and then decide how to use technology to accomplish the program's goals. In other words, planners need to focus on the relationship between themselves and those in the priority population, and the ways people connect with each other, because social media is really all about developing relationships. Thackeray and Bennion (2009) have adapted the strategic thinking acronym

Table 8.1 Using *POST* to Think Strategically About Social Media

POST	Li & Bernoff (2008)	Thackeray & Bennion (2009)
People	What are they ready for?	What technology do they use? Why?
Objectives	Why do you want to pursue the Groundswell?	What do you want to happen (i.e., a change in attitudes, knowledge, and/or behavior)?
Strategy	How do you want relationships to change (e.g., customers to carry your messages; customers to become engaged)?	How will you use the marketing mix (i.e., product, price, place, promotion)?
Technology	What technology to use?	What technology will you use, given what you are trying to accomplish?

POST, found in a book by Li and Bernoff (2008), to assist program planners in creating health promotion interventions that include social media (see **Table 8.1**).

Regardless of the communication channel used in creating a communication intervention, planners need to consider the literacy level of those in the priority population. **Literacy** "is the ability to use printed and written information to function in society, to achieve one's goals, and to develop one's knowledge and potential" (White & Dillow, 2005, p. 4). "Literacy can be thought of as currency in this society. Just as adults with little money have difficulty meeting their basic needs, those with limited literacy skills are likely to find it more challenging to pursue their goals—whether these involve job advancement, consumer decision making, citizenship, or other aspects of their lives" (Kirsch, Jungeblut, Jenkins, & Kolstad, 1993, p. xix). The last national assessment of adult literacy in the United States was conducted in 2003. That study, called the National Assessment of Adult Literacy (NAAL), assessed a representative sample of over 19,000 adults age 16 and older on *prose* (the knowledge and skills to perform prose tasks such as reading and comprehending a news story), *document* (the knowledge and skills to perform document tasks such as completing a job application), and *quantitative literacy*, sometimes referred to as **numeracy** (the knowledge and skills to perform quantitative tasks such as balancing a checkbook or calculating a tip) (USDE, n.d.). Results of the 2003 NAAL were reported using four literacy levels: *below basic* (indicates no more than the most simple and concrete literacy skills, e.g., searching a short, simple text to find out when to show up for an appointment), *basic* (skills necessary to perform simple and everyday literacy activities, e.g., finding specific information in a pamphlet), *intermediate* (skills necessary to perform moderately challenging literacy activities, e.g., consulting reference materials to determine which foods contain a particular vitamin), and *proficient* (skills necessary to perform more complex and challenging literacy activities, e.g., comparing viewpoints in two editorials). **Figure 8.2** provides a comparison of the percentage of adults in each literacy level for the two most recent national literacy assessments.

The 2003 NAAL included the first-ever national health literacy assessment of adults in the United States. The health literacy scale used in the assessment and the tasks that the adults were asked to perform were guided by the following definition of **health literacy**: the degree to which individuals have the capacity to obtain, process, and understand

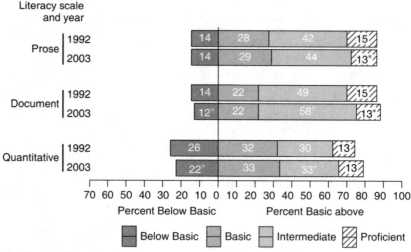

Literacy scale and year

Figure 8.2 Percentage of Adults in Each Literacy Level: 1992 and 2003
Source: White & Dillow (2005).

basic health information and services to make appropriate health decisions (USDHHS, 2000). "Health literacy is a complex phenomenon that involves skills, knowledge, and the expectations that health professionals have of the public's interest in and understanding of health information and services" (USDHHS, 2011b, p. 4). It is influenced by many things including "the language we speak; our ability to communicate clearly and listen carefully; and our age, socioeconomic status, cultural background, past experiences, cognitive abilities, and mental health. Each of these factors affects how we communicate, understand, and respond to health information" (USDHHS, 2011b, p. 5).

Like the general literacy assessment, health literacy results from the NAAL were reported using the same four literacy categories: below basic, basic, intermediate, and proficient. The results showed that 14% had below basic health literacy, 22% had basic health literacy, 53% had intermediate health literacy, and 12% had proficient health literacy (Kutner, Greenberg, Jin, & Paulsen, 2006). Stated a bit differently, this study showed "that nearly 9 out of 10 adults may lack the skills needed to manage their health and prevent disease" (CDC, 2009d, p. 2). Though the problem of limited health literacy affects people of all ages, races, incomes, and education levels, it "has been found to be even greater for older adults, those with limited education, minorities, the poor, and those with limited English proficiency" (CDC, 2009d, p. 2).

Though the NAAL assessment of health literacy included a quantitative component, in recent years health numeracy has emerged as a separate and important issue (Golbeck, Ahlers-Schmidt, Paschal, & Dismuke, 2005). As with health literacy, health numeracy is not at the levels it should be and may have a significant impact on health status (Estrada, Martin-Hryniewicz, Peek, Collins, & Byrd, 2004). **Health numeracy** has been defined as "the degree to which individuals have the capacity to access, process, interpret, communicate, and act on numerical, quantitative, graphical, biostatistical, and probabilistic health information needed to make effective health decisions" (Golbeck et al., 2005, p. 375). This definition recognizes that there are degrees of health numeracy that fall along a continuum, and "that health numeracy is not simply about understanding (processing and interpreting), but also functioning (communicating and acting) on numeric concepts in terms of health" (Golbeck et al., 2005, p. 375). **Box 8.2** presents the four functional categories of health numeracy identified by Golbeck and her colleagues (2005).

Because of the lack of health literacy and health numeracy in the United States, health education specialists need to work to ensure that the health communication interventions are appropriate for their priority population. **Box 8.3** presents practical tips from the Centers for Disease Control and Prevention for improving health literacy.

Box 8.2 FUNCTIONAL CATEGORIES OF HEALTH NUMERACY

- "Basic health numeracy involves sufficient basic skills to identify numbers, and make sense of quantitative data requiring no manipulation of numbers. Examples include identifying the appropriate number of pills to take from a prescription bottle, the date and time of a doctor's appointment, and using a phone book to find a clinic's phone number" (p. 375).

- "Computational health numeracy involves the ability to count, quantify, compute, and otherwise use simple manipulation of numbers, quantities, items, or visual elements in a health context so as to function in everyday health situations. Examples include determining net carbohydrates based on information on a nutritional label or determining fees based on a sliding scale" (p. 375).

- "Analytical health numeracy involves a higher level of literacy than the previous levels. It involves the ability to make sense of information, such as that presented in functional health numeracy, but also involves higher level concepts such as inference, estimation, proportions, percentages, frequencies, and equivalent situations. It often requires information to be pulled from multiple sources and in multiple formats. Examples of analytical health numeracy include determining whether cholesterol levels are within the normal range, understanding basic graphs, and comparing benefits from various insurance policies or programs" (pp. 375–376).

- "Statistical health numeracy involves an understanding of basic biostatistics involving probability statements, skills to compare information presented on different scales (probability, proportion, percent), the ability to critically analyze quantitative health information such as life expectancy and risk, and an understanding of statistical concepts such as randomization and a "blind" study. Examples of statistical health numeracy include determining preference of treatment based on probabilities of efficacy and side effects, interpreting complex graphs of health information, and making decisions based on relative versus absolute risk" (p. 376).

Source: "A Definition and Operational Framework for Health Numeracy." A. L. Goldbeck, C. R. Ahlers-Schmidt, A. M. Paschal, and S. E. Dismuke, from *American Journal of Preventive Medicine.* Copyright © 2005 by Elsevier. Reprinted with permission.

Box 8.3 TEN TIPS FOR HEALTH MARKETING AND COMMUNICATION PRACTITIONERS FOR IMPROVING HEALTH LITERACY

1. *Health literacy is a two way street.* In all outreach efforts, aim for shared understanding between you (public health professional) and the public. Don't assume everyone will understand your messages and/or how to manage their health. For example, if you want to include an illustration in your campaign materials, make sure to test it with your audience to ensure they understand its intended meaning.

2. *Know your audience.* Take an audience-centered approach. Who will do what differently as a result of your program/service? Who can you influence most effectively? What do they care about? What do they struggle with? Take time to learn about your audience and develop materials and programs accordingly. Avoid the one-size-fits-all approach. For example, older adults tend to rely on their health care providers to make medical decisions on their behalf. Therefore, health care providers may be an important audience to consider as a channel for reaching older adults with health information.

3. *Involve your target audience.* When members of the target audience participate in designing and testing communication, outcomes are more successful, including those for people with limited health literacy. Ask for feedback from your intended audience on everything you do from choosing the right words, colors, and visuals for a brochure to piloting a new training program or service.

4. *Don't stop at rewriting materials.* Health literacy is more than testing readability levels. Assessing whether your audience can actually apply and use your information is the important part. Your audience should be able to demonstrate the skills or explain in their own words (teach-back) what you are asking them to do. For example, if your brochure explains how to assemble an emergency home kit, have the audience show you what they have learned.

5. *Keep it simple.* Present audiences with no more than three or four main messages. Give specific actions in clear language and recommendations. Skip the "nice to know" details. For example, give specific steps for keeping foods safe. Detailed descriptions of bacteria that cause food-borne illness may not be necessary.

6. *Include resources for additional learning.* It is safe to assume that there are members of your target audience who have limited health literacy. Develop materials with the knowledge that everyone prefers health information that is clear and actionable. Provide a list of resources for those who may want to learn more.

7. *Develop key partnerships. Identify partners who know your audience.* Collaborate with traditional partners, as well as adult educators, journalists, and other nontraditional partners to help increase the dissemination of health information to the public. Partners can assist with gaining access to communities where issues of trust and fear may exist and offer expertise and knowledge of their communities.

8. *Consider their culture and language. Not ours.* Health professionals have their own culture and language as a result of their training and work environments. It is important to remember that our audiences do not speak our professional jargon and that culture influences how people communicate, understand, and respond to health information.

Box 8.3 (CONTINUED)

9. *Evaluate your environment.* Assess how easy it is to access and use your services, programs, and materials. For example, settings with a large number of signs can be intimidating and overwhelming for persons with limited health literacy skills. Consider internal changes to improve access and enhance navigation within your agency.

10. *Put it on your agenda.* Educate yourself and offer to educate senior leaders and staff on the importance and implications of health literacy. Advocate for all staff to participate in health literacy trainings and presentations.

Source: Centers for Disease Control and Prevention (CDC) (2009d).

Table 8.2 Guidelines for Preparing Written Materials

Guideline	Explanation
1. Needs and priority population identification	Identify the topic and the priority population (e.g., middle-aged women and mammography).
2. Plan the project	Develop a work plan and budget for your material.
3. Audience research	Segment your priority population using such factors as experience, attitude, culture, etc.
4. Material development	
a. Style	Use an active voice with familiar terms that highlight key points. If possible, develop a behaviorally oriented interactive message.
b. Organization	Sequence or prioritize the message.
c. Content	Use words and terms that are understandable to laypeople. Use short sentences and paragraphs.
d. Format	Make it appealing to the eye, making sure the reader can identify the main points.
5. Graphics and illustrations	Graphics and illustrations should be positive and easy to understand, and should summarize the message.
6. Pretesting	Make sure the materials work before you use them with the priority population. Also, make sure the reading level is appropriate.
7. Printing	Consider paper color, size, and cost.
8. Distribution and training	Develop a distribution system and instructions for use.

Source: "Guidelines for Preparing Written Materials." J. Meyer and J. Rainey in *American Journal of Health Education.*
Copyright © 1994 by American Alliance for Health, Physical Education, Recreation and Dance. Adapted with permission.

In addition, Meyer and Rainey (1994) created a set of guidelines for health education specialists to follow when creating health promotion materials for low-literacy populations. We find their guidelines to be useful regardless of the priority population. Their eight guidelines have been modified and are summarized in **Table 8.2**. The only addition we would make to their list would be to check the reading level of the written materials.

"For the general public, writing at the 6th grade reading level is usually safe. You can check if you're on target by using a readability test such as the SMOG (stands for Simple Measure of Gobbledegook), the Fog-Gunning Index, or the Fry Readability Formula" (USDHHS, OSAP, 1991, p. 3). You can find such formulas in most reading methods books and on selected computer word-processing programs. **Box 8.4** presents the steps in the process of testing readability using the SMOG.

Box 8.4   THE SMOG READABILITY FORMULA

To calculate the SMOG reading grade level, begin with the entire written work that is being assessed, and follow these four steps:

1. Count off 10 consecutive sentences near the beginning, in the middle, and near the end of the text.

2. From this sample of 30 sentences, circle all of the words containing 3 or more syllables (polysyllabic), including repetitions of the same word, and total the number of words circled.

3. Estimate the square root of the total number of polysyllabic words counted. This is done by finding the nearest perfect square, and taking its square root.

4. Finally, add a constant of 3 to the square root. This number gives the SMOG grade, or the reading grade level that a person must have reached if he or she is to fully understand the text being assessed.

A few additional guidelines will help to clarify these directions:

- A sentence is defined as a string of words punctuated with a period (.), an exclamation point (!), or a question mark (?).
- Hyphenated words are considered as one word.
- Numbers that are written out should also be considered, and if in numeric form in the text, they should be pronounced to determine if they are polysyllabic.
- Proper nouns, if polysyllabic, should be counted, too.
- Abbreviations should be read as unabbreviated to determine if they are polysyllabic.

Not all pamphlets, fact sheets, or other printed materials contain 30 sentences. To test a text that has fewer than 30 sentences:

1. Count all of the polysyllabic words in the text.

2. Count the number of sentences.

3. Find the average number of polysyllabic words per sentence as follows:

$$\text{Average} = \frac{\text{Total \# polysyllabic words}}{\text{Total \# of sentences}}$$

4. Multiply that average by the number of sentences *short of* 30.

5. Add that figure to the total number of polysyllabic words.

6. Find the square root and add the constant of 3.

Box 8.4 (CONTINUED)

Perhaps the quickest way to administer the SMOG grading test is by using the SMOG conversion table. Simply count the number of polysyllabic words in your chain of 30 sentences and look up the appropriate grade level on the chart.

SMOG Conversion Table*

Total Polysyllabic Word Counts	Approximate Grade Level (±1.5 Grades)
0–2	4
3–6	5
7–12	6
13–20	7
21–30	8
31–42	9
43–56	10
57–72	11
73–90	12
91–110	13
111–132	14
133–156	15
157–182	16
183–210	17
211–240	18

*Developed by Harold C. McGraw, Office of Educational Research, Baltimore County Schools, Towson, Maryland.

Source: National Cancer Institute (2002 & 2004).

Health Education Strategies

Earlier (Chapter 1) *health education* was defined as "any planned combination of learning experiences designed to predispose, enable, and reinforce voluntary behavior decisions conducive to health in individuals, groups, or communities" (Green & Kreuter, 205, p. G-4). You may be asking, "How is this definition different from the definition presented in the earlier section for health communication strategies?" There are some health communication strategies, because of the way they are designed, that could be classified as health education strategies. And, there are some health education strategies that could meet the definition of health communication strategies. There is no clear dividing line between these two categories of intervention strategies. That is, they are not mutually exclusive categories. In fact, it is for this reason that some authors have included health education strategies as part of the health communication strategies category or vice versa. Yet, we have decided to separate the two types of strategies. In general, we see health communication strategies as those that inform people (e.g., a brochure on skin cancer or a mass media campaign on preventing HIV), while health education strategies are those that are planned learning experiences that provide knowledge and skills to the learners in a more formal educational setting. We see health education strategies as those usually associated with settings such as classes, seminars, workshops, and courses, both face-to-face and online. Some examples include prenatal classes for expectant parents, a workshop for parents on how to better communicate with their teenager, or a first aid and CPR course for potential babysitters.

Prior to presenting information about creating health education interventions it is important to have some background in how people learn. Many theories/models have been put forth to help explain how people learn. While many of the theories/models include components that are unique to the theory/model, there is also much overlap in the content. Space does not allow for the review of those theories/models here. However, we are fortunate that other authors (Bryan, Kreuter, & Brownson, 2009; Minelli & Breckon, 2009) have reviewed those theories/models. Those reviewers have identified many of the common components and created lists of learning principles. Their lists can help guide planners as they create health education interventions. We present their lists here. Minelli and Breckon (2009) refer to their list as the 10 general principles of learning. For them, learning is facilitated: (1) if several of the senses (e.g., seeing, hearing, speaking) are used; (2) if the learner is actively involved in the process, rather than a passive participant; (3) if the learner is not distracted by discomfort or extraneous events; (4) if the learner is ready to learn; (5) if that which is to be learned is relevant to the learner and that relevance is perceived by the learner; (6) if repetition is used; (7) if the learning encountered is pleasant, if progress occurs that is recognizable by the learner, and if that learning is recognized and encouraged; (8) if the material to be learned starts with what is known and proceeds to the unknown, while concurrently moving from simple to complex concepts; (9) if application of concepts to several settings occurs, which generalizes the material; and (10) if it is paced appropriately for the learner.

The principles offered by Bryan and colleagues (2009) are specific to adult learners. The principles represent a synthesis of recurring themes that the authors found when reviewing existing theories/models related to adult education. Their adult learning principles include:

1. Adults need to know why they are learning.

2. Adults are motivated to learn by the need to solve problems.

3. Adults' previous experience must be respected and built upon.

4. Adults need learning approaches that match their background and diversity.

5. Adults need to be actively involved in the learning process. (p. 559)

With this brief overview of learning principles, let's look at the makeup of a health education intervention. Though health communication strategies may be the most frequently used health promotion intervention strategy, health education strategies are the ones that provide the opportunity for the priority population to gain in-depth knowledge about a particular health topic. Well-designed health education strategies take an understanding of the educational process and take a great deal of effort to create. In order to better understand this process, several terms must be defined. The first is the word *curriculum*. **Curriculum** refers to "a planned set of lessons or courses designed to lead to competence in an area of study" (Gilbert, Sawyer, & McNeill, 2011, p. 412). Examples include the health education curriculum of a school district or the curriculum for a hospital's diabetes education program. To further define a curriculum it is important to understand the terms *scope* and *sequence*. **Scope** refers to the breadth and depth of the material covered in a curriculum, whereas **sequence** defines the order in which the material is presented. To further clarify these definitions, scope has been referred to as the horizontal organization of the substance of the curriculum (Goodlad & Su, 1992), while the sequence is the vertical relationship among the curricular areas (Ornstein & Hunkins, 1998). It is not unusual for the scope of a health education curriculum to be presented as **units of study**. These units are defined as "an orderly, self-contained collection of activities educationally designed to meet a set of objectives. Other terms for this are *curriculum plans*, *modules*, and *strands*" (Gilbert et al., 2011, p. 188). Thus, a school health curriculum may have units on exercise, nutrition, chronic diseases, communicable diseases, and so forth, while the diabetes education curriculum might include units on self-management, working with a health care professional, and avoiding emergencies. And finally, units of study are further subdivided into **lessons**—the amount of material that can be presented during a single educational encounter, say for example the amount of material that can be presented in a one-hour class. The written outline of a lesson is referred to as a **lesson plan** and typically includes three components—introduction, body, and conclusion. The introduction provides an overview of what will be covered, the body presents the health content, and the conclusion reviews what was presented. There is an old saying that summarizes these three parts that states *tell them what you are going to tell them* [introduction], *tell them it* [body], *and tell them what you told them* [conclusion]. (See **Figure 8.3** for an example lesson plan format.)

Title of Program: _____ Title of Lesson: _____ Page ___ of ___ Unit: _____ Lesson No.: _____ Priority Population: _____ Length of Lesson: _____		
Resources & References	Content	Teaching Method
	Introduction: Body: 1. 2. 3. Conclusion:	
Evaluation:		

Figure 8.3 Example Lesson Plan Format

The heart of any lesson is the body or the content portion of the lesson. Gagne (1985) has created a framework, called the *Nine Events of Instruction*, for designing educational experiences that provides a nice outline for creating the body of a lesson. More recently, Kinzie (2005) modified Gagne's framework for application to health promotion applications. The modified framework includes five stages instead of the original nine created by Gagne: (1) *gain attention* (convey health threats and benefits); (2) *present stimulus material* (tailor message to audience knowledge and values, demonstrate observable effectiveness, make behaviors easy to understand and do); (3) *provide guidance* (use trustworthy models to demonstrate); (4) *elicit performance and provide feedback* (to enhance *trailability*, and develop proficiency and self-efficacy); and (5) *enhance retention and transfer* (provide social support and deliver behavioral cues) (Kinzie, 2005). **Table 8.3** provides an example of how these five stages can be applied to a health topic.

Table 8.3 Application of Instructional Design Framework to a Lesson on Breast Cancer

Stage	Content Covered	Method of Presentation
Gain attention	• Help participants identify personal risk to breast cancer • Share benefits of doing breast self-examinations (BSE), regular breast exams by physicians, and mammograms	• Use breast cancer risk appraisal or breast cancer pretest • Present a case study of women finding a lump in the breast early
Present stimulus material		
Tailor message to knowledge and values	• Using information from risk appraisal or pretest, tailor breast cancer information	• Lecture/discussion
Demonstrate observable effectiveness	• Explain importance of early diagnosis	• Use peer educators to role-play interaction with physician
Make desired behaviors easy to understand	• Present steps in BSE and making appointment with physician and for mammogram	• Use video showing correct steps for BSE or peer educators to demonstrate on models
Provide guidance	• Have others share experiences on how exams are conducted	• Use guest speakers who perform regular BSE and radiographers who do mammograms
Elicit performance and provide feedback	• Repeat steps in BSE and let participants practice BSE	• Use breast models for practice and provide critique
Enhance retention and transfer	• Encourage participants to share information learned with others and ways to remember to act	• Lecture/discussion • Brainstorm reminder ideas • Distribute BSE shower cards that explain importance of regular action for participants to place in their bathrooms

There are many different ways of presenting health education such as lecture, discussion, group work, audiovisual materials, computerized instruction, laboratory exercises, and written materials (books and periodicals). **Box 8.5** provides a more complete listing of educational activities, and Gilbert, Sawyer, and McNeill (2011) have provided a detailed discussion of these activities.

Box 8.5 COMMONLY USED EDUCATIONAL ACTIVITIES

A. Audiovisual materials and equipment
   1. Audiotapes, records, and CDs
   2. Bulletin, chalk, cloth, flannel, magnetic, and peg boards
   3. Charts, pictures, and posters
   4. Films and filmstrips
   5. Instructional television
   6. Opaque projector or Elmo
   7. Slides and slide projectors
   8. Transparencies, PowerPoint® slides, and overhead projector
   9. Video (DVDs and tapes)

B. Computer-based
   1. World Wide Web
   2. Desktop publishing
   3. Presentation programs
   4. Individualized learning programs
   5. Video conferencing
   6. Social media

C. Printed educational materials
   1. Instructor-made handouts and worksheets
   2. Pamphlets
   3. Study guides (commercial and instructor-made)
   4. Text and reference books
   5. Workbooks

D. Teaching strategies and techniques for the classroom
   1. Brainstorming
   2. Case studies
   3. Cooperative learning
   4. Debates
   5. Demonstrations and experiments
   6. Discovery or guided discovery

(Box 8.5 continues)

Box 8.5 (CONTINUED)

    7. Discussion

    8. Group discussion

    9. Guest speakers

   10. Lecture

   11. Lecture/discussion

   12. Newspaper and magazine articles

   13. Panel discussions

   14. Peer group teaching/coaching

   15. Poems, songs, and stories

   16. Problem solving

   17. Puppets

   18. Questioning

   19. Role playing and plays

   20. Simulation, games, and puzzles

   21. Tutoring

   22. Values clarification activities

  E. Teaching strategies and techniques for outside of the classroom

    1. Community resources

    2. Field trips

    3. Health fairs

    4. Health museums

    5. Health education centers

Health Policy/Enforcement Strategies

Health polices/enforcement strategies include executive orders, laws, ordinances, judicial decisions, policies, regulations, rules, and position statements. Though each of the different types of policy/enforcement strategies has its own definition, common to all of them is a decision made by an authoritative person, agency/organization, or body and that is presented in a statement or guidelines intended to direct or influence the actions or behaviors of others. Another way to think about them is as strategies that are mandated or regulated. Such strategies revolve around incentives, disincentives, or requirements to encourage or discourage actions by groups of individuals or society as a whole (Riegelman, 2010). This type of intervention strategy can regulate the behavior of individuals (e.g., use of safety belts and motorcycle helmets), organizations (e.g., paying taxes for certain activities), institutions (e.g., school board adopting a position statement that a district will only provide well-balanced meals in the cafeteria), or communities (e.g., housing codes for rental properties) (Brennan Ramirez et al., 2008). This type of intervention strategy can also be used to "affect the built environment, such as zoning related to new grocery stores or fast food restaurants, maintenance of sidewalks and streetscapes, or architectural design features such as neighborhood signage addressing the history and culture of the community" (Brennan Ramirez et al., 2008, p. 70).

This type of intervention strategy may be controversial. It has been criticized by some because it mandates a particular response from those governed by it. It takes away individual freedoms and sometimes plays on a person's pride, "pocketbook," and psyche. Stated a bit differently, "it runs counter to a fundamental emphasis on property rights, economic individualism, and competition in American political culture. The exceptionalism of the United States lies in its antistatist beliefs: Americans are less concerned with what government will do to benefit individuals than what government might do to control them" (Oliver, 2006, p. 196). This type of strategy must be sold on the basis of "common good." That is, the justification for this type of societal action is to protect the public's health. Health policy/enforcement strategies exist for the protection of the community and of individual rights.

> Officials are willing to intercede into the private activities and lives of people in order to protect the larger population. When such intervention occurs it is usually very narrow and very specifically defined. There also tend to be sanctions attached if people do not comply. For example, in the case of inoculations, if a mother and father did not have their child inoculated that child cannot attend school. If parents do not send their child to school they are in violation of the law, and there are criminal and civil penalties that are involved (Rich & Sugrue, 1989, p. 33).

Some would say that health policy/enforcement strategies do not allow for the "voluntary behavior conducive to health" suggested by Green and Kreuter (2005, p. G-4) in their definition of health education. But, at the same time, this kind of activity can get people to change their behavior when other strategies have failed. For example, before the passage of safety belt laws, most states were reporting about an 11% use rate by drivers of automobiles and were trying to attack the problem through communication strategies using the mass media (USDT, 2011). Now that safety belt laws are in effect in states, usage rates in those states are closer to 85%; in some states where there is strict enforcement, usage rates are as high as 88% (USDT, 2010). Another example comes from the work of Sorensen and colleagues (1991), which showed a 21% reduction in the number of employees who smoked in a company that put a nonsmoking policy in effect. Both of these examples show that health policy/enforcement strategies are necessary to reinforce and support prevention messages.

Block (2008) has identified six phases of policy making—agenda setting, policy formulation, policy adoption, policy implementation, policy assessment, and policy modification—that we feel can be adapted and applied to the creation of any of the health policy/enforcement strategies for a health promotion program. The first phase, *agenda setting,* deals with determining what the health problem is, analyzing whether the cause of the problem can best be solved with a policy/enforcement strategy, and identifying evidence to show that such a strategy will work. Phase 2, *policy formulation,* is the phase in which the policy or mandated action is actually developed. The actual wording of the policy is not easy work. It is difficult to move from a concept or idea to wording that effectively carries out the intent of the concept or idea and creates the most good for the most people. If the policy being created is a legal document (e.g., law, ordinance), it is not unusual for various interest groups to try to influence those writing the document so that the resulting work best represents their interests. In other words, there are likely to be both pro and con feelings toward the policy and thus this phase can be very political. The third phase, *policy adoption* or approval, takes place when the authoritative individual or group "approves" the formulated policy. Again, depending on the policy being considered, politics can impact the outcome.

Once the policy has been approved it must be *implemented*. This is the fourth phase of the process. In this phase, the necessary human and financial resources must be assembled to make the policy work. As a part of this phase, it is important that those who are implementing the new policy use good judgment and show respect for others when doing so. The fifth phase of the process, *policy assessment*, entails making sure that the policy is being carried out as written and that it is indeed working to solve the problem it was intended to solve. Based on the results of the policy assessment, the authoritative individual or group must consider the sixth and final phase—*policy modification*. In this phase some judgment and possible action must be made to determine whether the policy should be maintained, modified, or eliminated (Dunn, 1994). While working through these six phases, planners should bear in mind the following 12 points:

1. Have top-level support for the mandated action (ASTDHPHE, 2001; Emont & Cummings, 1989; Mikanowicz & Altman, 1995).

2. Have a representative group (committee) from the priority population help formulate the "mandatory" action.

3. Consider surveying those in the priority population to gain additional information regarding policy change (Mikanowicz & Altman, 1995).

4. Make sure expert advice on the subject of the mandated action is available to the group developing it.

5. Seek a legal opinion if necessary.

6. Examine the work of others and review the issues they faced when implementing "mandatory" actions.

7. Be sure that health policy/enforcement strategies are based on sound principles and, if possible, good research (ASTDHPHE, 2001).

8. Seek input and debate/discussion concerning the mandated action from the priority population while it is being formulated.

9. Develop health policy/enforcement strategies that are written simply and include a rationale, a general policy statement, specific areas affected, and clearly defined complaint, grievance, and enforcement procedures (Mikanowicz & Altman, 1995).

10. Consider phasing in the new regulation a little bit at a time. For example, if a no-smoking policy is going to be implemented, the planner may want to begin by restricting smoking in certain areas before banning it altogether. This not only helps people change gradually but it also expresses concern for them.

11. Provide education and behavior change programs to assist those in the priority population with the implementation of the "mandatory" actions (Mikanowicz & Altman, 1995).

12. Ensure that, once formulated, the "mandatory" actions:
    a. are actively communicated to those in the priority population.
    b. are reviewed on a regular basis for the purposes of evaluating and revising if necessary.
    c. apply to all in the priority population and not just to select groups.
    d. are consistently enforced. Be prepared to deal with the complaint and grievance processes (Mikanowicz & Altman, 1995).
    e. are enforced as a shared responsibility of all in the institution.

Environmental Change Strategies

Another group of strategies that has been used in meeting the goals and objectives of health promotion programs is environmental change strategies. Such strategies have been most useful in providing "opportunities, support, and cues to help people develop healthier behaviors" (Brownson, Haire-Joshu, & Luke, 2006, p. 342). As such, they help remove barriers in the environment. "Environmental barriers in a community can make modifying unhealthy behaviors challenging. Poor environmental quality; inadequate access to affordable, nutritious food; and safety issues often make healthy living impractical" (Flores, Davis, & Culross, 2007, para. 4). In other words, environmental change strategies are about creating health-enhancing environments (Hunnicutt & Leffelman, 2006). In the 1986 *Ottawa Charter for Health Promotion,* it was stated that the healthier choice should be the easier choice (WHO, 2009). Removing environmental barriers often helps to make the healthier choice the easier choice.

Environmental change strategies are characterized by changes "around" individuals and are not limited to the physical environment. Other environments include the economic environment (e.g., financial costs, affordability), service environment (e.g., accessibility to health care or patient education), social environment (e.g., social support, peer pressure), cultural environment (e.g., traditions of ethnic group), psychological environment (e.g., emotional learning environment), and political environment (e.g., support for healthy environments). Environmental change strategies have a close relationship to health policy/enforcement strategies because there are times when a policy change may be needed to make a change in the environment, for example a city or county ordinance that creates smokefree workplaces. Other examples of such strategies include equipping automobiles with safety belts, air bags, and child safety seats; placing speed bumps in parking lots by playgrounds to slow traffic where children are present; or installing fire and safety doors in apartment buildings to make them safer for the residents. Often environmental change strategies do not necessarily require action on the part of the priority population (CDC, 2003) as noted in the examples above. Yet, some of these strategies provide a "forced choice" situation, as when the selection of foods and beverages in vending machines or cafeterias are changed to include only healthful foods. If people want to eat foods from these places, they are forced to eat certain types of foods.

Other activities in this category may provide those in the priority population with health messages and environmental cues for certain types of behavior. Examples would be posting of no-smoking signs, eliminating ashtrays, providing lockers and showers, using role modeling by others, playing soft music in a work area, organizing a shuttle service or some other type of transportation system to get seniors to congregate for meals or to a health care provider, and providing point-of-purchase education, such as a sign on a vending machine or food labeling on the food options in the cafeteria.

Finally, like so many of the other intervention strategies, environmental change strategies often are more effective when combined with intervention strategies from the other categories. An example of such multiplicity is combining the mandating of safety belts in automobiles, which is important alone, with strict enforcement of safety belt laws (a health policy/enforcement strategy), which makes for a much more effective intervention.

Health-Related Community Service Strategies

Health-related community service strategies include services, tests, treatments, or care to improve the health of those in the priority population (CDC, 2003). Examples of this type of intervention strategy include, but are not limited to, completing a health risk assessment (HRA) form (see Chapter 4 for a discussion of HRAs); offering low-cost flu shots or child immunizations; providing clinical screenings (sometimes called biometric screenings) for diabetes, blood pressure, or cholesterol; and providing professional health checkups and examinations. Because a health-related community service strategy requires action on the part of those in the priority population, an important component of this type of strategy is to reduce the barriers to obtaining the service. Thus planners must be mindful of the affordability and accessibility of such services. Also, planners must weigh the consequences of including this type of strategy in an intervention. For example, if abnormal readings are found during a screening, those conducting the screening have an ethical obligation to follow up and make sure appropriate referrals for care are made. Chapman (2003a) has provided a nice review of many of the concerns associated with biometric screening.

Health-related community service strategies are often offered in settings such as grocery stores, shopping malls, health fairs, worksites, personal residencies, mobile units (e.g., vans equipped with mammography units), and easily accessible health care facilities. Such strategies usually have high credibility with priority populations because of their link with health care providers.

Community Mobilization Strategies

"Community mobilization strategies involve helping communities identify and take action on shared concerns using participatory decision making, and include such methods as empowerment" (Barnes, Neiger, & Thackeray, 2003, p. 60). In this book we present two subcategories of community mobilization strategies: (1) community organization and community building, and (2) community advocacy.

Community Organization and Community Building
Other than defining the terms *community organization* and *community building*, little will be presented here about

these terms because more information is presented elsewhere (Chapter 9). **Community organization** has been defined as "the process by which community groups are helped to identify common problems or goals, mobilize resources, and in other ways develop and implement strategies for reaching the goals they have collectively set" (Minkler & Wallerstein, 2005, p. 26). **Community building** is not so much a process as "an orientation to community that is strength based rather than need based and stresses the identification, nurturing, and celebration of community assets" (Minkler, 2005a, p. 4).

Community Advocacy   Community advocacy is a process in which the people of the community become involved in the institutions and decisions that will have an impact on their lives. It has the potential for creating more support, keeping people informed, influencing decisions, activating nonparticipants, improving service, and making people, plans, and programs more responsive (Checkoway, 1989). Community advocacy can have a big impact on social change issues, including those dealing with health. The community advocacy that deals with health issues is called **health advocacy**. This type of advocacy has been defined as "the processes by which the actions of individuals or groups attempt to bring about social, environmental, and/or organizational change on behalf of a particular health goal, program, interest, or population" (Joint Committee on Terminology, 2012). Galer-Unti, Tappe, and Lachenmayr (2004) have identified seven different ways of advocating for health and health education: (1) influencing voting behavior, (2) electioneering, (3) direct lobbying, (4) integrating grassroots lobbying into direct lobbying efforts, (5) using the Internet, (6) media advocacy—newspaper letters to the editor and opinion-editorial (op-ed) articles, and (7) media advocacy—acting as a resource person. They have further organized these seven advocacy strategies in a three-tiered approach to show the varying levels of involvement in the advocacy process. These levels and examples of each are presented in **Table 8.4**.

As noted in our earlier discussion of health communication strategies, the Internet and emerging technologies can be effective means to enhance advocacy efforts. Thackeray and Hunter (2010) have suggested that cell phones and social networking sites (SNS) on the Internet can be used for: (1) recruiting people to join the cause, (2) organizing collective action, (3) raising awareness and shaping attitudes, (4) raising funds to support the cause, and (5) communicating with decision makers. While both cell phones and SNS can be used for these advocacy-related purposes there are advantages and disadvantages to using one over the other in various situations. **Table 8.5** outlines the comparative qualities of each.

Auld (1997) offered a set of practical tips for influencing public policy. They are adapted here to apply to influencing public policy at the local as well as the state and federal levels.

1. *Opening doors.* Establish relationships that build trust and rapport with staff, legislative assistants, and, if possible, the elected officials themselves so that you can approach them for their support on an issue of concern. Know what committees your elected officials sit on and how they have voted on the issues.

2. *Identifying the players.* Identify who the stakeholders are on a particular issue and find out why they are.

Table 8.4 Advocacy Strategies: Good, Better, Best

Strategy	Good	Better	Best
Voting behavior	Register and vote	Encourage others to register and vote	Register others to vote
Electioneering	Contribute to the campaign of a candidate friendly to public health and health education	Campaign for a candidate friendly to public health and health education	Run for office or seek a political appointment
Direct lobbying	Contact a policy maker	Meet with your policy makers	Develop ongoing relationships with your policy makers and their staff
Integrate grassroots lobbying into direct lobbying activities	Start a petition drive to advocate a specific policy in your local community	Get on the agenda for a meeting of a policy-making body and provide testimony	Organize a community coalition to enact changes that influence health
Use the Internet	Use the Internet to access information related to health issues	Build a Webpage that calls attention to a specific health issue, policy, or legislative proposal	Teach others to use the Internet for advocacy activities
Media advocacy: Newspaper letters to the editor and op-ed articles	Write a letter to the editor	Write an op-ed piece	Teach others to write letters and op-ed pieces for media advocacy
Media advocacy: Acting as a resource person	Respond to requests by members of the media for health-related information	Issue a news release	Develop and maintain ongoing relationships with the media personnel

Source: "Advocacy 100: Getting Started in Health Education Advocacy" by Regina A. Galer-Unti, Marlene K. Tappe, and Sue Lachenmayr from *Health Promotion Practice, (3)*, pp. 283-288. Copyright © 2004 by Society for Public Health Education. Reprinted with Permission.

3. *Making the link.* Find out how the issues you are interested in are linked to the health problems of the population/constituency of the elected officials. For example, if you are interested in chronic diseases, show how they are linked to the elderly in the population/constituency.

4. *Crafting your position.* Make sure your position on the issue(s) is (are) developed on the best available science and data.

5. *Organizing the troops.* Organize others who may be interested in your issue to show broad representation from the population/constituency (see Chapter 9 for organizing techniques).

Table 8.5 Comparative Qualities of Social Networking Sites and Cell Phones in Advocacy

Technology	Advantages for Advocacy	Disadvantages for Advocacy
Social Networking Sites	Message sent on SNS can be stored indefinitely	Not all advocates may be able to attend in-person events because of geographic distances inherent in an online community
	Easy to invite friends and fans to join the advocacy cause	Older decision makers may not give as much credence to this form of communication
	Can organize events and post specifics about location, time, and purpose	Requires Internet access
	Reach a large number of people quickly	
	One central location for advocates to find information about the advocacy cause	
	Can post videos or photos	
	Unlimited space to post information	
	Can update posts from a Web-enabled cell phone or mobile device	
	Can check posts from a Web-enabled cell phone or mobile device	
Cell Phones	Reach a large number of people quickly in real-time	A text or video message may be quickly erased
	Text or video message will be received immediately	Decision makers may not be able to answer the phone when in a meeting
	Can use phones to take photos	Have to limit messages to 160 characters
	Decision maker can read a text message while in a meeting	Advocates' cell phone calling plans may be limited by the number of text messages they can send
	Can be used to send quick, brief reminders of events	Not all advocates may own a cell phone
	No need for Internet access	Cell phone numbers may be changed and contact with advocates is lost.
	Can talk to the other individual in person.	
	Can forward text or video messages to friends and other advocates	

Source: "Empowering Youth: Use of Technology in Advocacy to Affect Social Change." R. Thackeray and M. Hunter, M, from the *Journal of Computer–Mediated Communication, Volume 15*, pp. 575–591. Copyright © 2010 by John Wiley & Sons, Inc. Reprinted with permission.

6. *Visiting policy makers.* Schedule appointments with the elected official or staff to express your views on the issues. Take others with you who can help explain your views. Be on time, be brief, yet be prepared to educate by using practical examples.

7. *Demonstrating the power of press.* Demonstrate your link to the media and how you and your organization can get positive press for the elected official by activating (i.e., letters to the editor, etc.) your link.

8. *Reinforcing your message.* End your visit or follow up the visit with a packet that summarizes your position on the issues. Supporting scientific data should be included. Also, send a thank-you letter. As the issue moves through the legislative process, let your elected official know your views on its direction.

9. *Serving as a resource.* Stay in contact with the staff and elected official and offer to be a resource person to help them as needed on the issue.

10. *Responding quickly.* Be prepared to respond quickly when asked to be a resource person or testify to a legislative group. Requests often come at the last minute.

11. *Reaching the finish line.* Follow up on a piece of legislation after it has been passed to help those who have to implement it and to advocate for funding to help the implementation.

To further assist planners with community advocacy activities, the Coalition of National Health Education Organizations (CNHEO) maintains a Website for advocacy information. The Website features advocacy alerts, how to take action, health legislation, links to other advocacy sites, and other policy tools for health education and health promotion (CNHEO, 2011b). See the *Weblinks* at the end of this chapter for more information about the site.

Other Strategies

The other strategies category includes a variety of intervention activities that do not fit neatly into one of the six categories discussed above.

Behavior Modification Activities   Behavior modification activities, often used in intrapersonal-level interventions, include techniques intended to help those in the priority population experience a change in behavior. *Behavior modification* is usually thought of as a systematic procedure for changing a specific behavior. The process is based on the stimulus response and social cognitive theories. As applied to health behavior, emphasis is placed on a specific behavior that one might want either to increase (such as exercise or stress management techniques) or to decrease (such as smoking or consumption of fats). Particular attention is then given to changing the events that are antecedent or subsequent to the behavior that is to be modified.

In changing a health behavior, the behavior modification activity often begins by having those trying to make a change keep records (diaries, logs, or journals) for a specific period of time (24 to 48 hours, one week, or one month) concerning the behavior (such as eating, smoking, or exercise) they want to alter. Using the information recorded, one can plan an activity to modify that behavior. For example, facilitators of smoking cessation programs often will ask participants to keep a record of all the cigarettes they smoke from one class session to the next (see **Figure 8.4** for an example of such a record). After keeping the record, participants are asked to analyze it to see what kind of smoking habit they have. They may be asked questions such as: "What three cigarettes seem to be the most important of the day to you?" "In what three places or activities do you find yourself smoking the most?" "With whom do you find yourself smoking most often?" "Is there a primary reason or mood for your smoking?" "When during the day do you find yourself smoking the most and the least?" Once the participant has answered these questions, appropriate interventions can be designed to deal with the problem behavior. For example, if participants say they smoke only when they are by themselves, then activities would be planned so that they do not spend a lot of time alone. If other participants seem to do most of their smoking while drinking coffee, an activity would be developed to provide some type of substitute. If participants seem to smoke the most while sitting at the table after meals, activities could be planned to get them away from the table and doing something that would occupy their hands.

Another way of leading into a behavior modification activity is through a health status evaluation, or what is often referred to as a *health screening*. Such screenings could happen at home (e.g., BSE, TSE, hemocult), at a community health fair (e.g., blood pressure, cholesterol), or in the office of a health care professional (e.g., breast examination). Like record keeping via diaries, logs, or journals, health screenings can "grab the attention" (develop awareness) of those in the priority population to begin the behavior modification process.

Organizational Culture Activities   Closely aligned with environmental change strategies are activities that affect organizational culture. Culture is usually associated with norms and traditions that are generated by and linked to a "community" of people. Organizations, which are made up of people, also can have their own culture. The culture of an organization can be thought of as its personality. The culture expresses what is and what is not considered important to the organization. "Cultural norms are not statistical averages, but instead are related to social standards of appropriate behavior. Cultural norms are accepted and expected practice" (Golaszewski et al., 2008, p. 7). The nature of the culture depends on the type of organization—corporation, school, or nonprofit group and the importance that the organization's leadership places on it. For example, if organizational decision makers believe exercise is important, they may provide employees with an extra 20 minutes at lunchtime for exercise. Similarly, it is surprising to see how many young executives will use a corporation's exercise facility because the chief executive officer does. Other examples of organizational culture activities might include changing the types of foods found in vending machines, closing the "junk food" machines during lunch periods at school, offering discounts on the health foods found in the company cafeteria, and getting retailers to change the way they have done things in the past, such as moving their tobacco products from in front of a counter to behind a counter, so that an employee has to get them for the customer.

Like other health promotion strategies, the use of organizational culture activities should begin with an assessment. The term that has been given to assessments associated with organizational culture is a *culture* (or *cultural*) *audit*. A **cultural audit** is an evaluation of the assumptions, values, normative philosophies, and cultural characteristics of an organization in order to determine whether they support or hinder

Name _____

Date _____

Number of Cigarettes During the Day	Time of Day	Need Rating*	Place of Activity	With Whom	Mood or Reason
1.	_____	1 2 3	_____	_____	_____
2.	_____	1 2 3	_____	_____	_____
3.	_____	1 2 3	_____	_____	_____
4.	_____	1 2 3	_____	_____	_____
5.	_____	1 2 3	_____	_____	_____
6.	_____	1 2 3	_____	_____	_____
7.	_____	1 2 3	_____	_____	_____
8.	_____	1 2 3	_____	_____	_____
9.	_____	1 2 3	_____	_____	_____
10.	_____	1 2 3	_____	_____	_____
11.	_____	1 2 3	_____	_____	_____
12.	_____	1 2 3	_____	_____	_____
13.	_____	1 2 3	_____	_____	_____
14.	_____	1 2 3	_____	_____	_____
15.	_____	1 2 3	_____	_____	_____
16.	_____	1 2 3	_____	_____	_____
17.	_____	1 2 3	_____	_____	_____
18.	_____	1 2 3	_____	_____	_____
19.	_____	1 2 3	_____	_____	_____
20.	_____	1 2 3	_____	_____	_____
21.	_____	1 2 3	_____	_____	_____
22.	_____	1 2 3	_____	_____	_____
23.	_____	1 2 3	_____	_____	_____
24.	_____	1 2 3	_____	_____	_____
25.	_____	1 2 3	_____	_____	_____
26.	_____	1 2 3	_____	_____	_____
27.	_____	1 2 3	_____	_____	_____
28.	_____	1 2 3	_____	_____	_____
29.	_____	1 2 3	_____	_____	_____
30.	_____	1 2 3	_____	_____	_____

*Need rating: How important is the cigarette to you at this time?

    1 = Most important; I would miss it very much

    2 = Average

    3 = Least important; I would not miss it

Figure 8.4 Twenty-Four-Hour Cigarette Count

that organization's central mission (BusinessDictionary.com, 2011). When applied to health the audit would help determine whether the culture hinders or supports health promotion. There are companies that will perform health culture audits for organizations (Note: search the Internet with key words "health culture audit" for sources). In addition, the Wellness Council of America (WELCOA) has created a free WELCOA Quick-Inventory (Hunnicutt, 2009) as a means to help assess the environment of a workplace.

Once the status of the organizational culture has been determined there are several steps that can be taken to work toward a health supporting culture. Golaszewski and his colleagues (2008) have identified the following influences on an organization's health supporting culture: (1) shaping cultural health values (e.g., raise the visibility of benefits of healthy lifestyles, raise the visibility of leadership promoting healthy lifestyles, encourage employee forums where they can discuss health, showcase the organization's involvement in health promotion); (2) shaping cultural health norms (e.g., identify key norms for health promotion in the organization, conduct interviews of those in the priority population to determine support or lack thereof for a healthy culture, evaluate idea versus actual norm levels); (3) use cultural touch points (e.g., mechanisms that support a healthy culture like committing resources to health, leaders' modeling healthy lifestyles, rewards and recognitions for health, include health promoting ideas in organizational recruitment, orientation, training, communication, relationships, and rites, symbols, and rituals); (4) encourage peer support (e.g., mobilize existing support systems, develop mutual support systems); and (5) building a supportive cultural climate for wellness (e.g., foster a sense of community, foster a shared vision, foster a positive outlook, and foster cultural climate with health promotion).

Incentives and Disincentives   The use of incentives (sometimes referred to as "carrots") and disincentives (sometimes referred to as "sticks") to influence health behaviors is a common type of activity, especially in worksite settings. An **incentive** is "an anticipated positive or desirable reward designed to influence the performance of an individual or group" (Chapman, 2005a, p. 6). An incentive can increase the perceived value of an activity (Patton et al., 1986), motivate people to get involved, encourage health service use behavior (Chapman, 2005a), encourage compliance with professional health advice (Chapman, 2005a), remind program participants of their commitment to and goals for behavior change (Wilbur, 1983), promote short-term behavior change (French, Jeffery, & Oliphant, 1994; Robison, 1998), and maintain behavior change over time (Pescatello et al., 2001; Poole, Kumpfer, & Pett, 2001). The key to motivating people with incentives is knowing what will incite them to action. Thus for this type of activity to work, the planners need to match the incentives with the needs, wants, or desires of the priority population. However, this is not easy, for what is an incentive for one person may be a deterrent for another, and vice versa. If planners are not in touch with what program participants want, there is a chance of losing participant interest in the program (Hunnicutt, 2001). It has been suggested that incentives should even be tailored to the socioeconomic characteristics of the participants (Chenoweth, 1987) and, for that matter, the individual characteristics of each person. For example, a financial incentive will typically generate less response from wealthy participants than lower income participants (Haveman, 2010).

For program planners, the task becomes one of matching the needs of the program participant or potential program participant with available incentives. Two approaches can be used to accomplish this. The first is to include questions about incentives as part of any needs assessment conducted in program planning. For example, a workforce needs survey or focus group might include a question on incentives, such as "What incentives would entice you to participate in the exercise program?" or "What would it take to get you to participate in this program?" or "What would it take to keep you involved in a health promotion program?" or "Would you continue to participate in an exercise program if you knew you were going to be given a nice T-shirt after logging 100 miles running or walking, or participating for 50 days in a yoga class or swimming program?" The responses to these questions should provide some indication of the type of incentives that would be most appropriate for this priority population. The second is the shotgun approach, based on previous experience or the experience reported by others. The shotgun approach offers a variety of incentives to meet the needs of a large percentage of the program's priority population. However, the former approach is recommended as being more likely to meet the targeted needs and wants.

Based on the idea that incentives should meet the individual needs of those in the priority population, the possibility of different types of incentives is almost endless. Incentives are usually grouped into two major categories: financial and nonfinancial. Some examples of financial incentives include providing money in the form of extra pay, bonuses, or rebates (Chapman 2005a; Haveman, 2010; Pescatello et al., 2001; Poole, Kumpfer, & Pett, 2001); paying membership fees to health-related facilities (Chapman, 2005a); giving gift certificates; or reducing health insurance premiums or deductibles. Examples of nonfinancial incentives include giving special attention or recognition (e.g., name mentioned in a newsletter) (Chapman, 2005a; Haveman, 2010), social support, or providing additional vacation days or "well" days (Chapman, 2005a; Haveman, 2010).

Haveman (2010) has offered six principles that can assist program planners in creating effective incentives. His principles were intended for use with incentives associated with the delivery of health care, but we have adapted them to health promotion. Principle one is identifying the desired outcome. This may seem obvious but is often overlooked. For example, if the desired outcome is to have program participants stop smoking, the incentives should be tied to actually quitting and not just cutting back on the number of cigarettes smoked per day. The second principle is identifying the behavior change that will lead to the desired outcome. In the smoking cessation example, participants need to come up with a strategy to quit smoking, actually stop, and stay off cigarettes for a specified period of time. Principle three is determining the potential effectiveness of the incentive in achieving the behavior change. This is not easy because responsiveness to incentives varies greatly. "Understanding this response involves determining the extent to which the behavior targeted is amenable to change through the incentive. The size of the financial incentive should be appropriate to the effort required. If the perceived benefit of the action is exceeded by its perceived cost, the incentive will be ineffective" (Haveman, 2010, p. 2). (See **Box 8.6** for a list of factors that determine the effectiveness incentives.) The fourth principle is to link the incentive directly to the desired outcome or behavior. In the smoking cessation example, any incentive should be linked to either the final outcome—no smoking for one year after the quit date—or to the actions leading up to it, for example, setting a

> **Box 8.6** FACTORS THAT DETERMINE THE EFFECTIVENESS OF WELLNESS INCENTIVES

Major Factors	Minor Factors
Dollar value of the reward(s)	Importance to supervisor
Convertibility into item of personal value	Degree of fun experienced
Amount of effort needed to qualify	Language compatibility
Clarity of messaging	Convenience of record keeping
Timing and repetition of messaging	Amount of change in benefits
Extent of distrust in employers' motives	Availability of alternative standards
Supporting messages from management	Credibility of wellness staff
Ease of enrollment	Use of outside vendor
Perceived complexity of requirements	Adequacy of FAQs
Fairness and defensibility of requirements	Availability of FAQs
Group or competitive nature	Treatment of "gamers"
Desirability of required behavior	Utility of program documents
Readiness composition of population	Tax implications
Combination of pay values	Option to ask questions
Spousal eligibility	Time of the year
Compatibility of incentives with culture	Generational effects
Past wellness incentive performance	Reporting back to employees

Source: "The Changing role of incentives in health promotion and wellness." L. S. Chapman, D. Whitehead, and M. C. Connors, from *The Art of Health Promotion*. Copyright © 2008 by *American Journal of Health Promotion*. Reprinted with permission.

quit date, deciding on a strategy to quit, actually quitting, not smoking for six months, and not smoking for one year. If the second option is used, an incentive could be attached to each step. Further if this second option is used the incentives could be graduated so that incentives are worth more than the one given at the previous step. Principle five is identifying any possible adverse effects of the incentive. In the smoking cessation example, nonsmokers may say that they have no chance to receive a smoking cessation incentive. So how could those creating the incentive deal with this situation? The sixth, and final, principle is to evaluate and report changes in the behavior or outcome in response to the incentive. If a case is going to be made for using incentives as part of health promotion programs in the future, planners will need to document their work and show that the incentives, at least in part, were responsible for the outcomes or desired behavior.

The following advice is offered to planners who choose to use incentives:

1. Make sure the incentive will do no harm. "The golden rule of any policy is to ensure that its net result is salutary. Attention must first be devoted to understanding and assessing potential detrimental consequences, including consequences of inaccuracy and misuse, and taking steps to avoid them" (McGinnis, 2010, p. 3).

2. Make sure everyone can receive one, whatever the incentive may be (Kendall, 1984).

3. Make the incentives useful and meaningful (Kendall, 1984).

4. Ensure that the incentive ground rules are fair, understandable, and followed by everyone (Chapman 2005a; Kendall, 1984).

5. Develop (and refine) a communications plan for the incentives (Chapman, 2005a; Chapman, Whitehoad, & Connors, 2008).

6. Make a big deal of awarding the incentive; consider a special meeting or ceremony (Hunnicutt, 2001; McGinnis, 2010).

7. Use incentives that are consistent with health promotion philosophies. For example, avoid incentives of alcoholic beverages, high fat or high sugar foods, or other mixed-message prizes.

Just as incentives can be used to get people involved in behavior change, *disincentives* can be used to discourage a certain behavior. More formally, **disincentives** have been defined as "an anticipated negative or undesirable consequence designed to influence the performance of an individual or group" (Chapman, 2005a, p. 6). For example, "[s]ustained increases in excise taxes, constraining advertising and marketing, constricting use in public places, and penalizing the sale and distribution to minors have all worked to help drive down the use of tobacco" (McGinnis et al., 2002, pp. 88–89).

One final note that we need to mention before leaving this topic is the impact that federal legislation has had on incentives and disincentives. As we noted at the beginning of this section, though incentives and disincentives have been used in health promotion programs in a variety of settings, they have been used with great favor in worksite settings. Up until 1996, there were few limitations on how incentive and disincentives were structured (Chapman, 2005a) and because of this some employers were creatively tying incentives and disincentives associated with health to individual and group health insurance plans. However, Congress was concerned that employers were being unfair to some employees in order to reduce their health care costs. Accordingly, Congress enacted two pieces of legislation that have impacted the way incentives and disincentives can be used. They include the Health Insurance Portability & Accountability Act of 1996 (more commonly referred to as HIPAA) and the Genetic Information Nondiscrimination Act of 2008 (officially known as Public Law 110-233 and referred to as GINA). HIPAA has provisions in it that make it illegal for employers to discriminate against their employees because of a "health status related factor" with the outcome of affecting coverage or cost to the employee under a group or individual health plan (Chapman, 2005a). That is, those who offer and administer health insurance plans cannot deny health care claim expenses, charge some employees more for their health insurance premiums, or place a surcharge on their premiums because of health status related conditions like high blood pressure, high blood cholesterol, or poor vision. For example, an employer cannot require employees to pay higher premiums than their coworkers because they have high blood pressure. However, the law does not preclude offering incentives—in the form of premium discounts or rebates or modifying applicable co-payments or deductibles—to those who participate in health promotion programs. So an employer could reduce employees' co-payment on a visit to a doctor or on the cost of a prescription medication if the employees participated in the company's employee health promotion program.

GINA, which amends portions of HIPAA by treating genetic information as *protected health information* (PHI), prohibits discrimination in health coverage and employment based on genetic information. GINA went into effect for health care plans starting on or after December 7, 2009. Though the bulk of GINA is aimed at health care coverage provided by employers, it also impacts health promotion/wellness programs. The area of health promotion programming that it most affected is the use of health risk assessments (HRAs). HRAs cannot request genetic information prior to enrollment in a health care "plan, and no rewards or penalties may be offered in conjunction with an HRA that requests genetic information, even if the request is made after the enrollment" (Grudzien, 2009, para. 6). As a result of these regulations, planners "should review all wellness and disease management plans to determine how a HRA is used and what information is requested; remove any financial incentives or penalties if genetic information is collected in the HRA; and remove any genetic information from the HRA if financial incentives or penalties want to be offered" (Grudzien, 2009, para. 6).

Social Activities   The importance of social support for behavior change and its relationship to health are well recognized (e.g., IOM, 2001). Many people find it much easier to change a behavior if those around them provide support or are willing to be partners in the behavior change process. One of the major reasons why worksite health promotion programs were initially so well received is because of the built-in social support from coworkers (Behrens, 1983).

Reference has already been made to how social support could work as an incentive. That would be one form of a social activity. Other social interventions could include support groups or buddy system, social gatherings, and social networks.

Support Groups and Buddy System   The importance of support groups as part of comprehensive interventions has been well established. One need only look to the 12-step programs (such as Alcoholics Anonymous, Overeaters Anonymous, and Gamblers Anonymous) and commercial programs (such as Weight Watchers) to realize the importance of people coming together to share their experiences and support one another's efforts. A support group need not be large; it might be as small as just two people. A buddy system is an example of a two-person group. A buddy system can take one of two different forms. In the first, both individuals are trying to change a behavior. In such a relationship, the two individuals support each other, whether this means helping each other stay on a special diet or meeting each other at 6 A.M. for exercise. In the other form, only one of the two is trying to change a behavior. The one not changing the behavior may have already changed (e.g., has already quit smoking or is exercising regularly) and is acting as a mentor to the one trying to change, or may not be trying to change but provides support at regular intervals or as problems arise.

To enhance the motivation provided by support groups and buddy systems it is not uncommon for these activities to also use a *contest* (also referred to competitions or challenges) or a *contract*. A **contest** can be described as a challenge between two individuals/groups in which the object is to outperform the competitor. Examples of contests include the competition between two individuals to see who can lose the most weight, who can walk/run the most miles, or who can go the longest without a cigarette. Contests could also be based on teams within the priority population (such as two different companies, two schools, or departments within an organization), using similar criteria but now based on group total figures (pounds, miles, or cigarettes). Contests have been useful in introducing and promoting health promotion programs and achieving significant initial participation rates, but they have not been as useful as an ongoing recruitment tool (Wilson, 1990).

A **contract** is an agreement between two or more parties that outlines the future behavior of those parties. Contracts are a common part of everyday living. People enter into contracts when they sign a lease for an apartment or a residence hall agreement, take out an insurance policy, borrow money, or buy something over a period of time. The same concept can be applied to getting and keeping people motivated in health promotion programs. Program participants would enter into a contract with another person (the program facilitator, a significant other, or a fellow participant) and then work toward an objective or agreement specified in the contract. The contract would also specify **contingencies**—that is, what happens as a result of the contract's term either being met or not being met.

For an exercise program, this system might work as follows: The program participant and program facilitator would draw up a contract based on the participant's present status in the program (e.g., exercising for 30 minutes once a week) and on what would be a reasonable goal for the near future (e.g., eight weeks). Thus the contract might state that the participant will exercise for 30 minutes twice a week for the first week, 30 minutes three times a week for the second week, and so forth, building up gradually to the final goal of exercising for 60 minutes most days of the week at the end of eight weeks. The outcome should focus on a behavior that can be maintained at the end of the contract period. For a weight loss program, the goal might be written as eliminating snacking in the evening, increasing fruits and vegetables in the diet to five servings per day, and walking for 30 minutes three times a week. These are behaviors that can reasonably be maintained after the weight loss.

The parties to the contract then decide on what the contingencies will be. Thus the participant might offer to make a contribution to some local charity or state that she will continue in the program for another eight weeks if she does not meet the contract goal. The facilitator might promise the participant a program T-shirt if she fulfills the contract during the specified eight-week period. Other ideas for contingencies might include granting a kickback on fees for completing a certain percentage of the classes, or earning points toward products or services. No matter what the contingencies are, it seems to help if the contract is completed in writing.

Social Gatherings   Social gatherings can be an important type of social intervention. Bringing together people who may be confronting similar problems for the purpose of purely social interaction not related to the problem can indirectly help them deal with the problem. Examples of such activities might be single parents having a cookout or a group of senior citizens attending a play. Although these gatherings do not deal directly with these people's common problems, they do help fill voids in their lives and thus indirectly help with the problem.

Social Networks   Social networks are another type of social intervention. A *network* "is the web of social relationships that surrounds an individual and the structural characteristics of that web" (IOM, 2001, p. 145). The nature of the structural characteristics can be quite varied, consisting of almost anything that creates a special feeling: need, concern, loyalty, frustration, power, affection, or obligation, to name just a few. When people are "networking," they are said to be looking for relationships that would be useful in helping them with their concerns, such as problem solving, program development, resource identification, and others. As part of a health promotion intervention, social networking may take many different forms and can range from informal networking where participants create relations on their own to more formal networking where program participants are "assigned" others with whom to network. The actual networking itself may take place face-to-face, via the telephone, or through some type of social media. An example would be when program smoking cessation participants trade contact information (e.g., email address, telephone numbers, or "friend" another) for the purpose of connecting when trying to resist a cigarette or trying to locate a needed resource to solve a problem.

It should also be noted that although most social support and buddy systems take place between individuals, they can also be established at the institutional level. Like individuals, institutions can be paired up to help one another. For example, if two companies are interested in establishing health promotion programs, they could work together on their programs and share information and resources where appropriate. Or, if one company has a well-established program in place, then that company could mentor another company in setting up a program.

Creating Health Promotion Interventions

Once program planners have completed a needs assessment, written program goals and objectives, and considered different types of intervention strategies, they are in a position to begin designing an appropriate intervention.

Criteria and Guidelines for Developing Health Promotion Interventions

There is no one best way of intervening to accomplish a specific program goal that can be generalized to all priority populations. Each priority population has unique needs and wants that must be addressed. Nevertheless, successful and responsible health promotion programs generally adhere to some common set of guidelines, standards, or criteria around which their interventions are planned (Ad Hoc Work Group, 1987). Such guidelines help standardize and ensure the quality of the program, give credibility to a program, help with program accountability, provide a legal defense if a liability situation might arise, and identify ethical concerns that need to be addressed as a part of planning, implementing, and evaluating programs.

In 1987, the American Public Health Association (APHA), in collaboration with the Center for Health Promotion and Education of the Centers for Disease Control (CDC), developed a set of criteria to serve as guidelines for establishing the feasibility and/or the appropriateness of health promotion programs in a variety of settings (industrial, hospital, worksite, voluntary and official agencies) before making a decision to implement them. The criteria were not developed to assure successful programs, but rather to suggest issues that need to be considered in the decision-making process leading to the allocation of resources or the setting of program priorities (Ad Hoc Work Group, 1987, pp. 89–92). The five criteria suggested by the Work Group are:

1. A health promotion program should address one or more risk factors that are carefully defined, measurable, modifiable, and prevalent among the members of a chosen target group, and these factors that constitute a threat to the health status and the quality of life of target group members.

2. A health promotion program should reflect a consideration of the special characteristics, needs, and preferences of its target group(s).

3. Health promotion programs should include interventions that will clearly and effectively reduce a target risk factor and are appropriate for a particular setting.

4. A health promotion program should identify and implement interventions that make optimum use of the available resources.

5. From the outset, a health promotion program should be organized, planned, and implemented in such a way that its operation and effects can be evaluated.

In addition to the criteria set forth by APHA and CDC, other agencies and organizations have suggested criteria and guidelines. The Society of Prospective Medicine has developed the Ethics Guidelines for the Development and Use of Health Assessments (SPMBoD, 1999). Some organizations and professionals have set guidelines, criteria, or **codes of practice** for specific types of health promotion programs. Examples are the criteria set forth by the American College of Sports Medicine (ACSM, 2010) for exercise programs, the guidelines established by the American College of Obstetricians and Gynecologists for exercise during pregnancy, the clinical practice guidelines for smoking cessation available from the Agency for Healthcare Research and Quality (AHRQ, 2008), guidelines and criteria for the implementation of community-based health promotion programs for individuals with disabilities (Drum et al., 2009), and recommendations and guidelines for HIV/AIDS prevention (CDC, 2010d). Obviously, these guidelines and criteria are not all that are available. Prudent planners should seek out, through inquiry and networking, other criteria and guidelines that apply to programs they are planning.

Designing Appropriate Interventions

Selection of interventions for a health promotion program should be based on a sound rationale backed by the best available evidence as opposed to chance; a strategy should not be selected just because the planners think it "sounds good" or because they have a "feeling" that it will work. Too often, intervention decisions are "based on perceived short-term opportunities, lacking systematic planning and review of the best evidence regarding effective approaches" (Brownson, Fielding, & Maylahn, 2009, p. 175). As mentioned earlier, planners should choose or create an intervention that will be both effective and efficient. Although no prescription for an appropriate intervention has been developed, experience has indicated that the results of some interventions are more predictable than others. In this section, we present eight major questions that planners need to consider when creating health promotion interventions. **Figure 8.5** summarizes these major considerations.

1. *What needs to change? And, where is the change needed?* Designing an appropriate intervention begins by going back to the early steps in the program planning process and examining the results of the needs assessment and reviewing the goals and objectives of the proposed program. The needs assessment identified the behavioral, environmental, and genetic determinants or risk factors of the health problem. (Note: Remember that because genetic determinants either cannot be changed or often interact with behavior and environment, the planners' focus should be on behavioral and environmental factors.) For example, after identifying the determinants of a health problem, planners then determine the predisposing, enabling, and reinforcing factors that need to be addressed in their proposed program. These factors should be reflected in the program goals and objectives.

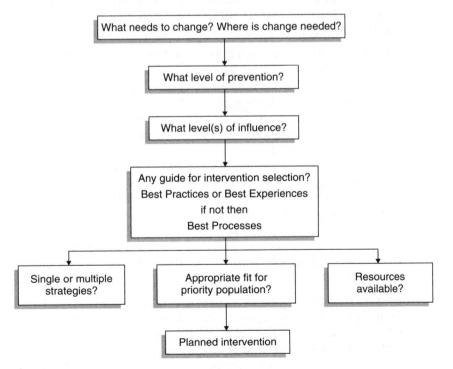

Figure 8.5 Items to Consider When Creating a Health Promotion Intervention

If the single purpose of a program were to increase the awareness of the priority population, the intervention would be very different from what it would be if the purpose were to change behavior.

Knowing what must be changed is critical to creating an intervention, but just as critical is understanding the context in which the change will take place. Understanding the context has been referred to as the *settings approach* (Baric, 1993) to health promotion. More specifically, a settings approach means addressing the contexts (physical, organizational, and social) "within which people live, work, and play and making these the object of inquiry and intervention as well as the needs and capacities of the people found in the different settings" (Poland, Krupa, & McCall, 2009, p. 505). Therefore when creating an intervention, planners need to analyze the setting—"who is there; how they think or operate; implicit social norms, hierarchies of power; accountability mechanisms; local moral, political, and organizational culture; physical and psychosocial environment; broader sociopolitical and economic context, etc." (Poland et al., 2009, p. 506)—to make sure the intervention is a good "fit" for those in the priority population. For those interested in more of what to consider when analyzing the setting, we recommend the questions posed by Poland et al. (2009).

2. *At what level of prevention will the program be aimed?* Because of the needs and wants of those in the priority population, planners need to consider at which level or levels of prevention—primary, secondary, and tertiary—the program will be aimed. For example, a program aimed at increasing the level of exercise is likely to be received differently by asymptomatic nonexercisers (primary prevention) than by a patient recovering from a heart attack (tertiary prevention).

3. *At what level(s) of influence will the intervention be focused?* Program planners must recognize that those in the priority population "live in social, political, and economic systems that shape behaviors and access to the resources they need to maintain good health" (Pellmar et al., 2002, p. 210). As such, planners need to decide at what level or levels of influence they can best obtain the goals and objectives of the program. For example, if the goal of the program is to increase safety belt use, can that be best accomplished by trying to intervene at an intrapersonal level with an individual education program, at the institutional level with a company policy, at the public policy level with a enhanced state safety belt law, or at multiple levels? Though it is possible that an intervention can be aimed at a single level of influence, the evidence is mounting that there is a greater chance of changing and maintaining health behaviors if interventions are aimed at multiple levels of influence (Glanz & Bishop, 2010). Therefore, planners need to ask and answer the question, "What levels of influence should be addressed to provide the best chances of achieving the program goal and objectives?"

4. *What types of intervention strategies are known to be effective (i.e., have been successfully used in previous programs) in dealing with the program focus?* In other words, what does the evidence show about the effectiveness of various interventions to deal with the problem that the program is to address? (Refer back to Chapter 2 for the definition of and available sources of evidence.) Using evidence does not mean

finding a specific intervention to deal with the problem but rather going through a process of decision making that is based on the evaluation of reliable data and previous work (Baker, Brownson, Dreisinger, McIntosh, & Karamehic-Muratovic, 2009). To assist planners in identifying the best available evidence, Green and Kreuter (2005) and Brownson and colleagues (2009) have put forth typologies for classifying interventions based on the level of scientific evidence. Green and Kreuter (2005) have suggested three sources of guidance for selecting intervention strategies—best practices, best experiences, and best processes. **Best practices** refer to "recommendations for an intervention, based on critical review of multiple research and evaluation studies that substantiate the efficacy of the intervention in the populations and circumstances in which the studies were done, if not its effectiveness in other populations and situations where it might be implemented" (p. G-1).

When best practice recommendations are not available for use, planners need to look for information on *best experiences*. **Best experience** intervention strategies are those of prior or existing programs that have not gone through the critical research and evaluation studies and thus fall short of best practice criteria but nonetheless show promise in being effective. Best experiences can be found by networking with other professionals and by reviewing the literature.

If neither best practices nor best experiences are available to planners, then the third source of guidance for selecting an intervention strategy is using *best processes*. **Best processes** intervention strategies are original interventions that the planners create based upon their knowledge and skills of good planning processes including the involvement of those in the priority population and appropriate theories and models (see Chapter 7). (See **Table 8.6** for a matrix of aligning objectives, program outcomes, methods, theory, intervention strategies, and activities.)

Whereas the Green and Kreuter (2005) typology for classifying interventions has three levels, the typology put forth by Brownson and colleagues (2009) has four— *evidence-based, effective, promising,* and *emerging.* The first level, evidence-based, includes interventions that are peer reviewed via a systematic or narrative review (e.g., those contained in the *Guide to Community Preventive Services* [CDC, 2011a]). This first level is parallel to the best practices level of Green and Kreuter (2005). The interventions found in the second level, *effective*, have been peer reviewed but are not part of a systematic or narrative review (e.g., article that appears in the scientific literature). Those interventions that are deemed effective via a program evaluation but without formal peer review make up the third level, *promising* (e.g., state or federal government reports that have not gone through peer review). Levels two and three, effective and promising respectively, are parallel to the best experiences described by Green and Kreuter (2005). The fourth and final level is *emerging*. This level includes ongoing works, practice-based summaries, or evaluation works in progress (e.g., pilot studies).

5. *Is the intervention an appropriate fit for the priority population?* Intervention strategies need to be designed to "fit" the priority population. Each priority population has certain characteristics that impact how it will receive an intervention. Two processes that help to "fit" an intervention to the priority population are tailoring and segmenting. The rationale for tailoring an intervention activity is based

Table 8.6 Matrix of Type of Objectives, Program Outcomes, Methods, Theory, Intervention Strategy, and Activities

Type of Objective	Program Outcome	Method	Theory—Construct*	Intervention Strategy	Possible Activities
Learning	• Awareness of risk perception/services/resources	Information	HBM—perceived susceptibility PMT—perceived severity TTM—processes of change	Health communication	• Informational session • Completion of HRA • Brochure on risks
	• Knowledge	Raising awareness Active learning	SCT—expectations SCT—behavioral capability HBM—perceived seriousness HBM—perceived benefits/barriers	Health communication Health education	• Classes, seminars, workshops • Printed materials
		Tailoring	PAPM—stages TTM—stages	Health communication and education	• Classes, seminars, workshops
	• Attitudes	Persuasive communication Processing information	SCT—expectancies TTM—decisional balance ELM—central route TPB—attitude toward the behavior SCT—reinforcement IMB—prevention motivation	Health communication and education	• Classes, seminars, workshops • Panel discussions • Guest speakers
	• Skills	Skills training and practice	SCT/HBM/TTM—self-efficacy TPB—perceived behavioral control SCT—self-control	Health communication and education Behavior modification	• Classes, seminars, workshops • Simulations

Level	Determinant	Construct	Theory	Strategy	Activities
Behavioral	• Behavior	Modeling	SCT—reinforcement		• Scenarios, role playing
		Coping response	C-BMRP—self-control	Incentives	• Determine and provide incentives
		Reinforcement	HBM—cues to action		• 24-hour behavior records
			SRT—punishment/reinforcement	Behavior modification	• Keeping journals
		Counter conditioning	TTM—processes of change	Health communication and education	• Classes, seminars, workshops
				Organizational culture	• Peer education
Environmental	• Physical environment	Modeling	SCT—reinforcement		• Regulations/ordinances
		Facilitation	SCT—reciprocal determinism	Health policy/enforcement	
		Barriers	HBM—perceived barriers	Environmental change	
			C-BMRP—high-risk situation		
	• Social environment	Organizational building	CRM—stages	Community mobilization	• Create a coalition
		Social support	TPB—subjective norm	Social activities	• Create networks/buddies
			SNT—ego/alter	Social Networks	

Abbreviations for theories: C-BMRP = cognitive-behavior model of relapse prevention; CRM = community readiness model; ELM = elaboration likelihood model of persuasion; HBM = health belief model; IMB = information—motivation—behavioral skills model; PAPM = precaution adoption process model; PMT = protection motivation theory; SCT = social cognitive theory; SNT = social network theory; SRT = stimulus response theory; TPB = theory of planned behavior; TTM = transtheoretical model.

on research that shows people pay more attention to information that is personally relevant to them (NCI, 2004). Because we presented information on tailoring earlier in the chapter in our discussion of health communication section, we will use this space to present information on segmenting. **Segmenting** is the process of dividing a broader population into smaller groups with similar characteristics that are likely to exhibit similar behavior/reaction to an intervention (see information in Chapter 11 about segmenting a priority population). Segmentation allows planners to create an intervention to fit the needs and characteristics of a priority population (Pasick, D'Onofrio, & Otero-Sabogal, 1996). Following are a few examples of how priority population segmentation can be applied. If program planners are developing written materials as part of their intervention, they need to make sure that the materials are written at an acceptable reading level for the priority population. From a developmental stage perspective, it is not reasonable to expect kindergartners to sit still for a one-hour lesson. Interventions also need to "fit" culturally within the priority population (Pérez & Luquis, 2008) and be culturally sensitive. Culturally sensitive interventions are those "that are relevant and acceptable within the cultural framework of the population to be reached" (Frankish, Lovato, & Shannon, 1998). In attempts to be culturally sensitive, because culture is often context specific, planners need to be careful not to perpetuate harmful cultural stereotypes.

One final item to consider when thinking about the appropriateness of an intervention strategy for the priority population is to ask if there is any chance that the strategy could cause any unintended effects in the priority population. For example, could the strategy threaten the physical safety or raise undue anxiety in the priority population (CDC, 2003)?

6. *Are the necessary resources available to implement the intervention selected?* Obviously some intervention strategies require more money, time, personnel, or space to implement than others. For example, it may be prudent to provide each person in the priority population with a $100 incentive for participating in the health promotion program, but it may not be possible because of budget limitations.

7. *Would it be better to use an intervention that consists of a single strategy or one that is made up of multiple strategies?* Again, we refer to the principle of multiplicity. A single-strategy intervention would most likely be easier and less expensive to implement and easier to evaluate. There are, however, some real advantages to using several strategies: (1) "hitting" the priority population with a message in a variety of ways from multiple levels of influence; (2) appealing to the variety of learning styles within any priority population; (3) keeping the health message constantly before the priority population; (4) hoping that at least one strategy appeals enough to the priority population to help bring about the expected outcome; (5) appealing to the various senses (such as sight, hearing, or touch) of each individual in the priority population; and (6) increasing the chances that the combined strategies would help reach the goals and objectives of the program (e.g., communication used to publicize a policy change) (CDC, 2003). Probably the biggest drawback to using multiple strategies is the difficulty of separating the effects of one strategy from the effects of others in evaluating the impact of the total

program and of individual components (Ad Hoc Work Group, 1987). However, Glasgow, Vogt, and Boles (1999) have developed an evaluation model titled RE-AIM (acronym for reach, efficacy, adoption, implementation, and maintenance) for use with multistrategy interventions.

Adapting a Health Promotion Intervention

As noted in the previous section of this chapter, planners should use the best available evidence to help create an intervention. Such evidence may show that an intervention was successful in another setting but that setting may be different (e.g., social context or other unique characteristics) than the one in which the planners are currently working. So the question for the planners becomes "Can the intervention that was successful in another setting (i.e., evidence-based intervention [EBI]) be adapted to work in the new setting?" To help answer this question, the CDC's Division of HIV/AIDS, along with some external partners, developed draft guidance to adapt EBIs. The guidance is titled the *Map of Adaption Process: A Systematic Approach for Adapting Evidence-Based Behavioral Interventions* (McKleroy et al., 2006). The approach of this framework emphasizes both the planners' experience working with the priority population and the resources available for adaption and implementation, while still maintaining fidelity to the core elements of the intervention, the theory on which it was based, and internal logic of the original intervention (McKleroy et al., 2006).

The adaptation framework is a five-step approach that is presented graphically in a linear format (see **Figure 8.6**). However, like other planning models presented in this book, the steps are interconnected and thus overlap in terms of their timing and ordering. McKleroy et al. (2006) have presented the following description of the five steps.

> The first action step, assess, involves assessing the target population, the EBIs being considered for implementation, and the agency's capacity to implement the intervention. The second, select, is determining whether to adopt the intervention without adaptation, implement the intervention with adaptation, or choose another intervention and repeating the assess action step before moving forward. The third action step, prepare, falls within the preparation phase and involves actually adapting the intervention materials, pre-testing the adapted materials with the target population, and increasing agency capacity and developing collaborative partnerships when necessary to implement the intervention. The fourth action step, pilot, is pilot testing the adapted intervention or its components if it is not feasible to pilot the entire intervention and developing an implementation plan. The fifth, implement, is conducting the entire adapted intervention with minor revision as needed. Additionally, the guidance includes feedback loops and checkpoints to ensure each action step is addressed adequately, and to provide an opportunity to revisit earlier action steps should difficulties occur. Process monitoring and evaluation, and routine supervision and quality assurance are also important considerations for the guidance. Credible evidence collected during the adaptation process should be evaluated to determine the success of the adaptation process as well as the effectiveness of the adapted intervention (p. 64).

If you are interested in adapting an EBI, we strongly recommend that you review McKleroy et al. (2006) for a more in-depth description and practical examples of the five-step framework.

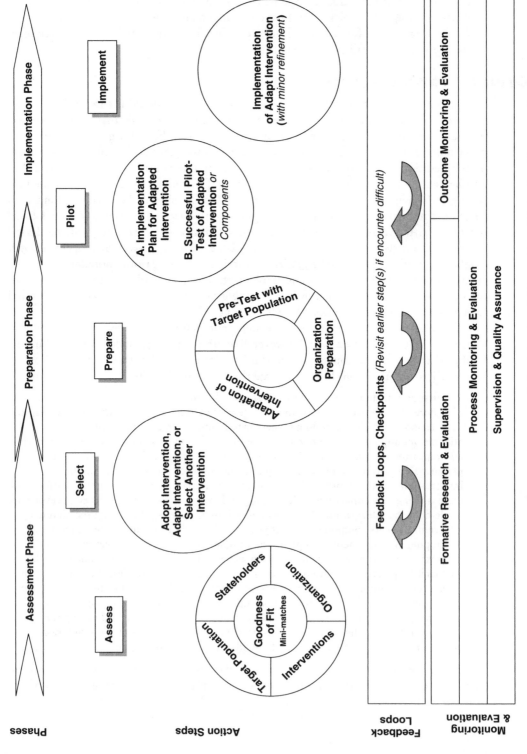

Figure 8.6 Map of Adaptation Process: A Systematic Approach for Adapting Evidence-Based Behavioral Interventions

Source: McKleroy et al. (2006).

SUMMARY

Interventions are strategies used by planners to bring about the outcomes identified in the program objectives. Interventions are also sometimes referred to as *treatments*. Although many times an intervention is made up of a single strategy, it is more common for planners to use a variety of strategies aimed at multiple levels of influence to make up an intervention for a program. In this chapter, intervention strategies were categorized into the following groups:

1. Health communication strategies

2. Health education strategies

3. Health policy/enforcement strategies

4. Environmental change strategies

5. Health-related community service strategies

6. Community mobilization strategies

7. Other strategies

Additionally, this chapter identified the need for program planners to be aware of recommended standards/criteria/guidelines when planning program interventions. Some examples of general, as well as program-specific, guidelines that have been set forth by professional organizations, other groups, and individuals were reviewed. This chapter also presented questions that planners need to consider when creating health promotion interventions. And, finally, the chapter provided an overview of a process for adapting evidence-based interventions for a new setting.

REVIEW QUESTIONS

1. What is an intervention?

2. What are the advantages of using a multistrategy intervention (i.e., principle of multiplicity) over one that includes a single strategy? Are there any disadvantages? If so, what are they?

3. What does *dose* mean in terms of an intervention?

4. What are the major categories of interventions? Explain each.

5. Define each of the following terms as they relate to health education strategies: *curriculum*, *scope*, *sequence*, *unit of study*, *lessons*, and *lesson plans*.

6. State and briefly describe the five stages of Kinzie's (2005) modified framework for instructional design.

7. Define *health literacy* and *health numeracy* and explain how they impact health promotion programs.

8. What is health advocacy?

9. What special issues are there related to incentives with which planners working in the worksite setting need to be concerned?

10. Why should program planners be concerned with program guidelines that have been developed by professional organizations and other groups?

11. What are some of the documents and sponsoring groups that have suggested standards, criteria, or guidelines for program development?

12. Briefly discuss the questions set forth in this chapter that should be considered before creating an intervention.

13. Identify and briefly explain the five steps in the framework for adapting an evidence-based intervention for a new setting.

ACTIVITIES

1. Create a multistrategy intervention for a program you are planning.

2. Create a multistrategy intervention for a program that has as its goal "to get third-grade students to wear helmets while riding their bicycles."

3. Using evidence found at the *Guide to Community Preventive Services* adapt a multistrategy intervention for a setting of your choice.

4. Create a multistrategy intervention for a program that has as its goal "the rehydration of young children in the small village of Y in the Third World country of Q."

5. Design and present on an 8½" x 11" piece of paper a bulletin board that could be used as part of the multiactivity intervention you are planning. Divide the piece of paper that represents the bulletin board into six equal sections and indicate what you will include in each section.

6. Interview a classmate to find out information about his or her health risks. Then, assuming you are a patient educator in a health clinic, create a one-page *tailored* letter to the person, urging him or her to seek an appropriate screening for the health risk(s).

7. Develop a three-fold pamphlet that can be used as an informational piece for a program you are planning.

8. With other students in your class, write a PSA script for a program you are planning. Then rehearse the script and record it.

9. Write a two-page, double-spaced news release that describes a program you are planning.

10. Write a letter to your state or federal senators or representatives and request their support of a piece of health-related legislation that is currently being considered.

WEBLINKS

1. **http://www.healtheducationadvocate.org**

   Health Education Advocate

   Sponsored by the Coalition of National Health Education Organizations (CNHEO), this Website is a timely source of advocacy information related to the field of health education and promotion. The site offers a number of items to help health planners with advocacy activities, including, but not limited to, information about how to identify and contact their senators and congresspersons, the status of specific bills, health resolutions and policy statements of sponsoring agencies, and advocacy resources.

2. **http://www.cdc.gov/socialmedia/**

   Social Media at CDC

   This page on the CDC's Website deals with the use of social media. From here you can link to the various social media tools of CDC and to a page that provides guidelines that have been developed to provide critical information on lessons learned, best practices, clearance information, and security requirements.

3. **http://nccc.georgetown.edu/index.html**

   National Center for Cultural Competence (NCCC)

   At this site you will find a lot of resource material dealing with cultural competence including a listing of publications, self-assessments, and current projects and initiatives.

4. **http://www.heart.org/HEARTORG/Advocate/Advocate_UCM_001133_SubHomePage.jsp**

   American Heart Association (AHA)

   This is the advocacy page of the AHA's Website. Like most other voluntary health organizations, the American Heart Association has an active advocacy program to support its mission. This site provides an overview of the advocacy work in which the AHA is involved.

5. **http://www2a.cdc.gov/phlp/**

   Public Health Law Program

   This page on the CDC's Website focuses on public health law and policy. From here you can link to public health law news and other materials and resources that examine the authority of the government at various jurisdictional levels to improve the health of the general population within societal limits and norms.

6. **http://www.thecommunityguide.org/index.html**

   Guide to Community Preventive Services

   This Webpage includes evidence-based recommendations for programs and policies to promote population-based health.

7. http://www.cancer.gov/cancertopics/cancerlibrary/pinkbook

Pink Book—*Making Health Communication Programs Work*

This Webpage for the *Making Health Communication Programs Work* book is a practical guide to developing specific communication strategies to promote health and prevent disease.

CHAPTER 9

Community Organizing and Community Building

After reading this chapter and answering the questions at the end, you should be able to:

- Define *community*, *community organizing*, *community building*, and *coalitions*.
- Outline the processes for organizing and building a community.
- Explain the term *mapping community capacity*.

active participants	gatekeepers	primary building blocks
bottom-up	grassroots	secondary building blocks
citizen-initiated	locality development	social action
coalition	mapping community	social planning
community	capacity	stakeholders
community building	occasional participants	supporting participants
community organizing	ownership	task force
executive participants	potential building blocks	

There are a number of different processes involved in planning health promotion programs and those processes vary based upon the circumstances of the planning situation. The processes selected and used to plan programs are in part predicated on the level of the influence (i.e., intrapersonal, interpersonal, and/or community), and the level of influence is often predicated on the size of the priority population. For example, certain processes are more useful when planning programs for relatively small groups or communities of people such as those found in worksites, clinics, and schools, whereas other processes must be considered when working with larger communities. By community, we do not mean only those groups of people within a certain geographic area, though that could define a community, but more specifically, a **community** is defined as "a group of people who have common characteristics" (Turnock, 2009, p. 502). Israel and colleagues (1994) have stated that communities are characterized by the following elements: (1) membership—a sense of identity and belonging; (2) common symbol systems—similar language, rituals, and ceremonies; (3) shared values and norms; (4) mutual influence—community members have influence and are influenced by each other; (5) shared needs and commitment to meeting them; and (6) shared emotional connection—members share common history, experiences, and mutual support. Thus communities can be defined by location, race, ethnicity, age, occupation, interest in particular problems (e.g., domestic violence), outcomes (e.g., breast cancer survivors), or other common bonds (e.g., people with a disability) (Turnock, 2009). Today, we can also talk about a cyber community (Minkler, Wallerstein, & Wilson, 2008).

Although many of the planning processes are applicable regardless of the size of the community, when working with large communities an additional process is needed in order to have a successful program. This additional process is organizing those in the community to come together to work as a group to deal with the needs of the community. This chapter addresses the fundamental elements of organizing communities for action. **Box 9.1** identifies the responsibilities and competencies for health education specialists that pertain to the material presented in this chapter.

Box 9.1 RESPONSIBILITIES AND COMPETENCIES FOR HEALTH EDUCATION SPECIALISTS

This chapter focuses on the fundamental elements of organizing communities. As such, the content presented cuts across several different areas of responsibility for health education specialists. The responsibilities and competencies related to these tasks include:

Responsibility I:	Assess Needs, Assets, and Capacity for Health Education
	Competency 1.1: Plan Assessment Process
	Competency 1.2: Access Existing Information and Data Related to Health
	Competency 1.4: Examine Relationships Among Behavioral, Environmental and Genetic Factors That Enhance or Compromise Health
Responsibility II:	Plan Health Education
	Competency 2.1: Involve Priority Populations and Other Stakeholders in the Planning Process
	Competency 2.2: Develop Goals and Objectives
	Competency 2.3: Select or Design Strategies and Interventions
Responsibility III:	Implement Health Education
	Competency 3.1: Implement a Plan of Action
Responsibility IV:	Conduct Evaluation and Research
	Competency 4.1: Develop Evaluation/Research Plan

Box 9.1 (Continued)

Responsibility V:	Administer and Manage Health Education
	Competency 5.2: Obtain Acceptance and Support for Programs
	Competency 5.3: Demonstrate Leadership
	Competency 5.4: Manage Human Resources
	Competency 5.5: Facilitate Partnerships in Support of Health Education
Responsibility VI:	Serve as a Health Education Resource Person
	Competency 6.2: Provide Training
	Competency 6.3 Serve as a Health Education Consultant
Responsibility VII:	Communicate and Advocate for Health and Health Education
	Competency 7.2: Identify and Develop a Variety of Communication Strategies, Methods, and Techniques
	Competency 7.5: Influence Policy to Promote Health

Source: NCHEC, SOPHE, & AAHE (2010).

Community Organizing Background and Assumptions

In recent years, there has been a shift in the focus of the work of planners and others in the helping professions. Where once the work of planners focused almost solely on the individual, today the focus is on broadening to the community. *Community-based, community empowerment, community participation,* and *community partnerships* are among the many terms that are being used more frequently by health agencies, outside funders, and policy makers (Minkler, 2005a). There are good reasons for the use of these terms and most revolve around the need for communities to organize.

With the evidence to show that interventions aimed at the community level (also referred to as *population-based approaches*) can have a positive affect on the health of a community, it is important that health education specialists have community organizing skills. In the early history of the United States, a sense of community was inherent in everyday life (Green, 1989). It was natural for communities to pool their resources to deal with shared problems. More recently, the need to organize communities has seemed to increase. "Advances in electronics (e.g., handheld digital devices) and communications (multifunction cell phones and Internet), household upgrades (e.g., energy efficiency), and increased mobility (e.g., frequency of moving and ease of worldwide travel) have resulted in a loss of a sense of community. Individuals are much more independent than ever before. The days when people knew everyone on their block are past. Today, it is not uncommon for people to never meet their neighbors" (McKenzie et al., 2012, p. 123). Because of these changes in community social structure and the resources necessary to meet the needs of communities, it now takes a concerted effort to organize a community to act for the collective good.

"The term *community organization* was coined by American social workers in the late 1880s to describe their efforts to coordinate services for newly arrived immigrants and the poor" (Minkler & Wallerstein, 2005, p. 27). More recently, *community organization* has been used by a variety of professionals, including health education specialists, and refers to various methods of intervention to deal with social problems. "Community organization is important in health education in part because it reflects one of the field's most fundamental principles, that of 'starting where the people are' (Nyswander, 1956)" (Minkler & Wallerstein, 2005, p. 27). "The health education professional who begins with the community's felt needs, is more likely to be successful in the change process and in fostering true community ownership of programs and actions" (Minkler et al., 2008, p. 288).

Community organizing has been defined as "a process by which community groups are helped to identify common problems or goals, mobilize resources, and develop and implement strategies for reaching their goals they have collectively set" (Minkler et al., 2008, p. 288). It is not a science but rather an art of building consensus within the democratic process (Ross, 1967). (See **Box 9.2** for definitions of related terms.) Although community organization may not be as "natural" as it once was, communities can still organize to analyze and solve problems through collective action. In working toward this end, those who assist communities with organizing must make several assumptions. Ross (1967, pp. 86–92) has stated these as follows:

1. Communities of people can develop the capacity to deal with their own problems.

2. People want to change and can change.

3. People should participate in making, adjusting, or controlling the major changes taking place in their communities.

4. Changes in community living that are self-imposed or self-developed have a meaning and permanence that imposed changes do not have.

5. A "holistic approach" can deal successfully with problems with which a "fragmented approach" cannot cope.

6. Democracy requires cooperative participation and action in the affairs of the community, and that the people must learn the skills that make this possible.

7. Frequently communities of people need help in organizing to deal with their needs, just as many individuals require help in coping with their individual problems.

Box 9.2	TERMS ASSOCIATED WITH COMMUNITY ORGANIZING
Citizen Participation	The bottom-up, grassroots mobilization of citizens for the purpose of undertaking activities to improve the condition of something in the community.
Community Capacity	"The characteristics of communities that affect their ability to identify, mobilize, and address social and public health problems" (Goodman et al., 1998, p. 259).

Box 9.2 (CONTINUED)	
Community Development	"A process designed to create conditions of economic and social progress for the whole community with its active participation and the fullest possible reliance on the community's initiative" (United Nations, 1955, p. 6).
Empowerment	"Social action process for people to gain mastery over their lives and the lives of their communities" (Minkler et al., 2008, p. 294).
Grassroots Participation	"Bottom-up efforts of people taking collective actions on their own behalf, and they involve the use of a sophisticated blend of confrontation and cooperation in order to achieve their ends" (Perlman, 1978, p. 65).
Macro Practice	The methods of professional change that deal with issues beyond the individual, family, and small group level.
Social Capital	"The relationships and structures within a community, such as, civic participation, networks, norms of reciprocity, and trust, that promote cooperation and mutual benefit" (Putnam, 1995, p. 66).
Participation and Relevance	"Community organizing that 'starts where the people are' and engages community members as equals" (Minkler & Wallerstein, 2005, p. 35).

The Processes of Community Organizing and Community Building

There is no single unified model of community organizing or community building (Minkler et al., 2008). In fact, Rothman and Tropman (1987, pp. 4–5) have stated, "We should speak of community organization methods rather than the community organization method." Over the years, several different community organization methods have been used, including revolutionary techniques (Alinsky, 1971). However, the best known categories of community organization were the three put forth by Rothman (2001) and include *locality development*, *social planning*, and *social action*. **Locality development** is most like community development and seeks community change through broad self-help participation from the local community. "It is heavily process oriented, stressing consensus, and cooperation and aimed at building group identity and a sense of community" (Minkler & Wallerstein, 2005, p. 30). **Social planning** "is heavily task oriented, focused on rational-empirical problem solving, usually by an outside expert" (Minkler & Wallerstein, 2005, p. 30). **Social action** "is both task and process oriented. It is concerned with increasing the community's problem-solving ability and achieving concrete changes to redress imbalances of power and privilege between the oppressed or disadvantaged group and the larger society" (Minkler & Wallerstein, 2005, p. 30). Although this model is not used as often as it once was, it was most useful during the civil rights and gay rights movements.

Though the concepts found in community organizing methods proposed by Rothman (2001) have been the primary means by which communities have organized over the years, they do have their limitations. One of the greatest limitations is that they are primarily problem-based and organizer-centered, rather than strengths-based and community-centered (Minkler et al., 2008). Some of the newer models are based more on collaborative empowerment and community building. Regardless of whether one talks about the "old models" or the "new models," they all revolve around a common theme: The work and resources of many have a much better chance of solving a problem or meeting a goal than the work and resources of a few.

Minkler and colleagues (2008) have done a nice job of summarizing the newer perspectives of community organizing with the older models by presenting a typology that incorporates both needs- and strength-based approaches. That typology is presented in **Figure 9.1**. This figure is divided into four quadrants with strength-based and needs-based on the vertical axis and consensus and conflict on the horizontal axis. Though this typology separates and categorizes the various methods of community organizing and building, Minkler and colleagues (2008) point out that

> Community organizing and community building are fluid endeavors. Although some organizing efforts primarily have focused in one quadrant, the majority incorporate concepts from multiple quadrants. It is important for organizing efforts to clarify their

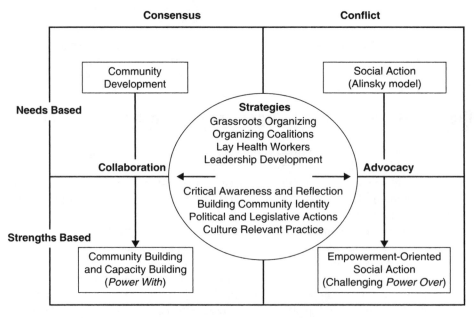

Figure 9.1 Community Organization and Community-Building Typology

Source: "Improving health through community organizing and community building." M. Minkler, N. Wallerstein, and N. Wilson, in *Health Behavior and Health Education: Theory, Research and Education*. K. Glanz, B. K. Rimer, and K. Viswanath (Eds.). Copyright © 2008 by Jossey-Bass. Reprinted with permission.

assumptions and decide on primary strategies based on group history, member skills, willingness to take risks, or comfort level with different approaches (p. 292).

Because the purpose of this chapter is to provide an overview of the community organizing and community-building processes, and at the risk of oversimplifying the processes, we would like to present a very general or generic approach to community organizing and community building (see **Figure 9.2**). It does not include everything planners need to know about community organizing and community building, but it does present the basic elements.

For further information about community organizing, refer to any of several references (Minkler, 2005; Minkler et al., 2008; Ross, 1967; Rothman 2001; Snow, 2001) that are devoted entirely to the subject. Also, there are several works that deal specifically with the application of community organization to health promotion activities (El-Askari & Walton, 2005; Minkler, 2005c; Minkler et al., 2008).

Before presenting the generic process for community organizing and community building, we would like to comment on the role of the planner in this process. For many years, the planner was seen as a "leader" of the community organizing effort. However, more often than not, the planner is an "outsider" with regard to the community being organized and, as such, has trouble gaining the credibility to serve as a leader. Yes, he or she may work in the community (remember that a community is often defined by something other than geographical boundaries) but often lives outside the community in which the organizing effort is needed. Thus, the role that the planner should take is that of a facilitator or assistant rather than the leader. Experience has shown that it is best if the leaders come from *within* the community. Keep this thought in mind as you read through the general model.

Recognizing the Issue

The processes of community organizing and building begin when someone recognizes that an issue exists in the community and that something needs to be done about it. This recognition may occur as a result of someone reviewing health data on the community and seeing a need (e.g., an unusually high number of teenage pregnancies), by someone actually observing a specific situation in the community that needs attention (e.g., injuries at a particular intersection), or as the result of a community crisis (e.g., lack of resources to deal with a natural disaster). "This person (or persons) is referred to as the initial organizer. This individual may not be the primary organizer throughout the community organizing/building process. He or she is the one who gets it started" (McKenzie et al., 2012, p. 125). For the purposes of this discussion, assume that the concern is a health problem, but remember that the community organization process may be used with any type of problem found in a community. Concerns can be as specific as trying to get a certain piece of legislation passed or as general as advocating for a drug-free community.

The recognition of an issue can occur from inside or outside the community. A citizen or a church leader from within the community may identify the issue, or it may first be identified by someone outside the community, such as an employee of a local or state health department, a state legislator, a politically active group, or someone from a local voluntary health agency. However, the community organizing efforts that have been most successful have been those that are recognized from the inside. "All historic

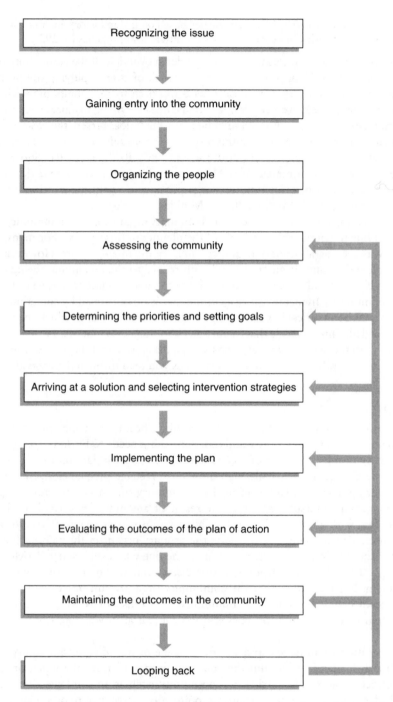

Figure 9.2 Summary of the Steps in Community Organizing and Building

evidence indicates that significant community development takes place only when local community people are committed to investing themselves and their resources in the effort" (Kretzmann & McKnight, 1993, p. 11). The primary reason for this is that those within the community are much more likely to take ownership of the effort. It is difficult for someone from the outside coming in and telling community members that they have problems or issues that need to be dealt with and they need to organize to take care of them. When there is internal recognition of the issue or concern, it is referred to as **grassroots, citizen-initiated,** or **bottom-up** organizing.

Gaining Entry into the Community

The second step of this generic process of community organizing and community building may or may not be needed. If the issue identified in the previous step is recognized by someone from within the community, then this step of the process will, more than likely, not be needed. We say "more than likely" because those within a community do not need to gain entry into it. But there may be some cases when someone from within a community may identify the issue but has not lived in the community long enough, lacks the political power, or does not know enough about the interactions of the community to proceed with the process. In these later cases, the person may be treated or feel like an "outsider" and may have to proceed as an outsider would.

If the issue is identified by someone from outside the community this becomes a most critical step in the process. Recognition of a concern does not mean that people should immediately set about correcting it. Instead, they should follow a set of steps to deal with it; gaining proper "entry" into the community is the first step. Braithwaite and colleagues (1989) have stressed the importance of tactfully negotiating entry into a community with the individuals who control, both formally and informally, the "political climate" of the community. These individuals are referred to as **gatekeepers.** The term infers that one must pass through the "gate" in order to get at the people in the community (Wright, 1994). These "power brokers" know their community, how it functions, and how to accomplish tasks within it. Longtime residents are usually able to identify the gatekeepers of their community. They may include people such as business leaders, education leaders, heads of law enforcement agencies, leaders of community activist groups, parent and teacher groups, clergy, politicians, and others. Their support is absolutely essential to the success of any attempt to organize a community.

Organizers must approach the gatekeepers on the gatekeepers' terms and "play" the gatekeepers' "game." However, before making this contact, organizers must first be familiar with the community with which they are working. "They must be *culturally sensitive* and work toward *cultural competence.* That is, they must be aware of the cultural differences within a community and effectively work with the cultural context of the community" (McKenzie et al., 2012, p. 125). Tervalon and Garcia (1998) stress the need for *cultural humility*—openness to others' culture. In other words, community organizers must have a thorough knowledge of the community and the people living there before they try to enter the informal boundaries of the community (Braithwaite et al., 1989). Having a thorough understanding of the community and tactfully approaching its gatekeepers will help community organizers develop credibility and trust with those in the community, and, as noted earlier, it is not easy to bring a concern to the attention of those in the community. Few people are glad to know they have a problem, and fewer still like others to tell them they have a problem. Move with caution, and do not be too aggressive!

When people from outside the community are working to facilitate the organizing efforts, they will find it advantageous to enter the community through an already established, well-respected organization or institution in the community, such as a church, a service group, or another successful local group. If those who make up an existing organization/institution in the community can see that a problem exists and that solving the problem will improve the community, it can help smooth the way to gaining entry and achieving the remaining steps in the process.

Organizing the People

Obtaining the support of the community members to deal with the concern is the next step in the process. It is best to begin with those individuals who are already interested in addressing the concern. This is not the time to try to convert people to the cause or to make sure that all the key players of the community are involved. The initial group must be made up of those people most affected by the problem and who want to see change occur. For example, if the identified problem is teenage drug use, then teens needed to be included in the group. If the issue is housing for individuals with low-incomes, then those individuals need to be included. If the problem is something that a community agency or organization (e.g., the local health department or a social service agency) has dealt with for a period of time but is unable to solve, then this group should be involved. Or, if a group of parents, or another defined group, has been struggling with the problem without resolution, then its leaders should be invited to participate. More often than not, this core group will be small and consist of people who are committed to the resolution of the concern, regardless of the time frame. Brager and colleagues (1987) have referred to this core group as **executive participants**. From among the core group, a leader or coordinator must be identified. If at all possible, the leader should be someone with leadership skills, good knowledge of the concern and the community, and most of all, someone from within the community. One of the early tasks of the leader will be to help build group cohesion.

Not everyone is cut out to be an organizer or a leader. Researchers have found that good organizers are successful because of a combination of skills and attributes. These skills and attributes fall into three main areas: change vision attributes, technical skills, and interactional or experience skills. *Change vision attributes* are closely aligned with an organizer's view of the world political terms. These people see a need for change and are personally dedicated and committed to seeing the change occur—so much so that they are willing to put other priorities aside to see the project through (Mondros & Wilson, 1994).

Technical skills include two areas: those related to efficacy on issues and those related to organizational health and effectiveness. The former includes being able to analyze issues, opponents, and power structure; develop and implement change strategies; achieve goals; and possess outstanding communication and public relation skills. Organizational health and effectiveness skills include building structures for the recruitment and involvement of others, forming and maintaining task groups, and implementing skills of fundraising and organizational management (Mondros & Wilson, 1994).

The third characteristic of a good organizer is possessing *interactional* or *experience skills*. These include an ability to respond with empathy, to assess and intervene with individuals and groups, and to be able to identify, develop, educate, and maintain organizational members and leaders (Mondros & Wilson, 1994).

With the core group and leader in place, the next step is to expand the group to build support for dealing with the concern—that is, to broaden the constituency. Brager and colleagues (1987) have noted that other group participants will include *active, occasional*, and *supporting participants*. The **active participants** (who may also be executive participants) take part in most group activities and are not afraid to do the work that needs to be done. The **occasional participants** become involved on an irregular basis and usually only when major decisions are made. The **supporting participants** are seldom involved but help swell the ranks and may contribute in nonactive ways or through financial contributions. When expanding the group, look for others who may be interested in helping, and ask current group members for names of people who might be interested. Look for

---

Box 9.3 UNDERSTANDING DIVERSITY

Members of a group come from many different backgrounds. Some members may be much older or much younger than other members; some may represent different cultural, racial, or ethnic groups; some may represent different educational levels and abilities. Extra awareness and flexibility are required for the facilitator and other group members to remain sensitive to different backgrounds. Below we suggest a few ways to improve your awareness of differences. In general, new information is acquired so that different perspectives can be understood and appreciated.

- Become aware of differences in the group by asking questions and getting involved in small group discussions.
- Seek involvement and input and listen to persons of different backgrounds without bias, and avoid being defensive.
- Learn the beliefs and feelings of specific groups about particular issues.
- Read about current and emerging issues that concern different groups, and read literature that is popular among different groups.
- Learn about the language, humor, gestures, norms, expectations, and values of different groups.
- Attend events that appeal to members of specific groups.
- Become attuned to cultural clichés, stereotypes, and distortions you may encounter in the media.
- Use examples to which persons of different cultures and backgrounds can relate.
- Learn the facts before you make statements or form opinions about different groups.

Source: Centers for Disease Control and Prevention, USDHHS, (no date), p. A2–15.

people who may already be dealing with the concern, affected by the problem through their present work, or who have resources to contribute. This search should include existing social groups, such as voluntary health agencies, agricultural extension services, religious organizations, hospitals, health care providers, political officeholders, policy makers, police, educators, lay citizens, or special interest groups. (See **Box 9.3** on tips for understanding the diversity in a working group.)

Over the last few decades, in many communities the number of people interested in volunteering their time has decreased. Today, if you ask someone to volunteer, you may hear the reply, "I'm already too busy." There are two primary reasons for this response. First, there are many families in which both husband and wife work outside the home. Between 1970 and 2010, the proportion of married women with preschool-aged children who were in the labor force more than doubled, from 30.3% to 63.9%. Also during this same period of time, the proportion of married women with children of school age who were working or looking for work jumped from 49.2% to 70.8%. In 2010, 58.1% of married couples with children reported that both husband and wife were employed outside the home (USDL, 2011). Second, there are more single-parent households. Today, they constitute over one-fourth (27%) of all family households with children, and most (84.9% vs. 15.1%) are headed by women (USCB, 2010). (See **Box 9.4** for tips on working with volunteers.)

Box 9.4   TIPS ON WORKING WITH VOLUNTEERS

Volunteers work for self-satisfaction, personal growth, fun, and other intangible rewards. Each volunteer should be treated as a colleague and recognized as an official part of the team. However, offer volunteers more flexibility than you can to employees, and adjust your expectations accordingly. For example, because volunteers cannot contribute as much time as paid, full-time workers do, they cannot complete tasks as quickly. When scheduling activities, be realistic about how long a busy participant will need to complete it.

Get to know each volunteer personally so that you can learn about special abilities and limitations and match responsibilities to skills. Vary responsibilities as desired by volunteers.

Be sure to assign specific and clearly defined tasks and to explain procedures and expectations. Develop a work plan or job description for the volunteer to help ensure that roles and responsibilities are understood. Provide training and give credit for work done. Give lots of feedback, encouragement, and signs of appreciation. Be willing to change the placement of volunteers, if that seems appropriate, or even dismiss a volunteer if necessary.

Keep in mind the following key points of working with volunteers. They want to be:

- appreciated for the work that they do.
- busy with worthwhile and varied tasks.
- provided with clear communication about tasks and expectations.
- developed through training.

Source: Centers for Disease Control and Prevention (no date), p. A2–17.

Sometimes these expanded community groups become *task forces* or *coalitions*. A **task force** has been defined as "a self-contained group of 'doers' that is not ongoing, but rather brought together due to strong interest in an issue and for a specific purpose. Task forces are sometimes convened at the request of an overseeing body or committee" (Butterfoss, 2007, p. 30). A **coalition** is "a formal alliance of organizations that come together to work for a common goal" (Butterfoss, 2007, p. 30)—often, to compensate for deficits in power, resources, and expertise. Coalitions "develop an internal decision-making and leadership structure that allows member organizations to speak with a united voice and engage in shared planning and implementation activities. Links to outside organizations and communication channels are formal. Member organizations are willing to pull resources from existing systems, as well as seek new resources to develop a joint budget. Agreements, benchmarks, roles, and assignments are often written" (Butterfoss, 2007, p. 30). The underlying concept behind coalitions is collaboration, for several individuals, groups, or organizations with their collective resources have a better chance of solving the problem than any single entity.

Box 9.5   CHARACTERISTICS OF SUCCESSFUL COALITIONS

- Continuity of coalition staff, in particular the coordinator position.
- Ownership of the problem by coalition members and the community.
- Community leaders support the coalition and its efforts.
- Active involvement of community volunteer agencies.
- High level of trust and reciprocity among members.
- Frequent and ongoing training for coalition members and staff.
- Benefits of membership outweigh the costs.
- Active involvement of members in developing coalition goals, objectives, and strategies.
- Development of a strategic action plan rather than a project-by-project approach.
- Consensus is reached on issues instead of voting.
- Productive coalition meetings.
- Large problems are broken down into smaller, solvable pieces.
- Steering committee of elected leaders and staff guides coalition.
- Task or work groups of members design and implement strategies.
- Rules and procedures are formalized.
- Local media are actively involved.
- Coalition and its activities are evaluated continuously.

Source: "Building and Sustaining Coalitions." F. D. Butterfoss, from *Community Health Education Methods: A Practical Guide*. R. J. Bensley and J. Brookins-Fisher (Eds.). Copyright © 2009 by Jones & Bartlett Learning. Reprinted with permission.

"Building and maintaining effective coalitions have increasingly been recognized as vital components of much effective community organizing and community building" (Minkler, 2005, p. 16). Aitaoto, Tsark, and Braun (2009) found that the key to sustaining coalitions include having a champion, a supportive organizational home, and access to technical assistance and resources. Butterfoss (2009) has created a longer list of characteristics of successful coalitions (see **Box 9.5**), while Kegler and Swan (2011) have tested the community coalition action theory (CCAT) for consistency of its constructs with working community coalitions. For those who want more information about coalition development, Butterfoss (2006, 2007, 2009), Goldstein (1997), and Wandersman, Goodman, and Butterfoss (2005) provide nice overviews of the processes of building and sustaining coalitions.

Assessing the Community

Earlier in this chapter reference was made to the Rothman (2001) typology of community organization: locality development, social planning, and social action. Each of these community organizing strategies operates "from the assumption that problems in society can be addressed by helping the community become better or differently organized, and each strategy perceives the problems and how or whom to organize somewhat differently" (Walter, 2005, p. 66). **Community building** "is an orientation to community that is strength based rather than need based and stresses the identification, nurturing, and celebration of community assets" (Minkler, 2005, p. 4). Asset-based community building is intended to affirm strong community-rooted traditions, and to build on the good work already going on in communities (Kretzmann & McKnight, 1993). One of the major differences between community organization and community building is the type of assessment that is used to determine where to focus the community's efforts. In the community organization approach, the assessment is focused on the needs of the community, whereas in community building, the assessment focuses on the assets and capabilities of the community. A clearer picture of the community will be revealed, and a stronger base will be developed for change, if the assessment includes the identification of both the needs and assets, and involves those who live in the community. Hancock and Minkler (2005, p. 139) provide this illustration:

> For example, a narrowly defined needs assessment designed and conducted by outside experts as a means of justifying and providing raw data for organizing around a predetermined community health need may be effective in achieving its objectives. But by failing to meaningfully involve community members in determining the goals of the assessment process, by focusing solely on needs rather than identifying and building on community strengths, and by failing to make empowerment of people a central goal of the assessment process, such an approach would fail to meet several critical criteria of community organizing and community building practice.

You may recall (in Chapter 4) we outlined the procedures for conducting a needs assessment and described how the resulting needs could be placed on a map (i.e., *mapping*) to provide a visual representation of the needs of a community. **Figure 9.3** provides an example of such a map. However, an assessment that focuses entirely on needs/deficiencies presents only half of the information that is needed in community organizing and building (McKnight & Kretzmann, 2005). Organizers also need to know the capacities and assets. McKnight and Kretzmann (2005) point out "communities have never been built upon deficiencies. Building community has always depended on mobilizing the capacities and assets of a people and place" (p. 170).

In order to map community assets—a process referred to as **mapping community capacity**—McKnight and Kretzmann (2005) have categorized assets into three different

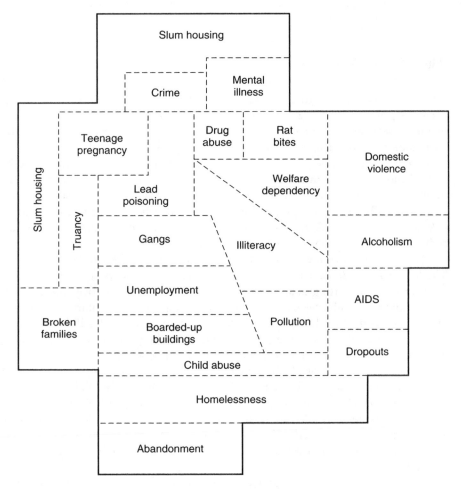

Figure 9.3 Neighborhood Needs Map

Source: "Mapping Community Capacity" by J. L. McKnight and J. P. Kretzmann from *Community Organizing and Community Building for Health*, Ed. M. Minkler. Copyright © 2005 by Rutgers, the State University Press. Reprinted with permission.

groups based on their availability to the community and refer to them as *building blocks.* **Primary building blocks** are the most accessible assets (see **Figure 9.4**). They are located in the neighborhood and are largely under the control of those who live in the neighborhood. Primary building blocks can be organized into the assets of individuals and those of organizations or associations. (See **Box 9.6** for examples of each.) The next most accessible building blocks are **secondary building blocks,** which are assets located in the neighborhood but largely controlled by people outside (see Box 9.6). The least accessible assets are referred to as **potential building blocks.** They are resources originating outside the neighborhood and controlled by people outside (see Box 9.6). Figure 9.4 presents an example of an asset map using the three types of building blocks. Knowing both the needs and assets of the community, organizers can work to identify the true concerns of the community and the capacity to deal with them.

Determining Priorities and Setting Goals

Once the community has been assessed, the community group is ready to develop its goals. The goal-setting process includes two phases. The first phase consists of identifying the priorities of the group—what the group wants to accomplish. The priorities should be determined through consensus rather than through formal voting. (See **Box 9.7** for tips on how to reach consensus.) The second phase consists of using the priority list to write the goals. To help ensure that the ideals of community organization take hold, the **stakeholders** (those in the community who have something to gain or lose from the community organizing and building efforts) must be the ones to establish priorities and set goals. This may sound simple, but in fact it may be the most difficult part of the process. Getting the stakeholders to agree on priorities takes a skilled group facilitator because there is sure to be more than one point of view.

When working with coalitions and task forces, one is likely to face some challenges (Clark, Friedman, & Lachance, 2006). One challenge that may surface when determining priorities and setting goals is *turf struggles* (disagreements over the control of resources and responsibilities). Even though individuals or representatives of their organizations have come together to solve a problem, many people will still be concerned with finding specific solutions to the problems faced by their organization. For example, in the case of drug abuse in the community, consensus may indicate that the majority of people believe the solutions lie in the educational system, but people who work in drug treatment centers may believe that they lie in the treatment of drug abuse. The facilitator will need special skills to keep these treatment center people involved after the priority-setting process does not identify their concern as a problem the group will attack. One means of dealing with this is to have subgoals that can be worked on by special interest subcommittees. Such an arrangement will allow the subcommittee to have a feeling of **ownership** in the process.

Miller (as cited in Minkler & Wallenstein 2005, p. 39) has identified five criteria that community organizers need to consider when determining priorities and setting goals. The concern/issue/problem: (1) must be winnable, ensuring that working on it does not simply reinforce fatalistic attitudes and beliefs that things cannot be improved; (2) must be simple and specific so that any member of the organizing group can explain it clearly

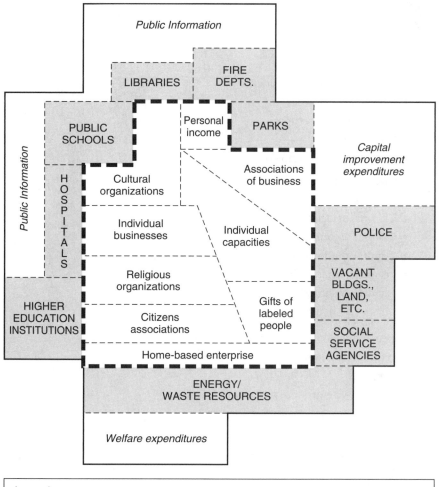

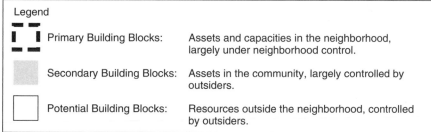

Figure 9.4 Neighborhood Assets Map

Source: "Mapping Community Capacity" by J. L. McKnight and J. P. Kretzmann from *Community Organizing and Community Building for Health*, Ed. M. Minkler. Copyright © 2005 by Rutgers, the State University Press. Reprinted with permission.

Box 9.6 BUILDING BLOCKS (ASSETS) OF COMMUNITIES

Primary Building Blocks

Individual assets

- Skills and abilities of residents
- Individual businesses
- Home-based enterprises
- Personal income
- Gifts of labeled (disabled) people

Organizational assets

- Associations of businesses (e.g., chamber of commerce)
- Citizens' associations (e.g., neighborhood watch)
- Cultural organization (e.g., Old West End Festival, British Club)
- Communications organizations (e.g., newspapers, TV, radio)
- Religious organizations
- Financial institutions

Secondary Building Blocks

Private and nonprofit organizations

- Higher education institutions
- Hospitals
- Social service groups (e.g., Rotary, Kiwanis)

Public institutions and services

- Public schools
- Police and fire departments
- Libraries
- Parks

Physical resources

- Vacant land, vacant commercial and industrial structures, vacant housing
- Energy and waste resources

Potential Building Blocks

Welfare expenditures

Public capital-information expenditures

Public information

Source: "Mapping Community Capacity" by J. L. McKnight and J. P. Kretzmann from *Community Organizing and Community Building for Health*, Ed. M. Minkler. Copyright © 2005 by Rutgers, the State University Press. Reprinted with permission.

Box 9.7   REACHING CONSENSUS

Groups sometimes find it hard to reach a consensus, or general agreement. Remind participants of the following guidelines to group decision making.

- Avoid the "one best way" attitude; the best way is that which reflects the best collective judgment of the group.
- Avoid "either, or" thinking; often the best solution combines several approaches.
- A majority vote is not always the best solution. When participants give and take, several viewpoints can be combined.
- Healthy conflict, which can help participants reach a consensus, should not be smoothed over or ended prematurely.
- Problems are best solved when participants try to both communicate and listen.

If a group has trouble reaching consensus, consider using some special techniques such as brainstorming, the nominal group process, and conflict resolution.

Source: Centers for Disease Control and Prevention (no date), p. A2-12

---

in a sentence or two; (3) must unite members of the organizing group and involve them in a meaningful way in achieving concern/issue/problem resolution; (4) should affect many people and build up the community; and (5) should be a part of a larger plan or strategy to enhance the community.

Arriving at a Solution and Selecting Intervention Strategies

To achieve the goals that it has set, the group will need to identify alternative solutions and—again, through consensus—choose a course of action. Most community problems/issues/concerns can be dealt with in any of several ways; however, each alternative has advantages and disadvantages. The group should examine the alternatives in terms of probable outcomes, acceptability to the community, probable long- and short-term effects on the community, and the cost of resources to solve the problem. Most of the intervention strategies discussed earlier (in Chapter 8) are means by which the group can address the problem/issue/concern.

Much of the work to identify the appropriate solution(s) can be accomplished through subcommittees. Subcommittees can complete specific tasks that will contribute to the larger plan of action. Their work should yield specific strategies that are culturally sensitive and appropriate for the community. The plan of action is usually written in a proposal format and will be given final approval at a meeting of the full committee or coalition. It is important to take care in putting together this proposal; as many as possible of the ideas of the various subcommittees should be included. This will help to ensure approval of the entire plan. In the end, the real test of the course of action selected is whether it can provide whatever it is the people are seeking (Brager et al., 1987).

Final Steps in the Community Organizing and Building Processes

The final four steps in community organizing and building processes include implementing the plan, evaluating the outcomes of the plan of action, maintaining the outcomes in the community, and, if necessary, "looping" back to the appropriate point in the process to modify the steps and restructure the work plan. Implementation of the intervention strategy includes identifying and collecting the necessary resources for carrying out the solution and creating an appropriate time line for implementation. Oftentimes the resources can be found within a community and thus *horizontal relationships* (the interaction of local units with one another) are needed (Warren, 1963). Other times the resources must be obtained from units located outside the community and in this case *vertical relationships* (those where local units interact with extra-community systems) are needed (Warren, 1963). An example of this latter relationship is the interaction between a local chamber of commerce and its state affiliate. More detailed information on implementation is presented later (Chapter 12).

The evaluation step of the community organizing and building process includes two types of evaluation: formative and summative evaluation. Briefly, formative evaluation deals with the measurement of the process used to improve the quality of the effort, whereas summative evaluation focuses on comparing the outcomes of the process to the earlier stated goals (see Chapters 13 and 14 for more on evaluation). When reporting on the work of coalitions, Clark and her colleagues (2006) stated process evaluation (a form of formative evaluation) "was the easier type of assessment to conduct. Effective tools are more available, data collection is more immediate, and problems of association and correlation are less daunting than those associated with outcome evaluation. Outcome evaluation requires time, patience, and the willingness to accept that in complex community settings, definitive conclusions are elusive" (p. 152S).

Maintaining or sustaining the outcomes may be one of the most difficult steps in the entire process. Maintaining or sustaining the outcomes are challenged by (1) the energy and effort necessary to stay organized, (2) continuing the interest and involvement of the members (Clark et al., 2006), (3) continuing need for funding to sustain the efforts, and (4) "ensuring the lasting impact of their work through policies, cross-facility agreements, standardized protocols, and so on" (Clark et al., 2006, p. 151S). At this point organizers need to seriously consider the need for long-term capacity for a lasting solution.

Through the steps of implementation, evaluation, and maintenance/sustainability of the outcomes, organizers may see a need to "loop back" to a previous step in the process to rethink or rework before proceeding onward in their plan. And finally, once the work of the group has been completed (that is, either the issue has been solved or community empowerment achieved), the group can either disband or reorganize to deal with other issues.

SUMMARY

Community organization refers to various methods of intervention whereby individuals, groups, and organizations engage in planned collective action to deal with social concerns. The literature on community organizing and building is not distinct; it is often intertwined with such terms as *community-based*, *community empowerment*, *community participation*, and *community partnerships*. The process of community organization has been used for many years in the area of social work, but its history in the area of health promotion is much more recent. This chapter presented generic processes for community organizing and building, which should be an adequate introduction to the process.

REVIEW QUESTIONS

1. What is meant by the term *community*?

2. How does community organization relate to community empowerment?

3. From which discipline did community organization originate?

4. What is the underlying concept of community organization?

5. What are some of the assumptions under which planners work when organizing a community?

6. What are the basic steps in the community organizing and building processes?

7. What is the difference between a task force and a coalition?

8. What is meant by the term *gatekeepers*?

9. What is the difference between a needs assessment and a capacities and assets assessment?

10. What is meant by *mapping community capacity?*

11. What are the differences among primary, secondary, and potential building blocks (assets)?

ACTIVITIES

1. Assume that a core group of individuals have come together to deal with concern about the high rate of teenage pregnancy in a community. Identify (by job title/function) others who you think should be invited to be part of the larger group. In addition, provide a one-sentence rationale for inviting each. Assume that this community is large enough to have most social service organizations.

2. Provide a list of at least 10 different community agencies that should be invited to make up an antismoking coalition in your home town. Provide a one-sentence rationale for including each.

3. Assume that you want to make entry into a community with which you are not familiar in order to help to organize and build the community. Describe such a community, and then write a two-page paper to tell what steps you would take to gain entrance into the community.

4. If you wanted to find out more about your community's resources regarding exercise programs, with whom would you network? Provide a list of at least five contacts, and provide a one-sentence rationale for why you selected each.

5. Ask your professor if he or she is aware of any community organizing or building efforts in a local community. If such exists, make an appointment along with some of your classmates to interview the organizers. Ask the organizers to respond to the following questions:

   a. What concern is the group tackling?
   b. Who identified the initial concern?
   c. Who makes up the core group? How large is it?
   d. Did the group complete an assessment?
   e. What type of intervention is being used?
   f. What type of community organizing or building model was used?

6. To get a feel for the process of mapping community capacity, obtain a map of your college/university and "map" the health-related assets on your campus. Try to identify the assets in terms of primary, secondary, and potential building blocks for the campus as defined by McKnight and Kretzmann (2005). After your map is complete, analyze what you have found. Where are most of the assets located? Did the results surprise you? If your campus were going to increase its health capacity, what would you recommend? Why?

7. The most common form of community organizing efforts found in most communities are coalitions. Ask your professor if he or she is aware of any coalitions in the community. If such exists, with some of your classmates make an appointment to interview the coordinator of the coalition. Find out about the general functioning of the coalition and specifically ask about the challenges the coalition has faced and how its members dealt with them. If possible, also attend a coalition meeting. Summarize your results in a three-page paper.

WEBLINKS

1. http://www.abcdinstitute.org

   Asset-Based Community Development (ABCD) Institute, Northwestern University

   The ABCD was built on the community development research of Jody Kretzmann and John L. McKnight. The Website provides background information on many of the projects sponsored by the ABCD Institute.

2. http://ctb.ku.edu/en/default.aspx

   The Community Tool Box (CTB), University of Kansas

   The CTB provides practical information to support work in promoting community health and development. This Website is maintained by the Work Group on Health

Promotion and Community Development at the University of Kansas in Lawrence, Kansas, and offers a list of chapters that provide step-by-step guidance for community-building skills. Within each chapter are a number of sections that include background information, examples, tools and checklists, and PowerPoint® slides.

3. http://www.nhlbi.nih.gov/health/prof/heart/obesity/hrt_n_pk/cm_gde.pdf

   National Heart, Lung, and Blood Institute (NHLBI)

   This is the NHLBI Webpage where you can find the *Hearts N' Parks Community Mobilization Guide*, developed by the NHLBI and the National Recreation and Park Association. The guide was created to assist planners at the community level with implementing a Hearts N' Parks program that is aimed at promoting heart-healthy lifestyles and changes such as increased physical activity and heart-healthy eating among children and adults. The guide provides all the necessary tools for implementing this program including background information and materials, techniques for creating and delivering heart-healthy activities to participants, tools and strategies for reaching targeted groups, forming partnerships, and working with the media, as well as assessment tools to measure program performance.

4. http://www.marininstitute.org/action_packs/community_org.htm

   Marin Institute

   The Marin Institute (TMI) is located in Marin County, California, and is supported by the Buck Trust (from the Leonard and Beryl Buck Foundation). TMI works to reduce alcohol problems through environmental prevention. This particular Webpage provides a detailed explanation of community organizing.

5. http://www.mediaengage.org/execute/mapping/index.cfm

   National Center for Media Engagement (NCME)

   NCME is funded by the Corporation for Public Broadcasting and is affiliated with the University of Wisconsin-Extension. The NCME Website provides resources for community mapping including a tutorial on how to map a community using Google Earth and a two-part Webinar on how to map a community.

PART II

IMPLEMENTING A HEALTH PROMOTION PROGRAM

The chapters in this section present information used in implementing a health promotion program. The chapters identify important components related to implementation and address the challenges one may face during the implementation process. The chapters and topics presented in this section are:

CHAPTER 10

Identification and Allocation of Resources

After reading this chapter and answering the questions at the end, you should be able to:

- Define *resources*.
- List the common resources used in most health promotion programs.
- Identify the tasks to be carried out by program personnel.
- Explain the difference between internal and external personnel.
- Explain how *technical assistance*, *volunteers*, *teamwork*, and *cultural factors* are related to program personnel.
- Define *culturally competent*.
- Explain what is meant by the term *canned health promotion programs*.
- Identify questions to ask vendors when they are selling their programs, products, and services.
- List and explain common means of financing health promotion programs.
- Identify and explain the major components of a grant proposal.
- Define *budget*.
- Explain what is meant by *direct* and *indirect costs*.

KEY TERMS

adjourning
budget
canned program
cultural competence
curriculum
expenditures
external personnel
flex time
forming

full-time equivalent (FTE)
gift
grant
grantsmanship
hard money
in-house materials
in-kind contributions
internal personnel

memorandum of
   understanding (MOU)
norming
ownership
peer education
performing
profit margin
proposal
reforming

Key Terms, continued

request for applications (RFAs)	sliding-scale fee	technical assistance
request for proposals (RFPs)	soft money	vendors
resources	speakers bureaus	volunteers
SAM	storming	
seed dollars	team	

For a program to reach its identified goals and objectives, it must be supported with the appropriate resources. **Resources** include the "human, fiscal, and technical assets available" (Johnson & Breckon, 2007, p. 296) to plan, implement, and evaluate a program. The quantity or amount of resources needed to plan, implement, and evaluate a program depends on the scope and nature of the program. Most resources carry a "price tag," which planners must take into account. Thus planners face the task of securing the financial resources necessary to carry out a program. However, several different resources are provided by organizations, mostly voluntary or governmental health organizations, that are free or inexpensive. This chapter identifies, describes, and suggests sources for obtaining the resources commonly needed in planning, implementing, and evaluating health promotion programs. **Box 10.1** identifies the responsibilities and competencies for health education specialists that pertain to the material presented in this chapter.

Box 10.2 lists the major categories of resources and accompanying questions that need to be answered in order to have the necessary resources to plan, implement, and evaluate a program. If you are currently planning a health promotion program, take a few minutes to read through the list and attempt to answer the questions as they pertain to the program you are planning *before* you read the rest of the chapter.

Personnel

The key resource of any program is the individuals needed to carry out the program. Instead of trying to identify all the individuals necessary to ensure a program's success (because many times the same person is responsible for several different program components), planners should focus on the tasks that need to be completed by the program personnel. These tasks include: planning; identifying resources; advertising; marketing; conducting the program, including having the necessary interpreters for those who speak a different language than the one in which the program is offered and accommodating those with disabilities; evaluating the program; making arrangements for space and program materials; handling clerical work; and keeping records (for program sign-up, collection of fees, attendance, and budgeting).

In some cases, the program participants themselves constitute a program resource. For example, in the case of a worksite health promotion program, planners will need to find out whether the employees will participate on company time, on their own time before or after work hours, on a combination of company time and employee time, or on their own anytime during the work day as long as they put in their regular number of work hours. This last option is known as **flex time**. The current trend in worksite health

---

Box 10.1   RESPONSIBILITIES AND COMPETENCIES FOR
HEALTH EDUCATION SPECIALISTS

This chapter focuses on identifying and allocating resources needed to plan, implement, and evaluate a program. Because resources are needed for all aspects of the
program, Chapter 10 cuts across several different areas of responsibility. The responsibilities and competencies related to these tasks include:

Responsibility I: Assess Needs, Assets, and Capacity for Health Education

                          Competency 1.1: Plan Assessment Process

Responsibility II: Plan Health Education

                          Competency 2.2: Develop Goals and Objectives

                          Competency 2.4: Develop a Scope and Sequence for the
Delivery of Health Education

Responsibility III: Implement Health Education

                          Competency 3.2: Monitor Implementation of Health
Education

                          Competency 3.3: Train Individuals Involved in Implementation
of Health Education

Responsibility V: Administer and Manage Health Education

                          Competency 5.1: Manage Fiscal Resources

                          Competency 5.4: Manage Human Resources

                          Competency 5.5: Facilitate Partnerships in Support of Health
Education

Responsibility VI: Serve as a Health Education Resource Person

                          Competency 6.2: Provide Training

                          Competency 6.3: Serve as a Health Education Consultant

Source: NCHEC, SOPHE, & AAHE (2010).

---

promotion programs is to ask the employees to participate at least partially on their own
time. The reasoning behind this trend is that this investment by the participant helps to
promote a sense of program **ownership** ("I have put something into this program, and
therefore I am going to support it") and thus build loyalty among participants.

Internal Personnel

When identifying the personnel needed to conduct a program, planners have three basic
options. One, referred to as **internal personnel,** uses individuals from within the planning agency/organization or people from within the priority population to supply the
needed labor. These individuals may be hired specifically to serve as program personnel
or existing employees may be trained to handle specific tasks. An example of using internal personnel would be when a local health department was planning a health promotion program in a community, the employees of the health department might handle the

Box 10.2 APPLICATION—WHAT RESOURCES ARE NEEDED TO PLAN, IMPLEMENT, AND EVALUATE A PROGRAM?

Personnel

- Who is needed to plan the program? Professionals? Advisory committee?
- Who is needed to implement the program? Facilitators? Support staff? Will you use a vendor?
- Who will evaluate the program? Someone associated with the program? Someone from outside?
- Is there a need for a partnership?

Curriculum and other instructional resources

- What educational materials are needed to implement the program? Will the planners create them? Will they be purchased? Will they be donated?
- Is there a need for a curriculum?
- Will a canned program be used?

Space

- What space is needed to implement the program? How will you obtain the space? Will there be a charge for the space? Will it be donated? If donated, are there hidden costs like paying for custodial services?

Equipment

- What equipment is needed to plan the program? Is office equipment such as computers and copy machines needed?
- Is equipment needed for implementation such as tables and chairs, instructional equipment (e.g., computer and projector), exercise equipment, etc.?

Supplies

- What supplies are needed for planning the program such as typical office supplies? Are postal and mailing supplies needed?
- What supplies are needed for implementation? Who will provide them? Planners? Participants? Outside group?

Financial resources

- How will the program be paid for? Will the planning group pay for it? Will the program participants pay for it? Will some third party pay for it (i.e., sponsoring group or agency, grant funded)? Or will it be paid for by a combination of sources?
- Who is responsible for creating and monitoring the budget?

planning, implementation, and evaluation of the program. If that same health department was planning a health promotion program for the faculty and staff of a school district, there would likely be many school employees (e.g., school nurse, health education specialist, physical education instructor, family and consumer science teacher) who have the expertise (knowledge and skills) to carry out much of the program. If the department was planning a worksite program, there would probably be some employees who would be qualified to conduct at least a portion of the program (for example, an employee who is certified to teach first aid or cardiopulmonary resuscitation).

Another internal resource that health promotion planners are using successfully in a variety of settings, especially in schools (from kindergarten to college), is **peer education.** The process is simple: Individuals who have specific knowledge, skills, or understanding of a concept help to educate their peers. For example, college students may work with other college students to help educate them about the dangers of drinking and driving. The major advantages of peer education are its low cost and the credibility of the instructor. Children, for example, are greatly influenced by slightly older peers.

External Personnel

A second source of personnel for a program are individuals from outside the planning agency/organization or priority population who would conduct part or all of the program. Such individuals are considered **external personnel.** Typically, these individuals are brought in when it is found that there is a gap between what can be provided internally and what ultimately must be provided to accomplish the program goals and objectives (Harris, 2001). Many companies now offer or sell programs, services, or consulting to groups wanting health promotion programs. These companies are referred to as **vendors.** Some vendors are for-profit groups—such as hospitals, consulting agencies, health promotion companies, or related businesses—whereas others are nonprofit organizations—such as voluntary health agencies, YMCAs, YWCAs, governmental health agencies, universities/colleges, extension services, or professional organizations. Planners must be careful when choosing vendors (see **Box 10.3**) because the quality of vendors can vary greatly.

Box 10.3   SELECTING HEALTH PROMOTION VENDORS
Planners must be careful when selecting vendors because the quality of vendors can vary greatly. Harris and McKenzie (2004) created a checklist to help planners screen potential vendors to ensure they are a good match for the program being planned. Eight major areas to consider before selecting and entering into a contract with a vendor include: 1. Initial experience with the vendor—Was the vendor prepared for the first meeting? Can the vendor show how his/her product meets your needs? Did the vendor listen to you? Will the vendor provide a proposal? Does the vendor have a good reputation? 2. Product quality—Does the vendor have evidence to show the product is good? Will the vendor customize the product to fit your needs? Is the product up to date with regard to professional standards? 3. Professionals involved in service delivery—Are those who deliver the product qualified to do so? Are their credentials up-to-date? Are those who deliver the product evaluated?

Box 10.3 (CONTINUED)

4. Product/service delivery and satisfaction—Is the information about the product/service provided in a written document? Is there a contract to sign? Can the product/service be delivered as needed?

5. Vendor technological capability—Does the vendor have the technology to deliver the product/service as needed?

6. Evaluation and reporting—Does the vendor have the capability to collect, analyze, and report the data needed for the program?

7. Product cost and value—Is the cost competitive? Are there any hidden costs? Does the price per unit go down when more product/service is purchased?

8. General concerns—Does the vendor carry liability insurance? Is the vendor the best fit for the program?

Adapted from: The Checklist for Selecting Health Promotion Vendors. J. H. Harris and J. F. McKenzie. Copyright © 2004 by the Wellness Council of America. Reprinted with permission. And "How to Select the Right Vendor for Your Company's Selecting Health Promotion Program." J. H. Harris, J. F. McKenzie, and W. B. Zuti, from *Fitness in Business 1.* Copyright © 1986 by American School Health Association. Reprinted with permission.

Experts available through **speakers bureaus** are an often untapped inexpensive source of personnel for health promotion programs. Most local offices of voluntary health agencies, hospitals, and other health-related organizations maintain speakers bureaus. The services of these experts are usually available at little or no cost to groups. With some inquiry and a little networking, it is not difficult for planners to identify organizations that have individuals available to speak on a variety of health-related topics, or health care organizations willing to send their medical experts into the community to share their knowledge. The speakers bureau is a win-win concept for both the group offering the service and the one receiving it. Groups that take advantage of a speakers bureau gain access to expert information, but those delivering the information gain in terms of public relations and recognition.

There are advantages and disadvantages connected with using either internal or external personnel to conduct health promotion programs. **Table 10.1** lists the pros and cons of each.

Combination of Internal and External Personnel

The third option for obtaining personnel to carry out a program is using a combination of internal and external personnel. This option is the most common because it allows program planners to make use of the advantages of the first two options, while avoiding many of the disadvantages. In fact, in worksite health promotion there is evidence (Elliott, 1998) to support the use of both internal and external personnel by those in best-practice (i.e., the most successful) organizations.

Items Related to Personnel

In addition to determining the source of personnel for a program there are other personnel matters to which planners must attend. Four of these—technical assistance, volunteers, teamwork, and cultural factors—are discussed below.

Table 10.1 Advantages and Disadvantages of Using Internal and External Personnel

	Advantages	Disadvantages
Internal Program Personnel	1. Reduced costs. 2. Internal arrangements can be made to free needed personnel from their work schedules. 3. More control over those involved.	1. Limited by the interest and abilities of those on staff. 2. May have to train personnel or be limited by the expertise of those on staff. 3. Might spend more time developing the program than implementing it, thus reaching fewer people.
External Program Personnel	1. Known expertise. 2. The responsibility for conducting the program becomes the work of another. 3. Can request product (program) guarantees. 4. Sometimes external personnel are more respected than internal personnel simply because they are from the outside. 5. Bring global knowledge to the program because they have worked with a variety of entities and cultures (Harris, 2001). 6. Have the resources for sophisticated tools and programs because they can spread the cost across many clients (Harris, 2001). 7. Can reach a priority population that is geographically dispersed (Harris, 2001).	1. Often more costly than using internal personnel. 2. Subject to the limitations of any given vendor. 3. Sometimes less control over the program.

Technical Assistance   Sometimes there are enough people willing and able to handle the tasks associated with planning, implementing, and evaluating a program but for whatever reason they do not have the capability (i.e., knowledge, skills, and know how) to carry out the tasks. Or personnel may have knowledge and skills but need help in completing the tasks more effectively. Such situations call for *technical assistance* to enhance group members' capacity to complete the work. **Technical assistance** (TA), also known as *capacity-building assistance* (CBA), can be defined as a relationship in which individuals with specific knowledge and skills share their expertise, via advice and training, with those who need it. TA often comes from consultants or may be a part of a support program offered by a funding agency. For example, it is not uncommon for the Centers for Disease Control and Prevention (CDC) to offer technical assistance to groups that receive CDC funding for their programs, or to state or local health departments that need to enhance their capabilities.

Technical assistance providers must be more than just experts. They must demonstrate that they are good listeners and effective helpers to the people who will be actually conducting the planning tasks (Butterfoss, 2007). For effective TA to take place there must be a collaborative working relationship between the two parties. TA is typically provided after some sort of needs assessment (i.e., completing a checklist or questionnaire) of those who need the assistance. Once the needs are known (e.g., priority setting, intervention planning and effectiveness, evaluation techniques) the actual TA can be planned and delivered. Delivery can be completed using a number of different training strategies and can range from providing information via a telephone call, to supplying written or self-help materials, to referring those in need to other resources, to pairing those in need with a peer group (i.e., another group of planners who have completed a similar project), to more elaborate face-to-face training sessions that may last from a few hours to a few days at one time.

Volunteers Because of the circumstances associated with a health promotion program there may be a need to identify, recruit, select, and train volunteers to be a part of the personnel that help plan, implement, and evaluate the program. **Volunteers** "are individuals who serve an organization or cause. By definition, a volunteer does not get paid or receive compensation for services rendered. In health promotion programs, volunteers perform many tasks from direct service delivery, to service on boards of directors or as program advocates" (Fertman, Spiller, & Mickalide, 2010, p. 237). Often volunteers contribute services that otherwise would have to be performed by paid employees (Kilingner, Nalbandian, & Llorens, 2010) or not at all.

As with other personnel, planners should create a job description that outlines the tasks that need to be performed before recruiting volunteers. (See **Box 10.4** for an example job description for a volunteer.) Do not reduce all the volunteer jobs to simply running errands; some volunteers are happy doing that type of work but "others want skilled work with more responsibility. Defining real jobs is very important: volunteers do not like to sit around doing nothing" (Wurzbach, 2002, p. 53). In identifying the tasks to be completed by and creating job descriptions for volunteers, program planners need to remember that volunteers are motivated by different factors than those that motivate paid employees (Issel, 2009). The reasons vary. Some individuals are interested in volunteering as a means of giving back, sharing of their gifts and talents, or just helping others in the community. Others volunteer to gain experience or "get their foot in the door" of an organization where they hope to work some day. Some volunteer to do something worthwhile, stay active, or just for the social interaction (Van Der Wagen & Carlos, 2005). Still others may volunteer to enhance their knowledge or learn a new skill. The key for planners is to match the potential volunteers' motivation to the volunteer opportunities.

Once a suitable job description has been created planners are ready to recruit volunteers. Depending on the how many and what type of individuals are needed, a variety of techniques can be used to recruit volunteers. The most traditional way of recruiting is via

Box 10.4   SAMPLE JOB DESCRIPTION FOR A VOLUNTEER

Position Title:	Health Education Volunteer
Reports to:	Senior Health Education Specialist
Responsible for:	Distribution of health education materials at the patient education desk
Position Summary:	To assist patients of the Stonecrest Clinic get the education materials they need.
Duties:	• Greet all patients and significant others who approach the patient education desk.
	• Use materials available at the patient education desk to "fill" the patient education prescription provided by the health care providers in the Stonecrest Clinic.
	• Help obtain appropriate educational materials for the Stonecrest Clinic.
	• Monitor and maintain inventory; help to re-stock the education materials at the patient education desk, as needed.
	• Provide excellent customer service as outlined in the core values of the Stonecrest Clinic.
	• Answer the phone at the patient education desk.
Qualifications:	• Education
	—High school diploma or equivalent
	• Knowledge
	—Basic medical terminology
	• Skills
	—Communication: Good verbal and nonverbal skills
	—Computer: Typing speed of 40 wpm; able to search Internet; use word processing and database programs
	—Problem solving
Desirable:	• Health education experience
	• Customer service experience

a mass media outlet (e.g., radio, television, and newspapers), but posting flyers in high-traffic areas where desired volunteers pass can be effective as well. In addition, today viral recruiting can be used via social media or via personal word-of-mouth invitations. Places where planners may find potential volunteers include religious organizations, community service organizations (e.g., Jaycees, Rotary), and colleges and universities. In fact, many of the educational institutions require community service or service learning as part of graduation requirements.

Potential volunteers should not be accepted automatically for a position; instead they should be interviewed, just as a prospective employee would be. It is important to make sure that the person is right for the job, and that the person's philosophy is consistent with that of the organization where they will volunteer (Wurzbach, 2002). After the interview process, planners may find that they have attracted good people but those individuals may not have all the knowledge and skills to complete the work. This makes training the volunteers particularly critical to the success of a health promotion program (Issel, 2009). Similar steps noted in the technical assistance section earlier can be used to train volunteers.

Once on the job volunteers need to be supervised and periodically evaluated. The person to whom they report could handle this. If a program needs a large number of volunteers, it may be necessary to hire a volunteer coordinator (Wurzbach, 2002).

Good volunteers are not easy to find so every effort should be made to retain them. For the most part, if volunteers are happy and satisfied with the work they will continue. To increase the chances of this happening, include volunteers in staff meetings and functions when it is appropriate, and show appreciation for their help by saying thank you often, providing positive feedback, and publicly recognizing their achievements and service through newsletters, news releases, and/or recognition ceremony (Wurzbach, 2002).

Before leaving our discussion of volunteers, we want you to be aware that volunteer help does not always work out as planned. Organizations have "the right to decide on the best placement of a volunteer, to express opinions about poor volunteer performance in a diplomatic way, and to release an inappropriate volunteer" (Van Der Wagen & Carlos, 2005, p. 180). And finally, when volunteers resign, always hold an exit interview with them to get their comments on the good and bad aspects of their volunteer work (Wurzbach, 2002) so that you can improve future volunteer experiences.

Working as a Team   Because of the multiple tasks associated with planning, implementing, and evaluating health promotion programs and the need for a variety of resources to have effective programs, health education specialists often work as part of a group or team. Further, *teamwork* is becoming a preferred approach in many work settings because "organizational problems and issues are so complex today that no one person can grasp all the information nor have all the skills to adequately and thoroughly analyze and choose the best solutions. The complexity of problems also requires innovations and diversity of viewpoints to see all the options and consequences involved" (Kilingner et al., 2010, p. 224). A **team** had been defined as "a small group of people with complementary skills who are committed to a common purpose, a set of performance goals, and an approach for which they hold themselves mutually accountable" (Gomez-Mejia & Balkin, 2012, p. 384). Teams differ from *working groups* in that in a working group members are accountable for individual work but are not responsible for the output of the entire group (Gomez-Mejia & Balkin, 2012). Teams can vary in size and be as small as two people; however, the sizes of high-performing teams range between 5 and 12 members (Gomez-Mejia & Balkin, 2012).

Lovelace and colleagues (2009) found in a study that health education specialists "participated in an average of four teams per individual; three of these were interorganizational teams. Moreover, 40% of the respondents participated in five or more teams" (p. 428). These authors further stated that in order to be effective, health education specialists "must be able to work collaboratively with community members and other professionals" (p. 429). "In fact, words like *boundary-spanning*, *collaborative public management*, *bridge building*, and *facilitative leadership* all attest to the way that contemporary work is conducted" (Kilingner et al., 2010, p. 224).

Team creation can come about in a couple of different ways. When teams are created within an organization, say within a local health department, member assignments may occur formally when a supervisor or manager organizes a team based on the people and their skills. If interorganizational teams are assembled typically the team is composed of whomever each organization assigns to the team. This is a more informal means of team composition in that no one individual selects team members for their individual knowledge and skills. Whichever way is used, each team will need a leader or leaders to guide the work of the team.

"Teams are not instantly functional and effective" (Butterfoss, 2007, p. 164); they take time to develop. Understanding how teams develop and what stage a team is in can help planners be more efficient in the planning process. To help explain the development, Tuckman (1965) identified the development sequence of small groups. He created a model based on the review of "50 articles, many of which were psychoanalytic studies of therapy or T groups" (Tuckman, 2001). The original model included four stages—*forming*, *storming*, *norming*, and *performing*. Several years later, Tuckman and Jensen (1977) added a fifth stage—*adjourning*. More recently, the fifth stage has been called *mourning* (Butterfoss, 2007) or *reforming* (UNCE, 2003). Over time, the "stages of group development" terminology has changed a bit and the five stages are now associated with team development.

The first stage, **forming**, can be thought as an orientation stage. As such, little real work is accomplished. In this stage members are introduced, meet, and get to know each other. During this stage the ground rules for the group are established, such as defining the purpose of the team, team structure (e.g., roles and responsibilities), logistics for operation (e.g., procedures, meeting times), and expectations (Gomez-Mejia & Balkin, 2012). As such, "two important things must be accomplished in this first stage: members must feel welcome and included and have a sense that their opinions will be respected; and they need to develop a consensus, or group agreement, about the basic mission or goal they are working toward" (Butterfoss, 2007, p. 164). In the second stage, **storming**, members will have different opinions about team goals, assigned tasks and responsibilities, and procedures (Gomez-Mejia & Balkin, 2012). The conflict may be uncomfortable, turf wars can occur, and some members may feel frustrated. Good teams with good leadership will be able to work through this stage, but if the conflict is too great and cannot be resolved, teams may disband.

The teams that emerge will enter into stage three, **norming**. In this stage, "team members finally understand their roles and establish closer relationships, intensifying the cohesion and interdependence of members" (Gomez-Mejia & Balkin, 2012, p. 390). In the fourth phase, **performing**, teams are involved in "constructive action" (Tuckman, 1965); they are working toward the team goals. "This is the stage where a great deal of work can occur, and the team may become creative. As new tasks emerge, members confidently tackle them. The whole team works together or may delegate work to task groups and individuals" (Butterfoss, 2007, p. 165). After the performing stage, teams may enter into the **adjourning** (or *mourning*) stage or decide to move to **reforming**. In the former, the team has reached its goal, thus completing its work. As such it may decide to disband. However, the disbanding may not be easy, thus the term *mourning*. In the latter, reforming, the team may continue on by refocusing its efforts on other tasks or problems. **Table 10.2** provides a summary of member behavior, climate, and task outcome during team development.

There is no single prescription for creating effective working teams; however, several authors have identified characteristics that are important. Gomez-Mejia and Balkin (2012) have identified five behavioral characteristics of effective teams: (1) cohesiveness, (2) selecting high-performance norms, (3) cooperation, (4) exhibiting interdependence, and (5) trusting one another. Getha-Taylor (2008) asserts that there are three factors associated with collaborative competencies that set exemplars apart from average performers. Those factors include interpersonal understanding, teamwork and understanding, and team leadership. In identifying these three factors Getha-Taylor indicated that interpersonal understanding is the most important and only comes about through time and experience.

Cultural Factors   Regardless of who is involved in planning, implementing, and evaluating a health promotion program, there is a need to be aware of the importance of cultural factors. Cultural factors arise from guidelines (both explicit and implicit) that individuals "inherit" from being a part of a particular society, racial or ethnic group, religious community, or other group. In order for planners to be effective, they need to strive to be culturally competent (Davis & Rankin, 2006; Luquis, Pérez, & Young, 2006; Pérez & Luquis, 2008; Selig, Tropiano, & Greene-Moton, 2006). **Cultural competence** is "a developmental process defined as a set of values, principles, behaviors, attitudes, and policies that enable health professionals to work effectively across racial, ethnic and linguistically diverse populations" (Joint Committee on Terminology, 2012). Luquis and

Table 10.2 Integration of Team and Group Development Theories

Stage of Development	Leader Behavior	Member Behavior	Emotional Climate	Task Outcome
Forming	Directs	Dependence	Uncertain	Committing
Storming	Persuades	Resistance	Conflict	Clarifying
Norming	Participates	Cohesion	Support	Developing rules
Performing	Delegates Negotiates	Interdependence	Pride	Achieving
Reforming	Evaluates Reviews	Maintaining	Satisfied	Consolidating Renewing

Source: Coalitions and Partnerships in Community Health. Frances D. Butterfoss. Copyright © 2007 by Jossey-Bass. Reprinted with permission.

Pérez (2003) and Martinez-Cossio (2008) have discussed some of the issues surrounding cultural competence and some strategies by which planners can become more culturally competent. One strategy is becoming familiar with Standards for Culturally and Linguistically Appropriate Services (CLAS) presented by the Office of Minority Health (OMH, 2004) (see Weblinks at the end of this chapter for the Website). In addition, if planners are not familiar with the culture of those in the priority population we would recommend that they work with indigenous health workers and/or those who are well trained and are bilingual and bicultural.

Curricula and Other Instructional Resources

Earlier (in Chapter 8), the word **curriculum** was defined as a "planned set of lessons or courses designed to lead to competence in an area of study" (Gilbert et al., 2011, p. 412). When it comes to selecting the curriculum and other instructional materials that will be used to present the content of the program, planners can proceed in four ways: (1) by developing their own materials (in-house) or having someone else develop custom materials for them; (2) by purchasing or obtaining various instructional materials from outside sources; (3) by purchasing or obtaining entire "canned" programs from outside vendors; or (4) by using any combination of in-house materials, materials from outside sources, and canned program materials.

Developing **in-house materials** or having someone else develop custom materials has the major advantage of allowing the developers to create materials that very closely match the needs of the priority population. The more "unique" the priority population, the more important this approach may be—especially if the priority population possesses cultural differences. Materials must be relevant and culturally appropriate to the priority population (Adeyanju, 2008). However, a serious drawback is the time, money, and effort necessary to develop an original curriculum and other instructional materials. The exact amount of time necessary would obviously depend on the scope of the program and the expertise of those doing the work. No matter who does the work, however, the commitment of time and resources is sure to be considerable. In putting together an in-house program, planners should be aware of several different sources from which they can obtain free or inexpensive materials to supplement the ones they develop. Planners might also find that there is no need to create in-house materials because of the wide array of materials available. For example, most voluntary and governmental health agencies have up-to-date pamphlets on a variety of subjects that they are willing and eager to give away in quantity. Also, most communities have a public library with a video/DVD section that includes some health videos and DVDs. If the public library does not carry health videos and DVDs, almost all local and state health departments offer such a service. Planners who are unsure about what sources of information are available in their community can begin by checking the Yellow Pages of the local telephone directory or on the Internet.

Planners need to remember that just because a piece of instructional material exists does not mean it is appropriate for the priority population with which they are working. To help ensure that materials are suitable for the priority population, we would recommend the use of **SAM**: a suitability assessment of materials instrument (Doak, Doak, & Root, 1996) (see **Figure 10.1**). This validated instrument "was originally designed for use with print material and illustrations, but it has also been applied successfully to video- and audiotaped instructions. For each material, SAM provides a numerical score (in percent) that may fall in one of three categories: superior, adequate, or not suitable" (Doak et al., 1996, p. 49). Here are the steps for using SAM (Doak et al., 1996):

1. Read through the SAM factor list and the evaluation criteria.

2. Read the material (or view the video) you wish to evaluate and write brief statements as to its purpose(s) and key points.

3. For short materials, evaluate the entire piece. For long materials, select samples that are central to the purpose of the document to evaluate.

4. Evaluate and score each of the 22 SAM items, rating them as "superior" and assigning a score of two, "adequate" and assigning a score of one, "not suitable" and assigning a score of zero, or marking an item "N/A" if the factor does not apply to the material.

5. Calculate the total suitability score by summing the scores from the rated items and dividing by the total number of items rated. Do not include the items marked N/A. Multiply the score by 100 to get a percentage.

   70–100% = superior material
   40–69% = adequate material
   0–39% = not suitable material

6. Decide on the impact of deficiencies of the material and what action to take about whether to use or not use the material.

   Purchasing or obtaining entire canned programs from vendors has become very popular in recent years because of the time and money needed to create programs. A **canned program** is one that has been developed by an outside group and includes the basic components and materials necessary to implement a program. Because some vendors are for-profit groups whereas others are nonprofit organizations, the cost of these programs can range from literally nothing at all to thousands of dollars.

   Most canned programs have five major components:

1. A participant's manual (printed material that is easy to follow and read and is handy for participants)

2. An instructor's manual (a much more comprehensive document than the participant's manual, which includes the program content, background information, and lesson and unit plans with ideas for presenting the material)

3. Audiovisual materials that help present the program content (usually including videotapes/DVDs and audiotapes, PowerPoint® presentations, charts, or posters)

4. Training for the instructors (a concentrated experience that prepares individuals to become instructors)

5. Marketing (the "wrapping" that makes the program attractive to both the participants and the planners who will purchase it to market to the participants)

2 points for superior rating
1 point for adequate rating
0 points for not suitable rating
N/A if the factor does not apply to this material

FACTOR TO BE RATED	SCORE	COMMENTS
1. CONTENT		
(a) Purpose is evident	_____	_____
(b) Content about behaviors	_____	_____
(c) Scope is limited	_____	_____
(d) Summary or review included	_____	_____
2. LITERACY DEMAND		
(a) Reading grade level	_____	_____
(b) Writing style, active voice	_____	_____
(c) Vocabulary uses common words	_____	_____
(d) Context is given first	_____	_____
(e) Learning aids via "road signs"	_____	_____
3. GRAPHICS		
(a) Cover graphic shows purpose	_____	_____
(b) Type of graphics	_____	_____
(c) Relevance of illustration	_____	_____
(d) List, tables, etc. explained	_____	_____
(e) Captions used for graphics	_____	_____
4. LAYOUT AND TYPOGRAPHY		
(a) Layout factors	_____	_____
(b) Typography	_____	_____
(c) Subheads ("chunking") used	_____	_____
5. LEARNING STIMULATION, MOTIVATION		
(a) Interaction used	_____	_____
(b) Behaviors are modeled and specific	_____	_____
(c) Motivation—self-efficacy	_____	_____
6. CULTURAL APPROPRIATENESS		
(a) Match in logic, language, experience	_____	_____
(b) Cultural image and examples	_____	_____

Total SAM score: _____

Total possible score: _____ , Percent score: _____%

Figure 10.1 SAM Scoring Sheet

Source: Teaching Patients with Low Literacy Skills, 2nd Edition. C. C. Doak, L. G. Doak, & J. H. Root. Copyright © 1996 by J. B. Lippincott Company. Reprinted with permission of the authors.

The advantages and disadvantages of canned programs are just the opposite of those for materials developed in-house. No time is spent on development; however, the program may not fit the needs or the demographic characteristics of the priority population. For example, using the same canned smoking cessation program with middle-aged adults who realize the long-term hazards of cigarettes and with teenagers who are required to attend a smoking cessation program for disciplinary reasons may not be advisable. Most adults who enter smoking cessation programs are there because they do not want to smoke. Obviously, this is not the case with teenagers who have been caught smoking. The approaches taken with these two programs would have to be very different if both are to be successful. Another example of when use of a canned program would not be advisable is use of a program that was designed for upper-middle-class suburban adults in a program for low-income inner-city populations. The lifestyles of the two groups are just too different for the same program to be appropriate in both situations. Because of the possible mismatch between the needs and peculiarities (i.e., age, culture, ethnicity, norms, race, sex, socioeconomic status) of a particular priority population, planners are urged to move with caution when deciding on the use of a canned program. Make sure there is a good fit.

Canned programs often come attractively packaged and seemingly complete, but this does not mean that they are well-conceived and effective programs. Before adopting canned programs for use, planners should consider the following seven questions:

1. Is the program based on best practices? If not, why not?

2. Is there evidence to show the program is effective?

3. Does the program include a long-term behavior modification component? There are no "quick fixes" with regard to many health behavior changes. If behavior modification is used, it should be based on sound health behavior practice over an appropriate time frame.

4. Is the program educationally sound? Not only should the program be based on sound psychological and sociological theory but it should also be based on valid educational theory.

5. Is the program motivational? Health behavior change is not easy to accomplish, and so all programs need to include activities that motivate people to get and stay involved.

6. Is the program enjoyable? Planned programs should be enjoyable. Some people like hard work, but it is difficult to sustain hard work for a long time without some enjoyment.

7. Can the program be modified to meet the specific needs and peculiarities of the priority population? As mentioned earlier, not all populations have the same needs, beliefs, traditions, and ways of approaching a problem.

Space

Another major resource needed for most health promotion programs is sufficient space—a place where the program can be held. Depending on the type of program and the intended audience, space may or may not be readily available. For example, an employer may make space available for a worksite program, or a school system may furnish space for a school program. If space is a problem, planners may be able to locate inexpensive space in local schools, colleges and universities, religious facilities, and in "community service rooms" (rooms that are available free of charge to community groups as a community service) of local businesses. In addition, planners may find educational institutions and local businesses that are willing to cosponsor programs and thus contribute the space necessary to conduct the program. It may also be possible to obtain space by trading for it. For instance, a planner might trade expertise, such as serving as consultant for a program, in return for the use of suitable space. Or it might be possible to trade one space for another, such as trading the use of classrooms for time in the local YMCA/YWCA pool.

One final note of caution about space: Even if space is provided free of charge for a program, make sure to ask if there are any associated costs for the "free space." It is not uncommon for an organization offering the space (e.g., a school district) to do so with the obligation to pay for the custodial time to clean up the space once it has been used. Thus, a charge such as two hours of overtime pay for the custodial staff may be an obligation in order to use the free space.

Equipment and Supplies

Most health promotion programs will need both equipment and supplies in order to be planned, implemented, and evaluated. Though oftentimes the words *equipment* and *supplies* are used to mean the same thing, from planning and budgeting perspectives they are usually considered two different types of commodities, and not all organizations define the words the same. Some organizations define equipment and supplies by costs. That is, equipment may be anything costing more than $500, whereas supplies are anything costing between $1 and $499. Thus, a computer may be equipment, while paper or even a chair may be a supply. These same organizations usually have a dollar amount definition for major equipment items (sometimes referred to as *capital expenditures* or *capital equipment*) as anything costing more than so many thousands of dollars depending on the nature of the organization. Other organizations may define equipment and supplies based on the "life" of the commodity. For example, equipment may be anything that will last three years or more, and supplies anything that lasts fewer than three years. Thus, under this type of classification a computer may be considered a supply. Or, an organization may define equipment as something that is not consumable, like a desk, and a supply to be something that is consumable like photocopy paper. It is not so important how the words are defined, but planners need to know how they are defined and work within those parameters.

Some programs may require a great deal of equipment and supplies. For example, first aid and safety programs need items such as CPR mannequins, splints, blankets, bandages, dressings, and video equipment. Other programs, such as a stress management program, may need only paper and pencils. Whatever the kinds and amounts of equipment and supplies required, planners must give advance thought to their needs so as to:

• Determine the necessary equipment and supplies to facilitate the program

• Identify the sources where the equipment and supplies can be obtained

• Find a way to pay for the needed equipment and supplies

Financial Resources

To hire the individuals needed to plan, implement, and evaluate a health promotion program and to pay for the other resources required, planners must obtain appropriate financial support. Most programs are limited by the financial support available. In fact, few programs are financed at such a level that planners would say they have all the money they need. Because of this, the planners are often faced with making decisions about how to allocate the funds that are available. Some typical financial questions that planners generally must address are the following:

- Is it better to run an adequately financed program for a few people or to run a poorly financed program for more people?

- If funds are limited where is the first place we should cut?

- Should we start a program knowing that we will be short of funds, or should we wait until we have appropriate funding before we begin?

- Is it better to have fewer instructors or to make do with fewer supplies?

Programs can be financed in several different ways. Some sources of financial support are very traditional, whereas others may be limited only by the creativity and imagination of those involved. Following are several established ways of financing programs.

Participant Fee

This method of financing a program requires the participants to pay for the cost of the program. Depending on whether the program is offered on a profit-making basis, this fee may be equal to expenses or may include a **profit margin**. Participant fees not only are a means by which programs can be financed but they also help motivate participants to stay involved in a program. If people pay to participate in a program, then they may be more likely to continue to participate because they have made an investment—that is, a commitment. This concept has also been referred to as *ownership*. Many participants who pay a fee feel like they are part "owners" of the program. However, it should be noted that not everyone shares in the ownership concept. There are some participants who still would prefer a free or almost free program that has been paid for by others. An example of the ownership and cost issue is the participant fees associated with smoking cessation programs. If planners were looking for vendors of smoking cessation programs, they would find that the costs of such programs range from zero (e.g., American Cancer Society's *FreshStart* program) to modest (e.g., American Lung Association's *Freedom from Smoking* program) to expensive (e.g., those offered by private health promotion companies).

Deciding to finance a program through a participant fee may sound easy, but planners need to give serious thought to how much they will charge and who will be charged. Often, those most in need of a health promotion program are the least able to pay. Planners do not want to create a barrier to program participation by charging a fee or setting the fee too high. If a fee is necessary, then planners should consider creating a fee structure on "ability to pay." One form of this is a **sliding-scale fee**—that is, the less one's income, the lower the participant fee. Or, planners may want to consider offering "scholarships" to those unable to pay.

Third-Party Support

Most individuals are familiar with insurance companies' acting as third-party payers to cover the costs of health care. Although health insurance is not often used to pay for health promotion programs, others can be third-party payers. Third-party means that someone other than participants (the first-party) or planners (the second-party) is paying for the program. Third-party payers that may cover the cost of health promotion programs are:

- Employers that pick up the cost for employees, as is often the case in worksite health promotion programs

- Agencies other than the groups sponsoring the program—for example, when local service or civic groups "adopt" a pet program

- A professional association or union that financially supports a program

The money used by third-party payers can be generated from a special fund-raising event, from sale of concessions, or with money saved from reduced health care costs, absenteeism, or the remodeling of employee benefit plans.

Cost Sharing

A third means of financing a program involves a combination of participant fee and third-party support. It is not unusual to have an employer pay 50% to 80% of a program's costs and have employees pay the remaining 50% to 20%. Or, an employer may have a reimbursement policy for program participation. With such policies, employees are responsible for paying the participation fee, and then based on either attendance at the program (e.g., the employee must attend at least 80% of the program sessions) or completion of the program (e.g., employee must produce a certificate of completion), the employer reimburses the employee for either all or a portion of the participant fee. Such arrangements have the advantages of both ownership and a fringe benefit.

Cooperative Agreements

There are times when two parties (e.g., groups, organizations, individuals, agencies) decide to share resources and work together to offer a program or service. Oftentimes these agreements do not involve the transfer of money from one party to the other, though they may, but rather access to and sharing of resources (Fertman et al., 2010). For example, one agency may be willing to provide educational literature to another agency in return for space to present a program or the use of an employee's time. It is not uncommon for such agreements to be spelled out in a written document and signed by an individual of each agency with authority to do so. The written document may be a *letter of agreement* (Fertman et al., 2010) or something more formal like a *memorandum of understanding*

(MOU) or *memorandum of agreement* (MOA). A **memorandum of understanding** is defined as "a document that describes the general principles of an agreement between parties, but does not amount to a substantive contract" (Dictionary.com, 2011). It is not unusual for such an agreement to help support a grant proposal (Fertman et al., 2011) (see the discussion of grants below).

Organizational Sponsorship

Many times, the sponsoring organization (health department, hospital, or voluntary agency) bears the cost of the program as a part of its programming or operating budget. For example, the American Cancer Society offers its smoking cessation program free of charge. That is, program materials are provided free and an American Cancer Society volunteer conducts the program. The program is paid for with the society's community service funds.

Grants and Gifts

Another means of financing health promotion programs is through grants and gifts from other agencies, foundations, groups, and individuals. A **grant** is an award of financial assistance, the principal purpose of which is to transfer a thing of value from the grantor to a recipient to carry out a specific purpose (USDHHS, 2011a), whereas a **gift** (or *contributions*) can be sums of money or non-monetary items that are given voluntarily without compensation in return. Nonmonetary gifts are known as **in-kind contributions** and include such things as equipment, supplies, vehicles, food, or even services that are used to operate programs (Fertman et al., 2010). Both grants and gifts are often referred to as *external money*, or **soft money**. The term *soft money* refers to the fact that grants and gifts are usually given for a specific period of time and at some point will no longer be received. This is in contrast to **hard money**, which is an ongoing source of funds that is part of the operating budget of an organization from year to year.

Grant money has become an important source of program funding, especially for those working in voluntary or governmental health agencies. It thus becomes necessary for planners to develop adequate **grantsmanship** skills. These skills include (1) discovering where the grant money is located, (2) finding out how to get (apply for) the money, and (3) writing a proposal requesting the money.

Locating Grant Money   There are four basic types of grant makers: foundations, corporations, voluntary agencies, and government. These grant makers are found at three different levels: local, state, and national. They are not the only grant makers, however. Planners may also find a variety of local organizations (such as service groups like the Lion's Club or the Jaycees, or a community group like the United Way) that may be willing to support specific local causes through a grant. Philanthropic foundations are not-for-profit organizations that award grants to serve the public interest. A number of large national foundations support health promotion (e.g., Robert Wood Johnson Foundation, Rockefeller Foundation, W. K. Kellogg Foundation), but planners may find state and local foundations as well.

Not all corporations have giving programs, but many do as a part of a community service or public relations program. Planners will need to contact the corporations to "ask who is in charge of charitable giving, what subjects they consider for grants, and how the company giving program operates" (Guyer, 1999, p. 1). Library or Internet searching will possibly help answer these questions.

Voluntary health agencies also have grant programs. Though most grants from voluntary organizations at the national level are specified for research efforts, planners may find the local or state offices of these organizations are willing to provide **seed dollars** (start-up dollars) or *in-kind* contributions (such as providing free materials or other resources) for local programs.

Government is the largest grant maker. Government, at all three levels—local, state, and federal—makes grants for many purposes. With the other three grant makers (foundations, corporations, and voluntary agencies), planners can ask them to fund any project. However, with the government, only grants that are in one of the subjects specified by the government have a chance of being funded (Guyer, 1999).

When looking for grant makers, planners need to look for a pattern in giving by asking key questions: Has this funder made grants in the past for subject areas like mine? In my geographic area? In the amount I need? For the things I need funded? (Guyer, 1999). The answers to these questions, often found at Internet Websites of the grant makers, will indicate whether it is a good idea to contact the funder. After doing this initial "research," planners should call or write funding sources to ask questions and to obtain any guidelines, grant request forms or applications, and printed material about their grant making. This contact will also help establish a relationship with the funder. Planners not only can obtain needed information but they can also introduce their organization to the funder. This can be done by sending publications about the planners' organization, making personal contacts, and staying in touch (Guyer, 1999).

Planners can identify possible funding sources in several different ways. The first is by networking with others who have been successful in obtaining grant funding in the past. Because seeking grant funding is a competitive process, planners may have to network with others who are not seeking funding from the same grant maker. A second means of identifying funding sources is through library "research." A variety of books on grants may be found in college and university libraries as well as many larger public libraries. For example, there are directories of grant makers for foundations and corporations, and there is usually a directory that lists grant funders that are specific to a state. Most of these books are indexed by subject area.

Three good places to begin searches for government grants are the *Catalog of Federal Domestic Assistance* (CFDA), the *Federal Register*, and Grants.Gov. (See the Weblinks at the end of the chapter.) The CFDA, which is updated biweekly, is an online catalog "database of all Federal programs available to State and local governments (including the District of Columbia); federally-recognized Indian tribal governments; territories (and possessions) of the United States; domestic public, quasi-public, and private profit and nonprofit organizations and institutions; specialized groups; and individuals" (GSA, 2011, para. 2). The *CFDA* allows planners to search the database for programs meeting their needs and for which they are eligible. However, to apply for one of the programs, planners need to contact the office that administers the program they are interested in.

The *Federal Register* "is the official daily publication for rules, proposed rules, and notices of Federal agencies and organizations, as well as executive orders and other presidential documents" (U.S. GPO, 2011, para. 1). It would list the latest grant opportunities. *Grants.Gov* is a Website where planners can find and apply for federal government grants. The site was created in 2002 to improve government services associated with grants. At this Website planners will find over 1,000 grant programs from 26 federal grant-making agencies.

A third way of identifying funding sources is through the Internet. There are several advantages to using the Internet for seeking grant makers: convenience, time saving, and being able to reach several grant makers at the same time. Planners do not have to leave their office to conduct a search; thus much "leg work" of finding out whether a grant maker is a good fit with the planner's organization can be found almost instantaneously. In addition, some Websites permit an applicant to complete one form for grant consideration at several different funders (Breen, 1999).

The fourth way of identifying grant makers is the least difficult. Planners should be alert for **request for proposals (RFPs)** or **request for applications (RFAs)**. Many times some funding agency would like to have a project conducted for it, so the group will issue an RFP. If you feel qualified to do the work, you can submit a proposal.

Submitting Grant Proposals   As noted in the previous section, most funding agencies have specific guidelines outlining who is qualified to submit a proposal (perhaps only nonprofit groups can apply, or only practitioners who hold certain certifications) and the format for making an application. Those seeking money can request or apply for the money by writing a proposal. A **proposal** can be thought of as a written document that represents a request for money. A good proposal is one that is well written and explains how the needs of the funding agency can be met by the group wishing to receive the money. To increase their chances of writing a good proposal, planners should call the funding agency first and speak with the grant officer to find out specifically what he or she is looking for and the format desired.

Because there is a great deal of competition for grant money, it is more than likely that proposals will be read by a busy, impatient, skeptical person who has no reason to give any one proposal special consideration and who is faced with many more requests than he or she can grant, or even read thoroughly. Such a reader wants to find out quickly and easily the answers to these seven questions:

1. What do you want to do, how much will it cost, and how much time will it take?

2. How does the proposed project relate to the sponsor's interests?

3. What will be gained if this project is carried out?

4. What has already been done in the area of the project?

5. How do you plan to do it?

6. How will the results be evaluated?

7. Why should you, rather than someone else, conduct this project?

As noted, funding agencies request proposals/applications in a variety of different forms. However, several components are contained in most proposals no matter what the funding agency. **Box 10.5** presents these components.

Box 10.5 THE COMPONENTS OF A GRANT PROPOSAL

1. **Title (or cover) page.** When writing the title, be concise and explicit; avoid words that add nothing.

2. **Abstract or executive summary.** Provides a summary of the proposed project. May be the most important part of the proposal. Should be written last and be about 200 words long.

3. **Table of contents.** May or may not be needed, depending on the length of the proposal. It is a convenience for the reader.

4. **Introduction.** Should begin with a capsule statement, be comprehensible to the informed layperson, and include the statement of the problem, significance of the program, and purpose of the program.

5. **Background.** Should include the proposer's previous related work and the related literature.

6. **Description of proposed program.** Should include the objectives, description of intervention, evaluation plan, and time frame.

7. **Description of relevant institutional/agency resources.** Should identify the resources the proposer's organization will bring to the project.

8. **List of references.** Should include references cited in the proposal.

9. **Personnel section.** Should include the résumés of those who are to work with the program.

10. **Budget.** Should include financial needs for personnel (salaries and wages), equipment, materials and supplies, travel, services, other needed items, and indirect costs.

Combining Sources

It should be obvious that planners should not be limited to any single source for financing a health promotion program. In fact, it is more than likely that most programs will be funded via a variety of sources—that is, any combination of the sources listed previously.

Preparing and Monitoring a Budget

Simply put, a **budget** is a "formal statement of the estimated revenues and expenditures" (Johnson & Breckon, 2007, p. 170) for a program. A budget represents the decision makers' intentions and expectations by allocating funds to achieve desired outcomes (program goals and objectives) (Fallon & Zgodzinski, 2012).

A budget can be prepared for any length of time. When programs are planned, budgets are usually created for the entire length of the program. However, when a program is projected to last longer than a year, the overall program budget is typically broken down into 12-month periods.

Developing a budget is an essential and critical step of the planning process (Johnson & Breckon, 2007; Fallon & Zgodzinski, 2012). Typically, a program budget is developed by those planning the program and any other key decision makers who control resources that will be used in the program. The process begins by examining the financial objective of the program. From a financial standpoint, programs can make money (a profit), lose money, or break even. If a program must make money, the revenue will have to be greater than the expenditures, and the intended profit (*profit margin*) will need to be included in the budgeting process. **Figure 10.2** presents a sample budget sheet that lists line items that are often included in health promotion program budgets.

Revenue and Support	Amount
Contribution from sponsors	_____
Gifts	_____
Grants	_____
Participant fee	_____
Sale of curriculum material	_____
Total income	_____
Expenditures	
Direct Costs	
Personnel	
Salary & wages	_____
Fringe benefits	_____
Consultants	_____
Supplies	
Instructional materials	_____
Incentives	_____
Meeting costs	_____
Equipment	_____
Travel	_____
Postage	_____
Advertising	_____
Total of direct costs	_____
Indirect costs (includes rent, insurance, telephone, & other utilities)	_____
Total of indirect costs	_____
Total expenditures	_____
Balance	_____

Figure 10.2 Sample Budget Sheet

Once the financial objective of the program is known, planners can then turn their attention to the estimated revenues of the program. In other words, from where will the income come? If a program is being paid for by a grant, gift, or contributions from sponsors, the planners may know exactly how much money they will have to work with. However, if the revenue for a program is coming, either in part or whole, from participant fees, an estimate will have to be made of how many participants are expected to take part. At this point budgeting becomes a bit more complicated. Hopefully, there may be some history from previous programs to guide planners in estimating participation and thus estimate revenue, but sometimes planners may have to make decisions based on "best guesses." Whether revenue is estimated based on previous programs or best guesses, it is not uncommon to see a budget line in the revenue portion of the budget for participants' fees as: 22 participants @ $50 each = $1,100.

After the revenue for the program has been determined, planners need to estimate what expenditures are necessary for the program. An **expenditure** is a cost incurred while planning, implementing, or evaluating a program. The labels given to the costs (see **Box 10.6**), the detail to which the expenditures are listed in a budget, and various categories of expenditures (e.g., personnel, instructional materials, equipment) will vary based on the accounting practices of the organization.

Oftentimes, the largest expenditure for any program is for personnel, and because salaries and wages are often included in a budget, the detail required to show personnel involved in a program may be very involved. For example, when including the cost of personnel, planners may have to account for salaries or wages, Social Security taxes, and

---

Box 10.6   TYPES OF COSTS

- Fixed costs—those that do not vary depending on the amount of product or service delivered* (e.g., salaries and fringe benefits)
- Variable costs—those that do vary depending on the amount of product or service delivered* (e.g., supplies for each participant)
- Capital costs—those used for obtaining assets with an expected long life (e.g., office building)
- Direct cost—the portion of cost that is directly expended in providing a product or service* (e.g., wages and salaries)
- Indirect costs—the portion of cost that is indirectly expended in providing a product or service* (e.g., utilities, insurance, space, equipment maintenance)
- Hard costs—the purchase price of actual assets* (e.g., copy machine, computers)
- Soft costs—additional fees for items* (e.g., extended warranties, service contracts for the new equipment)
- Unexpected costs—costs that are not budgeted for (e.g., repair bill, legal fees)

*Source: VentureLine. (2011). *Accounting terms/accounting dictionary/accounting glossary*. Retrieved June 6, 2011, from http://www.ventureline.com/accounting-glossary/

fringe benefits (e.g., health and disability insurance, vacation days, sick days). As well, the exact dollar amount of fringe benefits is not calculated for a budget, but rather a percent of an employee's salary or wage is used to express the cost of fringe benefits. Thus, a fringe benefit line of a budget may read: 0.30 of $30,000 = $9,000. This means that the person preparing the budget estimates that the value of providing fringe benefits to a full-time employee making $30,000 per year is an additional $9,000. Another complicating factor in calculating personnel expenditures for a program is that a person may not be dedicated full time to a program, but the program is just one of many duties assigned to the employee.

The term used to quantify the number of people working on a program is *full-time equivalent* (FTE). A **full-time equivalent** is a unit of measurement that is calculated by dividing the average number of hours a person works per week by the average number of hours worked by a full-time employee per week. Thus, a person who works full-time is counted as 1.0 FTE. If a full-time employee averages 40 hours per week and a part-time employee works 20 hours per week, the part-time employee would count as 0.5 FTE. FTEs can also express the amount of time a person works on a program. For example, an FTE of say 0.40 would indicate that a person is working 40% of his or her time on the program. Therefore in a budget, it is not uncommon to see a salary budget line presented as: 0.20 FTE of $40,000 = $8,000. This means that 20% of a full-time equivalent (FTE) employee who makes $40,000 a year is being charged to the program. Regardless of the format used to create a budget, the budget should be put together in sufficient detail that all revenue and expenditures are accounted for.

While the dollar value for many of the other items included in a budget are straightforward (e.g., cost of instructional materials or supplies), indirect costs associated with overhead expenses (e.g., telephone and other utilities) are more difficult to put an exact dollar value on. For example, an organization may be running several different programs at the same time, but using just one telephone line to service all of the programs. So what percent of the telephone bill should be associated with each program? To handle this situation in the budget it is typical to determine the indirect costs as a percentage of the direct costs. The actual percentage used varies depending on the practices of the organization; however the percentage typically ranges between 10% and 50%. Thus, a budget that has direct costs of say $50,000 and an indirect cost rate of 30% would enter $15,000 in the budget for indirect costs.

After a program is up and running, the budget must be monitored. This duty often falls to the person who oversees the financial resources of those planning the program. It may be one of the program planners, but will more than likely be a person who has financial responsibilities for the planning organization. This person may be responsible for both preparing and distributing the financial reports. At a minimum, those receiving the reports should include the decision makers and those responsible for the day-to-day operation of the program. The financial reports are usually generated and distributed on a regular basis (i.e., monthly, bimonthly, quarterly), and each report usually includes actual revenue and expenditures for the period, year-to-date totals on actual revenue and expenditures, and year-to-date budgeted revenue and expenditures. Such data allows decision makers and planners to know exactly where they are with regard to financial resources. (see **Figure 10.3**).

Note: 3 months = 25% of budget	Total Budget	YTD 3/31/12	Percent of Budget	Budget Balance
Revenue & Support				
Contributions	1,747.50	1,247.00	71.35%	500.50
Grant #0428	1,000.00	0.00	0.00%	1,000.00
Grant #1205	62,000.00	23,000.00	37.10%	39,000.00
Grant #1107	120,000.00	60,000.00	50.00%	60,000.00
Participant fees	4,500.00	3,505.00	77.89%	995.00
Interest Income	100.00	27.98	23.98%	72.02
Total Revenue & Support	189,347.50	87,779.98	46.36%	101,567.52
Expenditures				
Personnel				
Salary & Wages—Administration	10,000.00	2,400.00	24.00%	7,600.00
Salary & Wages—Educators	70,000.00	18,000.00	25.71%	52,000.00
Salary & Wages—Clerical	30,000.00	7,600.00	25.33%	22,400.00
Subtotal Salary & Wages	110,000.00	28,000.00	25.45%	82,000.00
Payroll Taxes	19,000.00	5,000.00	26.32%	14,000.00
Health Insurance	15,500.00	3,500.00	22.58%	12,000.00
State Unemployment Taxes	8,000.00	2,000.00	25.00%	6,000.00
Workers Comp. Insurance	500.00	125.00	25.00%	375.00
Subtotal Personnel	153,000.00	38,625.00	25.25%	114,375.00
Operating Expenses				
Supplies	1,300.00	600.00	46.15%	700.00
Instructional materials	2,500.00	2,000.00	80.00%	500.00
Incentives	750.00	200.00	26.67%	550.00
Meeting costs	1,200.00	400.00	33.33%	800.00
Equipment—copier lease	1,200.00	400.00	33.33%	800.00
Travel	4,000.00	1,800.00	45.00%	2,200.00
Postage	300.00	125.00	41.67%	175.00
Advertising	400.00	150.00	37.50%	250.00
Subtotal Operating Expenses	11,650.00	5,675.00	48.71%	250.00
Total Direct Costs	164,650.00	44,300.00	26.91%	5,975.00
Total Indirect Costs (rate=15%)	24,697.50	6,646.10	26.91%	18,051.40
Total expenditures	189,347.50	50,946.10	26.91%	138,401.40
Net Surplus or (deficit)	-.--	36,833.88	-.--	-.--

Figure 10.3 Example First-Quarter Budget Report

SUMMARY

This chapter identified and discussed the most often used resources for health promotion programs: personnel, curriculum and other instructional materials, space, equipment and supplies, and funding. In addition, information was presented on how to secure and allocate resources, how to obtain funding, and how to create and monitor a budget.

REVIEW QUESTIONS

1. What are the major categories of resources that planners need to consider when planning a health promotion program?

2. What are the advantages and disadvantages of using internal personnel? External personnel?

3. How are technical assistance, volunteers, teamwork, and cultural factors associated with program personnel?

4. Define the terms *ownership*, *flex time*, *vendor*, and *canned programs*.

5. What are some key questions that planners should ask vendors when they try to sell their product?

6. How might program planners obtain free or inexpensive space for a program?

7. What is the SAM? What is it used for?

8. List and explain the different means by which health promotion programs can be funded.

9. What is meant by the term *profit margin?*

10. What is a budget? What are the major components of a budget?

11. What is the difference between direct and indirect costs?

ACTIVITIES

1. Identify and describe the resources you anticipate needing to carry out a program you are planning. Be sure to answer the following questions that apply to your program:

    a. What personnel will be needed to carry out the program? List the individuals and the duties to be carried out.

    b. What curriculum or educational materials will you use in your program? Why did you select it or them?

    c. What kind of space allocation will your program require? How will you obtain the space? How much will it cost?

    d. What equipment and supplies do you anticipate using? How will you obtain them?

    e. How do you anticipate paying for the program? Why did you select this method?

2. Visit the local office of a voluntary agency and find out what type of resources it makes available to individuals planning health promotion programs. Ask for a sample of the materials. Also, ask if the agency offers any canned programs. If it does, find out as much as you can about the programs and ask for any available descriptive literature.

3. Collect information on a single type of canned health promotion program (e.g., smoking cessation or stress management) from vendors. Then compare the strengths and weaknesses of the programs.

4. Through the process of networking and using the Internet and/or local telephone book, find where in your community there is free or inexpensive space available for health promotion programs.

5. Call three different voluntary agencies and one hospital in your community and find out if they have a speakers bureau. If they do, find out how to use the bureaus and what topics the speakers can address.

6. Prepare a mock grant proposal for a program you are planning. Make sure it includes all the components noted in Box 10.5.

7. Outline the major sources of income and expenses that would be associated with the program you are planning by preparing a budget sheet.

WEBLINKS

Note to readers: Because this chapter focuses on the resources necessary to conduct a program additional *Weblinks* are provided.

1. **http://www.cancer.org/**

American Cancer Society (ACS)

The ACS Website presents the most up-to-date information on cancer including treatment and prevention. The site also provides information about the ACS and the resources it can provide for cancer survivors and program planners.

2. **http://www.heart.org/HEARTORG**

American Heart Association (AHA)

The AHA Website provides planners with a wealth of information and materials about many of the cardiovascular diseases and stroke.

3. http://www.lungusa.org

American Lung Association (ALA)

The ALA Website provides a wealth of information about various lung diseases including asthma, chronic obstructive pulmonary disease (COPD), and lung cancer.

4. http://www.plannedparenthood.org

Planned Parenthood Federation of America, Inc.

Planned Parenthood is the world's largest voluntary reproductive health care organization. Planners working on programs aimed at reproductive health should find the organization's Website useful.

5. http://www.welcoa.org

Wellness Councils of America (WELCOA)

WELCOA's Website provides a variety of resources for those interested in worksite wellness programs.

6. http://www.aarp.org

AARP

AARP is a nonprofit membership organization dedicated to addressing the needs and interests of persons 50 and older. The organization's Website provides information that is applicable to those planning programs for seniors. This site also has a special section on health and wellness.

7. http://www.nationaldairycouncil.org

National Dairy Council (NDC)

The NDC's Website provides a wealth of information about nutrition and weight management.

8. http://www.nih.gov/

National Institutes of Health (NIH)

The NIH's Website not only includes information about NIH and links to all the institutes, centers, and offices but also includes health information, grant opportunities, and scientific resources.

9. http://www.cdc.gov/learning

Centers for Disease Control and Prevention (CDC)

This page at CDC's Website provides a wealth of information about various products and resources developed by CDC and CDC partners for the public health community.

10. http://www.healthfinder.gov/

    healthfinder

    Of all the *Weblinks* provided in this chapter, the healthfinder Website offers information on the greatest variety of health topics. It includes information on prevention, wellness, diseases, health care, and alternative medicine. It also includes medical dictionaries, an encyclopedia, journals, and more.

11. http://www.cdcnpin.org/

    CDC National Prevention Information Network (NPIN)

    The NPIN houses the nation's largest collection of information and resources on HIV/AIDS, STD, and TB prevention, much of which can be accessed through its Website.

12. http://www.cfda/cfda.gov

    The Catalog of Federal Domestic Assistance (CFDA)

    This is the Webpage for the CFDA that provides information on federal grants. The site deals with all types of assistance, not just financial aid. The site uses *Assistance Program* as a generic term rather than speaking about specific grant, loan, or other sorts of programs.

13. http://www.grants.gov

    Grants.gov

    This Website allows planners to electronically find and apply for competitive grant opportunities from all federal grant-making agencies. The site provides all the information planners need to apply for a grant and walks them through the process, step-by-step to their preferred practice setting.

14. http://www.gpo.gov/fdsys/

    U.S. Government Printing Office (GPO)

    The GPO Website links to the *Federal Register* (*FR*). Published by the Office of the Federal Register, National Archives and Records Administration (NARA), the *FR* is the official daily publication for rules, proposed rules, and notices of federal agencies/ organizations, as well as executive orders and other presidential documents.

15. http://www.minorityhealth.hhs.gov

    Office of Minority Health (OMH)

    The OMH Website presents information on cultural competence. The OMH was mandated by the U.S. Congress in 1994, via P.L. 101–527, to develop the capacity of health care professionals to address the cultural and linguistic barriers to health care delivery and increase access to health care for limited English-proficient people. This site provides many different resources including, but not limited to, standards, materials, and links to other websites to assist health professionals in becoming more culturally competent.

CHAPTER 11

Marketing:

Developing Programs That Respond to the Wants and Needs of the Priority Population

After reading this chapter and answering the questions at the end, you should be able to:

- Define *market*, *marketing*, and *social marketing*.
- Explain the exchange process.
- Describe the segmentation process.
- List and explain the factors that are used to segment an audience.
- Explain the diffusion theory.
- Explain how diffusion theory can be used in marketing a health promotion program.
- Explain the relationship between a needs assessment and a social marketing program.
- Explain the marketing mix or four Ps of marketing.
- Explain the six elements that make the social marketing approach unique.

KEY TERMS

barriers	early majority	place
benefit	exchange	pretesting
brand	innovators	price
competition	laggards	product
consumer-based	late majority	promotion
consumer orientation	market	segmentation
diffusion theory	marketing	social marketing
early adopters	marketing mix	

As you read each chapter in this text, you are learning how to develop, implement, and evaluate health promotion interventions that will influence behavior and ultimately improve individual and community health status. In this chapter you will learn how you can use social marketing as a planning approach to develop **consumer-based** programs and interventions. In other words, how to design programs that are based on a priority population's wants, needs, desires, preferences, and so forth. Specifically, this chapter will focus on social marketing's unique contribution to health promotion by examining six key areas that makes this approach unique from other planning approaches: consumer orientation, audience segmentation, exchange theory, the marketing mix, competition, and continuous monitoring (Thackeray & McCormack Brown, 2005). **Box 11.1** identifies the responsibilities and competencies for health education specialists that pertain to the material presented in this chapter.

Marketing and Social Marketing

Social marketing uses marketing principles to design programs that facilitate voluntary behavior change for improved personal or societal well-being (Andreasen, 1995; Kotler & Zaltman, 1971). In contrast, commercial **marketing** is defined by the American Marketing Association

---

Box 11.1 RESPONSIBILITIES AND COMPETENCIES FOR HEALTH EDUCATION SPECIALISTS

The content of this chapter includes information on several tasks that occur during the social marketing process. These tasks are related to four areas of responsibility for the health education specialist and are centered on involving the priority population, collecting data, and designing a strategy.

Responsibility I: Assess Needs, Assets, and Capacity for Health Education

Competency 1.3: Collect Quantitative and/or Qualitative Data Related to Health

Responsibility II: Plan Health Education

Competency 2.1: Involve Priority Populations and Other Stakeholders in the Planning Process

Competency 2.3: Select or Design Strategies and Interventions

Responsibility IV: Conduct Evaluation and Research Related to Health Education

Competency 4.3: Collect and Analyze Evaluation/Research Data

Competency 4.5: Apply Findings from Evaluation/Research

Responsibility VII: Communicate and Advocate for Health and Health Education

Competency 7.2: Identify and Develop a Variety of Communication Strategies, Methods, and Techniques

Source: NCHEC, SOPHE, & AAHE (2010).

as a set of processes for creating, communicating, and delivering value to customers. It is concerned with outcomes, typically financial, that benefit the organization or its stakeholders. Regardless of the intended outcome, the key marketing principles that ensure success are the same for marketing and social marketing. One fundamental principle is a continual focus on the wants and needs of the individual, also called the *consumer*, in a predetermined priority population. Other key principles include making sure that there is a product (i.e., a tangible item or service) that meets the consumers' needs, that offers a benefit that they value, at a price they can afford, available in places that are convenient, and is promoted in a way that attracts the consumers' attention and prompts them to action. This chapter discusses these basic marketing principles and how to apply them to developing a marketing strategy that results in the consumer using or purchasing a product to help them modify their behavior.

When people hear the word *marketing*, what often comes to mind are images such as highway billboards, humorous television commercials aired during the Super Bowl, or colorful advertisements in their favorite magazines. While these communication materials are an important part of a marketing strategy, they represent only the promotion piece of the marketing mix, also known as the four Ps. Marketing, as it relates to health promotion programs, is really a *consumer-based planning approach* (Neiger, Thackeray, Barnes, & McKenzie, 2003). The key factor that makes it different from other approaches is the consumer orientation, that is, there is a dedicated effort to understanding the priority population prior to developing an intervention and then keeping this knowledge of the priority population at the center of all program planning decisions.

Planners can choose from several different types of interventions (see Chapter 8). When using a social marketing approach to design interventions, planners do not rely on educational or communication campaigns or other persuasion techniques to facilitate the behavior change. In addition, laws and policies are not enacted that would coerce people to change behavior. Although these are all viable intervention methods, and often a multifaceted approach is needed to effectively address a community health problem, when planners use marketing principles to design a social marketing-based intervention they make it easy and convenient for the priority population to do the behavior. They do this by providing the priority population with opportunities and choices, also known as products, or tangible items and services (Rothschild, 1999). For example, if the program focus is on protecting the environment through reducing carbon emissions, an educational approach would teach school-aged children the benefits of saving energy. A mass media health communications campaign would encourage people to take public transportation as a way to reduce a person's carbon footprint. A law or policy approach would require people who exceed their allotment of energy each month to pay higher prices for the excess electricity they consumed. In contrast, a marketing strategy would make it easy and convenient to conserve energy by providing products and services that make it easy to do the behavior, such as providing recycling bins at a low cost to all homes in the neighborhood.

Exchange

The basic idea of marketing is that there are sellers who have a product and buyers who want to purchase or obtain the product because the product fills a need. In health promotion, the priority population is the buyer, also called the *consumer, target audience,* or *market*. Kotler and Clarke (1987, p. 108) define **market** as "the set of all people who have an actual or potential interest in a product or service." The seller (program planner) has a product, which is either a tangible item or service that meets consumers' needs, provides a benefit that they value, and will help support their efforts to make a positive behavior change. The seller's goal is to make it possible for consumers to get the product and the associated benefits at a reasonable cost and with minimal effort. This process is referred to as the **exchange**. Said another way, "strip away all the fancy language, and marketing comes down to offering benefits that an identified group of potential consumers will pay a price for and be satisfied with" (Novelli, 1988, p. 7). The process of marketing operates on this underlying concept of exchange theory (Bagozzi, 1975).

Applying the *exchange* concept to health promotion suggests that planners would like to have an exchange with the priority population whereby the program planner offers products and the associated benefits that the priority population values in exchange for the priority population giving some financial or nonfinancial cost. For this exchange to occur between the buyer and seller, the benefits offered by the product must be greater than what it costs consumers to obtain the product. Additionally, the benefits must be outcomes that are important and of value to the priority population. For example, a women's health program may have as one of its impact objectives to increase the number of working women who breastfeed their children. To help women to do this behavior, the program offers a breast pump rental service. The program is offering the breast pumps (a product) in exchange for women paying a small rental fee. This provides women with the benefit of providing the highest-quality nutrition to their children while continuing to work. In addition, it would be important for planners to know that what women consider an even greater benefit to breastfeeding is an opportunity to bond with their children (Lindenberger & Bryant, 2000). This benefit or outcome is of more importance than benefits program planners often promote, such as "your baby will be healthier," or "breastfeeding will cost less money." Although those benefits are true, the outcome or benefit that matters most to women is "bonding with my child."

The Marketing Process and Health Promotion Programs

Consumer Orientation

To successfully facilitate a product exchange, planners must have an understanding of the priority population (consumers). This **consumer orientation** means that all marketing-related program decisions—including the type of product that is developed, how it is offered, how much it will cost, how it is promoted, and the benefits promised—are based on what planners know about the priority population and their preferences. If planners are making decisions without knowing who is in the priority population and something about them, including things such as how they see the world, what makes them tick, how they spend their time, and what is important to them, then planners are not practicing marketing.

The process of knowing and understanding the priority population is part of the formative research process (see Chapter 3). The goal with formative research is to know enough about the priority population that a product can be created that meets the consumer's needs and provides a benefit they value. This formative research may be included as part of the needs assessment process (see Chapter 4). However, while similar data collection methods are used for gathering primary and secondary data, the focus of formative research as performed in social marketing is a bit different than that of a traditional needs assessment for a program. The types of data planners try to uncover in formative research are, as described in the SMART model (see Chapter 3), related to consumer analysis (wants, needs, and preferences of the priority population, barriers and facilitators to behavior change as well as using the product), market analysis (identifying competing behaviors, messages, and programs), and channel analyses (communication preferences).

Competition   People always have choices for how they are going to fill a need. These alternative choices are the **competition**. If people need to quench their thirst, they can drink water, milk, soda pop, or fruit juice. If people need new running shoes, they can choose different brands such as Nike, Adidas, or New Balance, and so forth. In social marketing, people also have choices for what behaviors they will participate in and products they will use to fulfill their needs. For instance, if people want to lose weight so that they can wear a new swimsuit during their summer vacation in Hawaii, they can choose from two behaviors to lose weight: (1) eat fewer calories and/or (2) engage in more physical activity. There are several products that could help them do this behavior, including purchasing a book that outlines a specific diet plan, attending a weight management class offered by the American Heart Association, hiring a personal trainer, buying a gym membership, using a pedometer to keep track of steps walked each day, and so forth. Each of these alternative choices and products comes with both costs and benefits.

On another level, competition can come from other programs or services that are offering similar programs or products or that are sending messages that are in conflict with the behaviors program planners are trying to promote (Wayman et al., 2007). For weight loss, competitive messages might come from fast food restaurants advertising low-cost, convenient foods (products) that are high in fat and calories. Competing programs would be any number of different organizations or agencies that offer similar weight loss classes. Competing products would include ways other than a pedometer to track steps of physical activity.

Planners should identify the competition during the formative research phase. Knowing what the priority population perceives is the competition and the benefits that they get from choosing that option can help planners make strategic decisions about products to offer that will provide a greater benefit at a lower cost than the competitive option. Understanding the competition also helps planners to know how to price products and how to frame messages for a promotional campaign. For example, Jane Chen and the social enterprise group *Embrace* discovered that newborn infants in developing countries were dying due to the lack of access to incubators. As part of their formative research they interviewed women, health care providers, and others in the community. The data revealed that women lived too far from the hospital and an incubator was too expensive for villages to purchase. Researchers found that as an alternative choice (the competition) parents were engaging in unsafe and ineffective behaviors including putting their babies under a light bulb or using a water bottle to keep them warm. The solution to this problem that met the parents' need to keep their infants alive was a new product called the Warm Embrace. The Warm Embrace is an infant-sized sleeping bag equipped with meltable wax that keeps the baby's body at a constant temperature for four to six hours. It costs less than 1% of a regular incubator and is saving lives (see http://embraceglobal.org/).

Planners conducting formative research may want to consider asking the following questions.

- What would make it easy for the priority population to obtain the product?
- What makes it difficult for or keeps the priority population from doing the desired behavior?
- What benefit does the priority population want as a result of doing the desired behavior?
- What would the priority population be willing to give up to obtain the product and accompanying benefits?
- What type of health promotion programs would the priority population participate in if they were offered in the community?
- Where would the priority population like the product offered?
- On what days of the week would the priority population like a service offered?
- At what time of the day would the priority population like the service offered?
- Would the priority population prefer individual attention or small group participation?
- How much would the priority population be willing to pay to receive the product?
- What is the best way to communicate information to the priority population about the product?
- What are the members of the priority population choosing to do right now to fill their needs?

Information about consumers gathered as part of formative research will be used to make strategic decisions about other aspects of the marketing strategy including selecting segments, determining which products to offer, where to offer the products and at what price, as well as the type of promotional strategy as discussed in the following sections.

Segmentation

Program planners may think that everyone can benefit from health promotion interventions, so they should try to reach everyone. However, not everyone is interested in responding, or even ready or willing to respond. Additionally, motivations for responding to interventions vary by individuals. **Segmentation** is a way to divide the priority population into smaller, more homogeneous groups. The goal of *segmentation* is to create groups of people who share similar characteristics or qualities that are associated with being at risk for certain health problems and who will respond in a similar way to the intervention.

There are several advantages to segmenting the priority population. Segmentation helps planners to narrow the focus of their marketing strategy. It is more likely that the right product will be developed to meet the specific needs and desires of the priority population, thus greatly increasing the chances for an exchange between the two parties. It helps planners to be more effective and efficient with limited resources because they are able to identify groups of the priority population who have similar needs and will respond to the marketing strategy in a similar way. Segmentation also helps planners to make the best decisions in terms of where to offer a product, how to make the price affordable, and how to tailor the promotional strategy including messages and communication channels to the priority population.

For example, a segmentation process discovered that among women who did not regularly receive mammograms, a lack of knowledge about how often they should get a mammogram was a key factor. One group did not know that they should have an annual mammogram, while the other one did (Forthofer & Bryant, 2000). Therefore, each segment of the population needed a unique marketing strategy. For those who already knew about the importance of an annual mammogram, the strategy might include providing a mobile mammography screening unit in places that are convenient for the women, such as their workplace. The marketing strategy for the segment who were not aware that they need an annual mammogram may include a promotional strategy with messages to first increase awareness that annual mammograms are recommended for women of their age and then offer mobile mammography screening units at their workplace.

Planners can segment groups of people using information gathered from secondary data such as literature and epidemiological data (*a priori*) or after collecting primary data using focus groups, interviews, and surveys (*a posteriori*). In this chapter you will learn a simple process that you can use as a framework for conducting audience segmentation that begins with a priori segmentation.

Factors or variables on which to base segmentation include demographics, geographics, geodemographics, lifestyle/psychographics, benefits sought, and behavior (readiness to change, knowledge, attitudes, beliefs, or behaviors) (see **Box 11.2**). Planners will need to experiment with several variables to determine what works best for them.

Planners most often start the segmentation process by using secondary data that include demographic variables such as age, gender, income, marital status, occupation, religion, ethnicity, and socioeconomic status. Nevertheless, just because people share similar demographics does not mean that they will engage in the same behavior. So while these data are usually the most accessible and may describe who is at greatest risk, these data do not always explain why people engage in behaviors or predict whether they will respond to the marketing efforts. Variables related to consumers' motives, personality attributes, and lifestyles can be "the most powerful segmentation variables in social marketing" (Slater, Kelly, & Thackeray, 2006, p. 171). For example, one segmentation study found that the most important factor that influenced the number of hours a person spent watching television was the lifestyle of eating dinner in front of the television (King et al., 2010). Demographic factors such as ethnicity or where they lived in the country did not make a difference. Knowing this information would help planners to create interventions to increase physical activity and reduce screen time.

Box 11.2   SEGMENTATION CATEGORIES AND VARIABLES

1. Geographic segmentation
   a. Nations
   b. States
   c. Regions
   d. Service areas
   e. Counties
   f. Cities, towns, villages
   g. Neighborhoods

2. Demographic segmentation
   a. Age
   b. Stage of life cycle
   c. Disease or diagnostic category
      • Health history
      • Risk factors
   d. Gender
   e. Health insurance
   f. Income
   g. Education
   h. Religion
   i. Race/ethnicity

3. Psychographic segmentation
   a. Social class
      • Upper upper (less than 1% of population)
      • Lower upper (2%)
      • Upper middle (12%)
      • Lower middle (30%)
      • Upper lower (35%)
      • Lower lower (20%)
   b. Lifestyle
   c. Attitudes
   d. Values
   e. Personality
      • Self-image
      • Self-concept

4. Behavioral segmentation
   a. Purchase occasion
   b. User status
   c. Usage rate
   d. Loyalty status
   e. Stages of buyer readiness
   f. Health behavior

5. Benefits sought

6. Constructs of behavior theories (e.g., stages of change)

Source: Adapted from Hertoz et al. (1993); Kotler & Clarke (1987); Romer & Kim (1995); Williams & Flora (1995).

Ideally, planners use multiple variables to identify audience segments. This requires use of statistical programs that can analyze data and create clusters or groups of people based on shared characteristics. For example, in a study of African American and white adults in St. Louis, researchers found that using demographics (i.e., age, race, sex, income, and years of education) was only slightly better at helping them identify a homogenous segment than doing no segmentation at all. They were able to get groups that were more similar when they used health status factors (i.e., general health status, number of chronic diseases, and whether the participant had been advised by a doctor or nurse to exercise more) or psychosocial variables (i.e., barriers to physical activity and the self-efficacy, intrinsic motivation, and social support scales). However, the best segmentation happened when they combined all three variables—demographics, health status, and psychosocial (Boslaugh, Kreuter, Nicholson, & Naleid, 2005). However, simple segmentation using primary and secondary data is still possible as described in the following steps.

Before beginning the segmentation process planners should have completed the needs assessment process (see Chapter 4), selected a priority topic, and written a goal statement (see Chapter 6). In addition, planners should have conducted formative research, as noted earlier, to gain an understanding of the health topic, including who is most affected and the associated risk factors. This information provides the foundation and will be used in decision making throughout the segmentation process.

The first step in segmentation is to review the formative research data to identify behaviors that influence whether people experience morbidity or mortality associated with the health topic. For example, if a program is focused on reducing diabetes-related morbidity, planners would review the secondary data and determine which behaviors influence whether someone experiences diabetes-related illnesses. They may find out that daily monitoring of blood glucose, regular physical activity, eating five servings of fruits and vegetables a day, and visits to the doctor for an annual eye exam are all behaviors that reduce the risk for diabetes complications. Once planners have identified all the possible behaviors, program staff and other stakeholders must decide which behavior will be the program's focus. This will become the impact objective.

Questions to consider when choosing between the possible behaviors include: (1) Is the behavior modifiable? (2) What is the relative impact that changing the behavior will have on the health status or risk factor; in other words, does the literature suggest that changing one behavior will result in greater outcomes than another behavior? (3) What are the current rates of the behavior in the priority population? (4) Is it possible to create a product that will make it easy or convenient to change the behavior, or are education or laws and policies more effective approaches?

The second step is to again review the data and literature, this time to identify which segmentation factors (see Box 11.2) are associated with and influence whether people participate in that particular behavior. If the behavior is a visit to the health care provider for an annual eye exam, planners may discover that having health insurance, making less than $25,000 dollars a year, being of Hispanic ethnicity, and a belief that eye exams are not important are all associated with whether or not someone receives an annual eye exam.

The third step is to group people together who share similar characteristics as it relates to the behavior. There is no right or wrong way to identify population segments.

Planners will want to choose factors that distinguish how the priority population will respond to the marketing strategy. The segmentation process planners develop for the priority population must be useful to the organization and relevant for program planning decisions. If planners have used statistical methods to create clusters then groups are naturally created. If planners are using primary and secondary data, they can simply group people by one or two variables that most influence or are associated with the behavior.

In one study, researchers were interested in creating segments of the population for a global warming engagement campaign (Maibach, Leiserowitz, Roser-Renouf, & Mertz, 2011). The variables they used to create their segments were global warming motivations (including beliefs about the issue and degree of involvement), behaviors, and policy preferences. The segmentation process revealed six distinct segments of the population with varying levels of beliefs about whether global warming is actually happening and if it is a problem, steps they are personally taking to reduce global warming, and what actions they think the government, businesses and individuals should take.

At this point, planners may decide that they need to have additional information about these potential audience segments so they collect primary data. These data may include psychographics (attitudes, values, and lifestyle), risk factors, health history, or personal health behaviors. Additional a posteriori segmentation could be completed after the primary data are collected and analyzed.

Once planners have identified potential segments, they have to choose one segment to focus on. There is no right or wrong, or simple and easy, way to choose between segments. Planners must weigh the data against the organization's abilities and its goals or what they are trying to achieve, then make the best decision. One approach to take—once all the possible segments are identified—is to review the segments by considering the extent to which segments exhibit each of the following five criteria (Kotler & Keller, 2007):

1. **Measurable.** With this criterion planners consider how many people are in the segment and whether important characteristics (or factors) can be measured.

2. **Substantial.** This criterion includes whether the segment is large enough and profitable enough, meaning will enough people be reached with the intervention to make a difference. Will the efforts be effective and efficient? The segmentation process for mammography discussed earlier actually resulted in seven segments, but they found that the majority of the population was in only two of the segments (Forthofer & Bryant, 2000). **Figure 11.1** shows the concept of audience segmentation, identifying African American teenagers for a dietary intervention. This figure illustrates that the priority population, African American teenagers, is a unique but potentially small segment when considering the total population and all of its health problems.

3. **Accessible.** This criterion assesses whether or not planners will be able to reach the segment and then deliver the services. Perhaps the product is a mobile mammography unit. One segment identified is located in a remote area of the state. Due to time and distance factors program staff are not able to reach them to deliver the service.

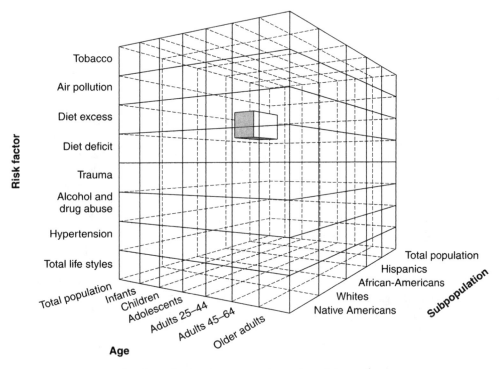

Figure 11.1 Example of Audience Segmentation, Identifying African American Teenagers for a Dietary Intervention

Source: U.S. Dept. of Health and Human Services (1986), p. 41.

4. **Differentiable.** Are the segments unique or different enough so that each segment responds in its own way to the marketing strategy? If the segments will respond the same, then they are really not unique groups. In developing a program to increase use of folic acid by women of childbearing age, planners found that women 18–24 were not receptive to messages about pregnancy whereas older women were more amenable to discussing the possibility of becoming pregnant (Lindsey et al., 2007). A marketing strategy for these two groups would be different and unique.

5. **Actionable.** Here planners decide whether programs can be developed that will attract and serve segments. Because of segment characteristics or organizational abilities, planners may not be able to create a product that adequately meets a segment's needs or benefits its members want. Planners in the United Kingdom learned that one of the main reasons that low-income people smoked was that smoking was a way to cope with stress and anxiety and it was one of their only pleasures in life (MacAskill, Stead, MacKintosh, & Hastings, 2002). In evaluating this segment, planners would have to decide whether they could develop a smoking cessation intervention that would be appealing and provide a benefit that helped people cope with stress and gave them greater pleasure.

Another alternative to choose between segments is to use the criteria suggested by Andreasen (1995) that share similar items: segment size, problem incidence, problem severity, defenselessness, reachability, general responsiveness, incremental costs, response to marketing mix, and organizational capability.

Marketing and the Diffusion Theory

A theory that can help planners in segmenting the priority population is the diffusion theory (Rogers, 1962). **Diffusion theory** provides an explanation for the spread of innovations (something new, such as a product) in populations; stated another way, it provides an explanation for the pattern of adoption of the innovations. If one thinks of a health promotion program as an innovation, the theory describes a pattern the priority population will follow in adopting the program. The pattern of adoption can be represented by the normal bell-shaped curve (Rogers, 2003) (see **Figure 11.2**). Those individuals who fall in the portion of the curve to the left of minus 2 standard deviations from the mean (this would be between 2% and 3% of the priority population) would probably become involved in the program just because they had heard about it and wanted to be first. These people are called **innovators**. They are venturesome, independent, and daring. They want to be the first to do things, though they may not be respected by others in the social system.

The second group of people to adopt something new includes those represented on the curve between minus 2 and minus 1 standard deviations. This group, which composes about 14% of the priority population, is called **early adopters**. These people are

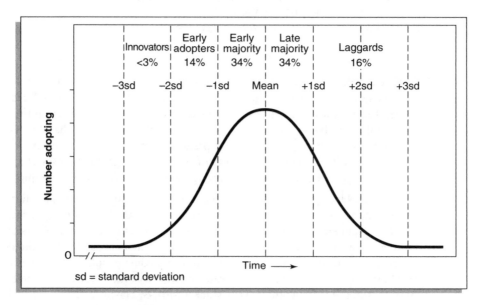

Figure 11.2 Bell-Shaped Curve and Adopter Categories

Source: Diffusion of Innovations. Everett M. Rogers. Copyright © 1962, 1971, 1983 by Simon and Shuster, Inc. Reprinted with permission.

very interested in the innovation, but they are not the first to sign up. They wait until the innovators are already involved to make sure the innovation is useful. Early adopters are respected by others in the social system and looked upon as opinion leaders.

The next two groups are the **early majority** and the **late majority**. They fall between minus 1 standard deviation and the mean and between the mean and plus 1 standard deviation on the curve, respectively. Each of these groups comprises about 34% of the priority population. Those in the early majority may be interested in the health promotion program, but they will need external motivation to become involved. Those in the early majority will deliberate for some time before making a decision. It will take more work to get the late majority involved, because they are skeptical and will not adopt an innovation until most people in the social system have done so. Planners may be able to get them involved through a peer mentoring program, or through constant exposure about the innovation.

The last group, the **laggards** (16%), are represented by the part of the curve greater than plus 1 standard deviation. They are not very interested in innovation and would be the last to become involved in new health promotion programs, if at all. They are very traditional and are suspicious of innovations. Laggards tend to have limited communication networks, so they really do not know much about new things.

Figure 11.3 presents an *S*-shaped curve showing the cumulative prevalence of adopters at successive points in time. At first, only a few people adopt (innovators). However, over time, the curve begins to climb as additional individuals decide to adopt the innovation (early adopters, early majority, and late majority). The curve then levels off

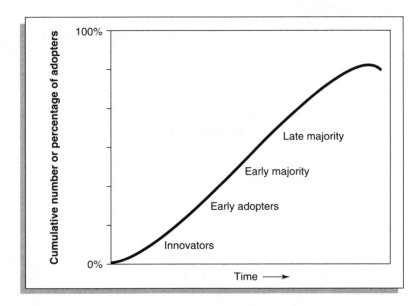

Figure 11.3 *S*-Shaped Curve and Cumulative Adoption

Source: Diffusion of Innovations. Everett M. Rogers. Copyright © 1962, 1971, 1983 by Simon and Shuster, Inc. Reprinted with permission.

as adoption of the innovation ceases, leaving a few who have not adopted (laggards) (Goldman, 1998; Rogers, 2003).

The real advantage of using diffusion theory when trying to market a health promotion program is that "the distinguishing characteristics of the people who fall into each category of adopters from 'innovators' to 'early adopters' to middle majority categories to 'late adopters' [laggards] tend to be consistent across a wide range of innovations" (Green, 1989). Therefore, different marketing techniques can be used depending on the type of people the planners are trying to reach with a program. For example, program planners want rapid diffusion of innovations. They know that although innovators will adopt the program or product first, the key subgroups of the priority population are the early adopters and early majority. It is especially important to identify the early adopters (opinion leaders) as soon as possible in the implementation process since, according to diffusion theory, the sooner they adopt the innovation the sooner the rest of the population will follow. The challenge is how to identify and reach the early adopters.

The application of diffusion theory to health promotion programs is quite common now (Haider & Kreps, 2004). To learn more about the concept and its application to health promotion programs, review some of the following references to see how they have applied the concept in a variety of health promotion and health education settings: Backer and Rogers (1998); Bertrand (2004); Berwick (2003); Borras, Fernandez, Schiaffino, Borrell, & La Vecchia (2000); Ferrence (1996); Goldman (1998); Hallfors & Godette (2002); Murphy (2004); Rogers (2002); Ruof, Mittendorf, Pirk, & von der Schulenberg (2002); Svenkerud & Singhal (1998); and Taylor, Elliott, & Riley (1998).

One of the more interesting uses of diffusion theory has been to "conceptualize the transference of health promotion programs from one locale to another" (Steckler et al., 1992). Steckler and colleagues (1992) developed a series of six questionnaires to measure the extent to which health promotion programs are successfully disseminated. Planners should refer to this work if they are interested in using and measuring diffusion.

Marketing Mix

Once audience segments are selected, planners are ready to make strategic decisions related to four marketing variables: product, price, place, and promotion—the four Ps. These variables are what planners use to design interventions that will help achieve their objective(s) and are referred to as the **marketing mix**. To realize the greatest effect in a marketing strategy there must be a combination of all market mix components, not just promotion (Belch & Belch, 2007).

Product   The **product** is what the planners are offering that will meet the consumers' needs, make it easy and convenient to do the behavior, and provide a benefit that consumers value. Products can be either tangible items or services and are sometimes referred to as *augmented products*. See **Box 11.3** for examples of social marketing–related products. These products provide the priority population with choices to help them change their behavior.

The benefits that are associated with using a product or service are called "core products" or the "bundle of benefits" (Kotler & Lee, 2008). People choose to buy certain

Box 11.3	PRODUCTS (TANGIBLE ITEMS AND SERVICES) IN SOCIAL MARKETING PROGRAMS

Insecticide treated nets

Contraceptives

Nutritional supplements

Food

Battery collection cage

Bike helmet

Clay pot

Glasses

Hand-washing facilities/containers

Medicine

Mosbar soap

Recycling container

Software program

Water disinfectant

Testings or screenings

Exams

Source: Thackeray, Fulkerson, & Neiger (2012).

products for the value or **benefit** the product provides. A common illustration of this point is the person who goes to a home improvement store and buys a drill; what he or she is really purchasing is the benefit of using that drill to have a hole in the wall. Similarly, a person who buys a hotel room is purchasing a restful night's sleep. The products or services provided by planners as part of a social marketing program must also provide a value that is of benefit to the priority population. Those values are determined during the formative research process. These core benefits are one of the most important things to discover, as they will become the motivation for people using the products to help them change behavior. These core benefits will also become part of the promotional strategy, discussed later in this chapter. See **Box 11.4** for examples of core products in social marketing campaigns.

The following two social marketing case studies illustrate products and their associated benefits. The Road Crew offered a transportation service to young males in rural Wisconsin to encourage them to not drive after a night of drinking alcohol (Rothschild, Mastin, & Miller, 2006). The Road Crew used older luxury vehicles to provide transportation for the men to and from the town as well as between bars during the night. The price for this service was $15 per night. The benefits that it provided the men included a fun way to get around town, the opportunity to have a last drink while going home, and less worry about getting a ticket or being in a crash as a result of drinking, all things that were important to the priorty population.

Box 11.4	EXAMPLE OF BENEFITS OR CORE PRODUCTS IN SOCIAL MARKETING STUDIES

"Don't lose your dreams"

"Have iron. Have power"

Makes us healthy

Avoid costly fines and penalties from noncompliance

Close loving bond; emotional benefits

Crew dependability on fire scene

Avoidance of HIV infections

Keep the family healthy and energetic; women charming; children more intelligent

Don't worry about getting home at end of the evening; continue to enjoy themselves; a way to have more fun during an evening out

Enhance women's beauty and health; decreased anemia

Financial savings; health and energy to spend with children and grandchildren; more fit, so able to do leisure activities

Find and develop relationships

Harvest without fear of injury or daily irritation

Hope and peace of mind

Maintain pride and self-esteem as they earn WIC benefits and learn about nutrition and other ways to help their families

Well-being; energy; ability to perform their roles better

Opportunity to keep their relationship (family) intact by ending the violence toward their partner

Peace of mind and life-saving benefit of early detection

Protect individual health; sense of altruism; information provision

Reduce traffic congestion; defer need to build road infrastructure; reduce environmental consequences of car use; increase physical activity and health outcomes; increase use of walking and cycling infrastructure and public transport

Safety of family or workers, financial concerns, impact of debilitating injuries

Spending time with friends, playing having fun, have opportunity to be active with parents, recognition from peers and adults; opportunity to discover and explore world around them

Source: Thackeray, Fulkerson, & Neiger (2012).

In Florida, program planners were concerned with reducing eye injuries among local citrus workers while harvesting fruit. They discovered that among the barriers that kept the workers from wearing protective eyewear was a belief that most workers expected the glasses would reduce their productivity and therefore reduce their income. Their solution was to provide safety goggles that were comfortable and did not fog up or fall off while being worn. The core benefit they provided was "pick rapidly without fear of daily irritation" (Monaghan et al., 2008, p. 80).

Price Price is what it costs the priority population to obtain the product and its associated benefits. It is what they have to "give up." In other words, price is the sum of costs the consumer must accept to engage in the exchange process (Neiger & Thackeray, 1998). The cost to the priority population may be financial, but often with health promotion interventions the costs are nonfinancial, that is, they involve social, mental, emotional, behavioral, or psychological costs. For example, if a program focused on getting Hispanic women with diabetes to regularly check their glucose, a low-cost glucometer could be offered to the priority population. In order to get this product and the associated benefits of a peace of mind that their blood sugar is in range so they will be less likely to damage their eyesight, the women would have to pay a certain amount of money. In addition to this financial cost, the women would have to give up time to go purchase the glucometer and learn how to use it. They would also have to take time every day to check their blood glucose.

In designing a marketing strategy, planners must make sure that the benefits the priority population receives are greater than what it costs them to obtain the product. Even if the costs are not actually less, planners have to make them appear less than what they are getting in return. Likewise, as part of the promotional strategy, planners must convey how the benefits received are much greater than what they cost. For example, for a mother to bring her child in to be immunized might cost her time away from other tasks, time to drive to the clinic, the effort to get to the clinic, and being willing to put up with a cranky baby for a few hours after the immunization is received. In communicating about this product (immunizations), the health education specialist has to convey that the benefits of knowing that her child is safe from childhood diseases are greater than a few minor inconveniences (her cost).

Price is not the same thing as barriers. **Barriers** are what keep people from responding to an intervention or doing a behavior. The cost or price of the product may be one factor that keeps people from obtaining it and using it to make a desired behavior change. But there may be other factors as well. Planners in the Marshall Islands found that barriers to people making healthy food choices included a lack of choices at the local supermarket, the perception that a can of meat (e.g., Spam) could feed more people than a piece of fresh fish, that fresh meat costs too much money and took too long to prepare and then cook, and a lack of skills for cooking foods in different ways (Gittelsohn et al., 2006).

In another example, when planners asked people about what would keep them from attending a nutrition education class, they said that the major reasons were that they lacked transportation and there was nobody to babysit their children (John, Kerby, & Landers, 2004). These are barriers but not costs: the people do not have to give up transportation or childcare to participate in the exchange. However, either thing will keep them from obtaining the product. They would have to give up money for transportation or to pay a sitter. In designing the product or intervention, planners have to make sure that they reduce the barriers and lower the cost—both for the same purpose—to make it easy for people to obtain the product or service and engage in the desired behavior.

In this case, the planners may want to offer a baby-sitting service at the same location where the class is being held.

From an economic standpoint, *price* refers to charging the appropriate amount for the product being provided. There are many ways to finance a program (see Chapter 10). The price must match the consumer's ability and willingness to pay and should not be so high that it becomes a barrier to them using the product or service. When considering the amount to be charged for a product, planners should answer seven questions:

1. Who are the clients?
2. What is their ability to pay?
3. Are co-payers involved?
4. Is the program covered under an insurance program?
5. What is the mission of the planner's agency?
6. What are competitors charging?
7. What is the demand for the program or product?

The price of a program and who pays for it help determine how a program should be marketed. Whether the program is intended to make a profit will have a great impact on the price. Does the program have to make money? Break even? Or can it lose money? It is a real art not to overprice or underprice the program. Demand and location (*place*) will also influence price. If a program is in high demand, obviously the price can be raised. For example, a stress-management program in a large metropolitan area may be able to command a higher price than one located in a small rural area.

Not only do the demand and the location influence the amount one might charge for a program, but so can the psychological mindset of those in the priority population. Some individuals would not participate in a free or inexpensive program because they question how such a program could be any good. Others believe they have to spend a lot of money to get anything of worth. Also, sometimes when programs are offered free of charge, people are less likely to attend regularly because they have not invested financially in the program. On the other hand, there are some people who, if given the choice of a free program versus one with a cost, will always take the free program, even if they are financially able to pay. Being able to segment the priority population with regard to these economic issues can help set the right price.

Place   The third marketing variable is **place**, which can be thought of as where the priority population has access to the product. When considering place, planners make sure that it easy for the consumer to obtain the product or service. In addition, it is important to avoid areas where people do not normally go or places where they would not feel comfortable or safe. For example, a local health department decided that they would make it easy for the senior-aged population to get their influenza vaccination. To do so, they offered a Saturday morning drive-up service where people could drive their cars to the health department parking lot and get a vaccination. Another example is a partnership between bar owners and public health researchers who aimed to make it easier for people to get a taxi ride home, thereby discouraging drinking and driving. They provided cab drivers with a special spot to wait (which also guaranteed them passengers). The area was well-lit, covered, and in a generally safe place, all important things to the customers (Bhatt, 2006).

When a product is offered it is closely associated with its place. If the priority population has to go to a specific location to obtain the product, planners might think about when it will be most convenient for the priority population to do so. For example, if consumers have to come to the local health department to have their car seat checked to ensure that it is properly installed, making the service available at times that are convenient for the priority population will reduce a barrier and make it more likely that consumers will take action to use this service. If it is a program, then planners might consider the optimum time of day to offer the program. If a worksite program is offered in the evening, so that the workers have to return to the worksite after dinner, that probably would not be much different from driving across town from work to attend a program. Offering a program right after a shift or on a lunch hour would probably be much more appealing to most workers. Obviously, planners should be concerned about placing their program in a desirable locale (where they are wanted and needed) at the best possible time.

Promotion The fourth marketing variable is **promotion**. As mentioned at the beginning of this chapter, promotion is what most people think of when they hear the word *marketing*. But promotion is just one component of the overall marketing mix. Promotion is the communication strategy, including the message and associated visuals or graphics as well as the channels, used to let the priority population know about the product, how to obtain or purchase it, and the benefits they will receive. Promotion is not about a general awareness campaign or related health communication intervention strategies. Promotion, also referred to as marketing communications, has four primary purposes (McDonald & Wilson, 2011):

1. Inform—increase product awareness or inform consumers

2. Persuade—convince people to purchase the product

3. Reinforce—remind them that the product exists

4. Differentiate—position the product as being different from the competition

There are various tools and associated channels that planners can use to achieve these purposes. Traditionally, promotional tools have included advertising, direct marketing, digital communications, sales promotion, personal selling, and publicity/public relations (Belch & Belch, 2007; McDonald & Wilson, 2011). The following section gives a general overview of these tools.

Advertising is marketing communication that is paid and nonpersonal, meaning it is not trying to reach one person but rather large groups of people. Common channels for advertising have included broadcast media (television and radio), print media (newspapers and magazines), outdoor media (billboards, bus wraps, and so forth). The national 5-a-day campaign used point-of-purchase advertising in grocery store produce departments to remind people to eat five servings of fruits and vegetables. Local coalition members developed a summer VERB program where they increased the number of places in the community for tweens to be active. They developed a card on which tweens could keep track of places they went to be physically active. Advertising space was paid for in the local newspaper, in a local family magazine, and on the radio. In addition, they got free publicity from the local media outlets and word of mouth from program partners and coalition members (Courtney, 2004). The National Bone Health Campaign used advertising including print ads and 30-second radio spots (Lefebvre, 2006).

Direct marketing involves communicating directly with consumers about a product with the purpose of getting them to purchase the product or service (Belch & Belch, 2007). Common channels for direct marketing include direct mail, direct selling, or telemarketing. Direct contact with specific groups that might be at high risk and in need of the programs (contacting recent heart attack patients about a program on the need to eat in a heart healthy manner), distributing mailbox stuffers or door-to-door flyers, or inserts with employee paychecks are examples of direct marketing. One of the most common ways that healthcare providers in the United States informed patients about the safety and effectiveness of genetic tests was through distributing pamphlets (Cho, Arruda, & Holtzman, 2006).

Personal selling refers to person-to-person interaction intended to persuade the customer to buy the product. Personal selling is used regularly in health care marketing. Pharmaceutical companies have representatives who meet one-on-one with health care providers for the purpose of convincing them to use a certain prescription drug. Another example of personal selling is the use of *lay health workers*, or *promotoras*. In rural South Carolina, promotoras were used to give information, assistance, and referral to services (Sherrill et al., 2005). One way these lay health workers could engage in personal selling is by going to individual homes and encouraging people with diabetes to attend the health clinic screening and have their blood glucose tested.

Sales promotions are incentives that entice consumers to try the product. Types of sales promotion include coupons, premiums (e.g., prizes with purchase), contests and sweepstakes, rebates, or samples (Clow & Baack, 2007). This tool is probably used less often in social marketing. However, a common tactic would be to use sales promotions for services such as a coupon for a reduced-cost mammogram, a coupon for a free bike helmet, or a reduced fee at the local fitness center.

Public relations, also called publicity, represents both internal and external marketing communications. The news media coverage that external public relations activities generate is typically not paid for by the organization (as compared with advertising). Typical public relations tools include the use of ongoing news media outreach and sponsorship of large events that draw attention and exposure such as a special kickoff, countdown, ribbon-cutting, or health party to get a program started. Public relations activities can also be used to increase awareness about new products. When the National Cancer Institute personnel released results from the Prostate Cancer Prevention Trial, one of their strategies was to hold a press conference and provide video news releases. This resulted in hundreds of news stories reaching millions of viewers (Croker et al., 2004).

Finally, there is digital communication. In recent years, the availability of the Internet has increased the options available for planners to use these traditional tools across a spectrum of channels. This form of promotion can generate a great deal of interest in the product for a relative low cost and in a short period of time. The availability of electronic media in addition to the Internet, including cell phones, MP3 players, or personal digital assistants has expanded promotional alternatives. For example, social marketers can use podcasts, PDA downloads, and the Internet to promote their products. Websites are probably the most common channel for Internet promotion. For example, advertising can now be part of a home page or social networking site, or included as banner ads in an online newspaper. The National Bone Health Campaign developed a Website specifically for teen girls (Lefebvre, 2006), and they placed banner ads on other Websites that the priority population often visited.

There are several factors to consider when deciding which of the promotional tools and channels to use. Two of the most critical are the communication objectives and the communication preferences for the priority population. If the objective is to increase awareness of a product, the tools and channels are different than if the purpose is to demonstrate how to use the product, or to illustrate key attributes, or provide in-depth details about the product features. The priority populations' communication preferences are also critical. For example, formative research for a disaster preparedness campaign in Vietnam found that the majority of respondents owned a radio, fewer people owned a television, and almost nobody had subscriptions to the newspaper or magazines (Ramaprasad, 2005). Therefore, in selecting a promotional strategy and materials, planners probably would not place an advertisement in the newspaper, but might consider a radio spot. The National Bone Health Campaign found that the most common ways for girls grades 6–12 to stay in touch with their friends was through text messages, instant messaging, and cell phones. In addition, the most popular magazines were *Seventeen* and *Teen People* (Lefebvre, 2006).

Additional questions that planners may want to ask when selecting a promotional tool and channel include:

1. What are the costs of each tool or channel versus the benefits?
2. Can the tool's or channel's capability build on or multiply the effects of another tool or channel?
3. Will the message reach a significant portion of the priority population?
4. Can the message be sent through several different channels?
5. Through how many intermediaries must the message travel to reach the priority population?
6. Can a tool be overused to the point that it will "turn off" the priority population to the message?

Messages include the words and graphics that are used to convey information about the product, where to obtain it and the benefits it will provide. The process for developing appropriate messages is both an art and a science. Many communication theories and models can be used to develop effective messages. A good place to start is with consumer-based health communications as described in the National Cancer Institute's book *Making Health Communication Programs Work* (NCI 2002; 2004), otherwise known as the "Pink Book" (see http://www.cancer.gov/cancertopics/cancerlibrary/pinkbook). In order to develop effective messages, planners must know what is motivating the priority population. This is learned while conducting formative research. They must know how to frame the message so that it will cut through the clutter, capture the priority population's attention, and motivate them to action. Key parts of the message should be that the product will offer a benefit that the priority population desires, that the product costs less than the benefits it provides, and how they can obtain the product.

For example, after performing formative research related to diet and physical activity among a group of public employees, planners learned that preferences for message content included "helping employees understand that the desired changes could be inexpensive, fun and easy, and that changes would require only a minimal amount of time." Based on these preferences, messages through email, public announcements, posters, and direct supervisor contacts (all preferred channels) were successfully used to recruit a large group of participants in a successful intervention (Neiger et al., 2001).

Another example of this concept was the segmentation process that resulted from focus groups conducted with teenage girls as part of a physical activity project (Staten, Birnbaum, Jobe, & Elder, 2006). The process resulted in seven main segments that described the girls: athletic, preppy, quiet, rebel, smart, tough, and other. In addition, they discovered preferences for the types of images that would be best for communication materials.

> Respondents provided the following suggestions: (a) for athletic girls, pictures should show girls participating in organized, competitive activities; (b) for preppy girls, pictures might show girls cheerleading, well-dressed individuals, groups of friends being active, girls being active with boys watching (with positive affect, not leering or jeering), and organized sports with "cute" uniforms; (c) for quiet girls, pictures should show girls alone or in small groups doing activities (don't focus on competitive sports); (d) for rebel girls, pictures might include girls on skateboards, perhaps with some visible body piercing, girls wearing dark clothes, images implying dancing to punk rock music; and (e) for smart girls, pictures should show girls who are not too muscular or strong being active in small groups, and positive attitudes and neat but not trendy dress may be appealing. Small group images that show some smart girls and some preppy girls being active together may be appealing. And (f) for tough girls, pictures might show girls doing stepping or hip-hop dance or girls playing basketball (not necessarily in uniform; show street games, pick-up games). Images of girls should not be conservative. Groups of friends would be appealing. (p. 76)

An important component of any marketing strategy is ensuring that you have a strong brand. A **brand** is "a name, term, design, symbol, or any other feature that identifies one seller's good or service as distinct from those of other sellers" (American Marketing Association, 2007). The brand can be considered the image, reputation, or how the organization wants people to think or feel when they hear about or see the brand (Kotler & Lee, 2006). A strong brand can increase competitive advantage. This means that when given a choice, consumers are more likely to choose the organization's product because of what they associate with the brand. Elements that contribute to the brand include the logo, tag line, colors, images, and even the product name. For example, when planning a vacation and thinking about lodging options, what words, images, or feelings come to mind when you hear "Motel 6" or "Days Inn." In contrast, what comes to mind when you hear "Marriott" or "Hilton." Each of these companies has a distinct brand.

The choice of a program name is an important element in its brand and promotion, since the name can make a difference in whether someone from the priority population will be interested in the program. Creating a name is part of the marketing process used to develop informative and persuasive communication flows between the providers of a program and those in the priority population. More likely than not, a program name will be the first contact that someone in the priority population will have with the product (health promotion program). A program name is analogous to the headline of a newspaper article. When most people read a newspaper, they do not read every article; rather, they skim the headlines of the articles and then read those articles that appeal to them. It is the headlines that grab their attention. The same concept applies in advertising a product. A good headline ought to compel members of the priority population to read the rest of the message (Granat, 1994), or, in the case of a health promotion program, create enough interest that those in the priority population want to find out more about the program.

In addition to creative names, acronyms are useful in bringing attention to a program. For example, Foldcraft, a company in Minnesota, uses the acronym H.E.A.L.T.H. as the name of its health program. It stands for "Hey Everyone Always Learns The Hard way." Program titles and acronyms seem to be limited only by the planners' creativity. **Box 11.5** shows additional examples of past and current program names.

Working with Creative Teams to Help Execute the Promotional Strategy   Depending on the agency and the available budget, planners may be responsible for developing and executing the promotional strategy or they may hire a marketing or public relations firm to do some of the creative work including creating messages, materials, or brand logos and tag lines. If planners are working with a creative agency, the following suggestions will help ensure that the process is successful. Keep in mind that the actual process may vary depending on the creative team and their agency policies. At all phases of the process, planners should make sure to have open and honest communication with the creative team. It is important to trust their creative skills and abilities, but planners need to make sure that they are on track with the program objectives.

The first step is to identify a public relations or marketing agency. The organization that a planner works for may require all outside work to be solicited through a specific procurement or bid process. In other instances, planners may be able to work directly with an agency of choice. In either circumstance, the first step is to identify a list of possible agencies. Consider getting recommendations from other health promotion programs or health-related organizations that have hired creative agencies. Ask the agency for samples of their previous health-related campaigns.

Once an agency has been selected, hold a meeting with members of the program planning team and the creative team. This is sometimes referred to as a *discovery meeting*. At this meeting the creative team will assess what needs to be accomplished. Planners should bring to this meeting all the research about the priority population and the program goals and objectives. A concise way to convey this information is by using a creative brief, which is a synopsis that describes the priority population, the benefits they seek, the barriers they face, the purpose of the communication, and potential communication channels. (See **Box 11.6** for an outline of a creative brief.)

Box 11.5   SAMPLE PROGRAM NAMES

Title (topic)	Organization/Company
A Plan for Life (general health)	IBM
Awakening the Spirit (diabetes)	American Diabetes Association
For Your Health (general health)	CNO Financial Group
Freedom from Smoking (smoking cessation)	American Lung Association
FreshStart (smoking cessation)	American Cancer Society
Health e Strategies (e-health)	Wellness Councils of America
Health Miles Health Rewards Program (general health)	Virgin Life Care
Health Track (general health)	Union Pacific
Healthy Balance Program (general health)	Caterpillar
Heart at Work (cardiovascular health)	American Heart Association
Hey Everyone Always Learns The Hard way	Foldcraft (Minnesota)
Live for Life (general health)	Johnson & Johnson
Live Well—Be Well (general health)	Quaker Oats
STEPS to a Healthier U.S.	U.S. Department of Health and Human Services
Time Out for Life (general health)	Colonial Life and Accident Insurance Company
Total Life Concept (general health)	AT&T
United Way at Work (general health)	United Way
StayWell (general health)	Control Data
Up with Life (general health)	Dow Chemical

After the discovery meeting, the creative team will come back to the agency with recommendations for how to proceed, including the type of appeal (e.g., humor, slice of life) and the type of communication materials. They should also provide a cost estimate for how many person-hours it will take to develop the materials and the cost of material production.

The next step is to sign an estimate agreement. Before doing so, planners need to make sure that they agree with the creative team's recommendations. That is, does the recommended approach on strategy correspond to program goals and communication objectives? At this point planners want to clarify what work and deliverables are included in the fees.

Once the agreement is signed, the creative team will begin their work. Based on the budget, they will flesh out a limited number of concepts, also known as draft ideas. After reviewing the

| **Box 11.6** | CREATIVE BRIEF FOR A PROMOTIONAL STRATEGY |

1. Background (overview about the topic and project):

2. Priority Population/Segment (concise description of the priority population):

3. Purpose of Promotion (increase awareness of product, remind them product exists, encourage them to act):

4. Core Benefit to Highlight:

5. Place (where the people will access the product):

6. Price (both tangible and intangible):

7. Communication Preferences (tools and channels):

concepts, planners can choose which one(s) they want to be part of their campaign. A limited number of modifications (sometimes just one) is included in the original cost estimate. Other major changes beyond that may require another fee. Knowing that several modifications can increase the cost of a promotional campaign is one reason that the discovery meeting is so important and why planners want to be prepared with formative research about the priority population. Planners should also make sure to build in time and money for pretesting materials and messages with the priority population, as discussed in the next section.

Pretesting

Though planners conduct formative research and learn as much about consumers as they can prior to developing the marketing strategy, planners need to make sure that they are still on track with consumer preferences before offering products or launching the promotional campaign. The process of getting this feedback is called **pretesting**. Pretesting ensures that planners have developed program components in response to, and are reflective of the priority population's needs, wants, and expectations.

Ideally, planners should test all components of the marketing strategy including products, messages, materials, and selected promotional tools. However, the breadth and depth of pretesting is usually determined by the budget. It is important to include in the project time line, as well the budget, adequate time and financial resources to complete pretesting.

Pretesting can be completed in two phases, both of which occur during the development process when products and promotional materials are in draft form, before ideas finalized or any promotional materials are produced. Phase one involves testing the product concepts. Think of concepts as a prototype or draft form of products and services. Pretesting concepts gives planners the opportunity to get feedback on the design of the product as well as the product-related benefits. The topics planners would want to receive feedback on when pretesting the product or service may include:

- How likely they would be to use the product
- What they see as benefits to using the product
- What they see as the barriers; what factors would keep them from using it

- What products features they like
- What product features they would change, and why
- If the places selected to offer the product are convenient
- If the product price is reasonable
- If the benefits associated with product use are believable
- If the product functions as designed
- If instructions for how to use the product are clear

The second pretesting phase is testing the promotional strategy messages and materials. It is best to test messages and materials separately because planners will not know if the priority population is responding to the message or the material. For instance, do they think the message is not very motivating because of the content of the message or because the brochure design influenced how they understood the message? **Box 11.7**

Box 11.7 TOPICS FOR MESSAGE AND MATERIAL PRETESTING

Show *a copy of draft messages and ask:*

What is the main idea that you get from this message?

What else are they trying to say?

What do you think they want you to know?

What do you think they want you to believe or think?

What action do you think they want you to take?

Where is the best place to reach you with this message?

Where would you most likely notice it and pay attention to it?

What words are confusing or hard to understand?

Describe what type of person this message is trying to reach.

The main purpose of this message is to persuade you and people like you to [describe action related to the product].

How likely do you think it is that this message will influence you to take this action?

What about this message is motivating?

Show a draft of a promotional material and ask:

What do you like about this [material]?

What don't you like about this [material]?

What stands out to you?

How attention-getting is this [material]? *(Note: Use a Likert scale here to measure response.)*

Source: Adapted from Kotler & Lee (2008); National Cancer Institute (2002).

outlines aspects of the promotional messages and materials about which planners may want to get feedback during the pretesting process.

Pretesting allows planners to identify red flags or, in other words, facets of the strategy that may reduce the chances of success. However, positive feedback from the priority population during the pretesting phase cannot indicate the degree to which the consumers will like the product or service, or how successful the promotional messages and materials will be at influencing people to use the product or service. The inability to generalize pretesting results to a larger population is due to a small sample size and selection methods (see Chapter 5).

The methods planners can use for pretesting depend on what aspect of the marketing strategy is being tested, the topics being explored, the amount of money available for pretesting, and the timeline. In general, focus groups and central location intercept (grab sampling) interviews are common pretesting methods. These qualitative methods are preferred because they allow the planners to interact with the priority population, get in-depth reactions to products, messages and materials, and follow up with clarifying questions or probes. Considerations for when to use each of these methods for pretesting are presented in **Box 11.8**.

Pretesting should always be completed with members of the priority population. Planners can use probability or nonprobability (also called purposive) samples (see Chapter 5) to select the participants. In addition, planners may want to obtain reviews from subject matter experts or gatekeepers. Subject matter experts are people who have advanced knowledge about the health topic. Having subject matter expert review ensures that the promotional messages are factually and technically correct, thereby reducing the chance of conveying false information. Gatekeepers are people who control whether messages, materials, or products reach the priority population. Gatekeeper review enables the planners to get buy-in from individuals who are influential in distributing the product or disseminating promotional materials. Examples of gatekeepers are nurses at doctors' offices, radio station owners, newspaper editors, or individuals whom the priority population identifies as community leaders.

Continuous Monitoring

Continuous monitoring conducted as part of a marketing strategy is somewhat analogous to aspects of both formative and process evaluations (see Chapter 14). What makes continuous monitoring unique is its focus on getting reaction and comment from the priority population about all aspects of the program during the implementation phase. The monitoring function determines if things are going as planned, if the program is operating below expectations, and whether changes noted indicate that the program is moving in the right direction (Andreasen, 1995). This continuous monitoring provides program planners with data regarding level of program acceptance by the priority population, reach of messages, product distribution sites, and in general, what is working and what is not working. Overall, continuous monitoring improves the effectiveness of the program by continually integrating feedback from the priority population.

Box 11.8   ISSUES TO CONSIDER WHEN CHOOSING BETWEEN FOCUS GROUPS AND INTERCEPT INTERVIEWS FOR PRETESTING

Issue to Consider	Use Focus Groups When:	Use Intercept Interviews When:
Group Think or Peer Pressure*	Group discussion will generate additional feedback or will stimulate new ideas.	Group discussion or presence of other individuals will keep respondents from being open and honest about their feelings.
Depth of Responses*	More in-depth discussion and responses about pretesting topic is desired.	Quick responses and reactions to pretesting topic will be sufficient.
Demonstration of product or viewing of messages and materials	Respondents can be shown the product prototype or storyboards with messages and materials.	Respondents can be shown the product prototype or storyboards with messages and materials.
Number of topics to be pretested	A moderate number of topics is being tested.	A limited number of topics is being tested.
Access to Priority Population*	An adequate number of priority population members can be assembled at the same time in one location.	An adequate number of priority population members can be found in a central location.
Length of Respondent Availability	Respondents are available for approximately 1–2 hours.	Respondents are available for approximately 15–20 minutes.
How the Priority Population Uses the Product	The priority population may use the product or service as a common public experience (e.g., taxi ride service).	The priority population uses the product on a personal level (e.g., a new glucometer to measure blood sugar).
How the Priority Population Receives the Communication	The priority population may receive the communication in a public setting (e.g., billboard).	The priority population receives the communication individually (e.g., text message on their cell phone).

*Adapted from: *Marketing Public Health: Strategies to Promote Social Change.* M. Siegel and L. Doner. Copyright © 1998 by Jones & Bartlett Learning. Reprinted with permission.

SUMMARY

An important aspect of any health promotion program is being able to design a product that will attract the priority population initially and keep them involved once they have begun a new behavior. All products must provide a benefit or outcome that the priority population values. Using marketing principles can help planners develop successful programs. Understanding the priority population, including their wants and needs, is at the heart of the marketing process. An important step in the process is identifying segments that share similar characteristics. The marketing mix should take into account the four Ps of marketing: product, price, place, and promotion. These elements together become the basis for the marketing strategy that will facilitate the exchange between the program planner as the marketer and the priority population as the customer. Before launching the program, products, messages, and materials should be pretested with the priority population. After the program starts, continuous monitoring and getting feedback from the priority population will help keep the program on track.

REVIEW QUESTIONS

1. Define the following terms: *market, marketing* , and *social marketing.*

2. What is the relationship between formative research and needs assessment?

3. How does segmenting your priority population help you in planning?

4. What are some factors to use when segmenting your priority population? Which ones are most important?

5. How does diffusion theory relate to marketing a program?

6. What are the five different groups of people described in diffusion theory? When would each group most likely join a health promotion program?

7. What has to happen in order for an exchange to take place between a planner and the priority population?

8. Describe the six elements that make a social marketing approach unique from other planning approaches?

9. What are the four Ps of marketing? Explain each one.

10. What are the purposes for pretesting?

ACTIVITIES

1. Respond to the following statements/questions with regard to a program you are planning:

   a. Describe your product (i.e., tangible item or service). What benefit is it providing to your customer?

   b. Describe your segmented population. What segmentation factors did you use to identify segments?

   c. What will it cost the priority population to obtain the product? Explain the rationale on which you based your decision.

   d. Where will the product be placed? What is your reason for placing it this way? If you have a service product, when will it be offered (location, days, and time)?

   e. What promotional tools will you use to promote your program? How, when, and where will you let the priority population know about the item or service?

2. Create a promotional piece that could be used to promote your product through advertising, direct marketing, personal selling, or sales promotions. This promotional piece should include both text and graphics and highlight the core benefit being offered.

3. Survey members of the priority population to find out what would motivate them to begin a specific health behavior. Make sure to ask about products and services that would help them make that change.

WEBLINKS

1. http://www.marketingpower.com

   American Marketing Association

   The American Marketing Association is one of the largest professional associations for marketers. This Website provides best practices related to marketing strategies, including marketing tools and templates and marketing services directories.

2. ctb.ku.edu/en/tableofcontents/chapter_1045.aspx

   Community Tool Box

   This Website provides excellent resources on promoting participation and social marketing. Topic sections include step-by-step instruction, examples, checklists, and related resources.

3. http://www.hc-sc.gc.ca/ahc-asc/activit/marketsoc/index_e.html

   Social Marketing Network

   This Website provides the latest information on social marketing and lessons learned by Health Canada's Marketing and Creative Services Division. Current case studies provide step-by-step instructions for the marketing process.

4. http://www.social-marketing.com

   Weinreich Communications

   This Website contains social marketing-related articles, resources, conference calendar, and extensive lists of links to pertinent sources of information.

5. www.nsmcenter.org/uk/content/nsmc

   National Social Marketing Centre (NSMC)

   The NSMC is a center for excellence in behavior change and social marketing located in the United Kingdom. This Website provides tools and resources for designing social marketing programs as well as case studies from around the world.

6. LISTPROC@LISTPROC.GEORGETOWN.EDU

   Georgetown Social Marketing Listserv

   This is an active social marketing listserv with discussions centering on a variety of social marketing topics. Subscribers can elect to receive a daily digest of emails or receive each one as it is posted. To subscribe, send an email message to the URL listed above. In the body of the message write "SUBSCRIBE SOC-MKTG [insert your own name]."

CHAPTER 12

Implementation:
Strategies and Associated Concerns

After reading this chapter and answering the questions at the end, you should be able to:

• Define and explain a logic model.
• Define *implementation*.
• Identify the different phases for implementing health promotion programs.
• Define *management*.
• Identify and briefly explain the major resources that must be managed during implementation.
• Identify major pieces of federal legislation that impact human resource management.
• List and briefly describe the concerns that need to be addressed before implementation can take place.

accounting	external audit	logic model
act of commission	financial management	management
act of omission	fiscal accountability	negligence
anonymity	fiscal year	news hook
audit	Gantt chart	nonmaleficence
beneficence	HIPAA	outcomes
confidentiality	implementation	outputs
critical path method	informed consent	PERT
disability	inputs	phased in
ethical issues	internal audit	pilot testing

Key Terms, continued

program kick off	prudent	Type III errors
program launch	task development time line	
program rollout	technical resources	

arlier (in Chapters 1–10) we discussed the steps necessary to plan a solid health promotion program, and presented information (in Chapter 11) that would assist planners in marketing the program they planned. As a part of the marketing process we presented information on the process of program adoption using diffusion theory (Rogers, 2003). It is the adoption of a program (or stated differently, the decision to participate) by those in the priority population that is the beginning of the program implementation process. Yet many other things need to be considered in the implementation process that are critical to a successful program. The eventual impact of a program will be judged not only by the effectiveness of the interventions but also by the quality of the implementation (Parcel, 1995). In fact, Timmreck (2003) has stated "implementation is the most critical part of the planning process; a plan that is not implemented is no plan at all" (p. 171). In this chapter, we present the key phases in implementing a program and identify the many concerns that must be addressed as implementation unfolds. **Box 12.1** identifies the responsibilities and competencies for health education specialists that pertain to the material presented in this chapter.

Logic Models

Before discussing implementation, we will present information here on logic models because of their usefulness in the implementation process. Logic models have been widely used in community health programs (Helitzer, Willging, Hathorn, & Benally, 2009). In the previous edition of this book we presented information on logic models in Chapter 1, but that may have been too early to fully appreciate their usefulness in the planning process. Logic models can help all stakeholders understand the "big picture" of how planning, implementing, and evaluating all fit together. "A logic model attempts to convey visually the connection between program activities and the program's desired outcomes; that is the logic of the program" (Lando, Williams, Sturgis, & Williams, 2006, p. 2). Or stated a bit differently, a **logic model** "is a systematic and visual way to present and share your understanding of the relationships among the resources you have to operate your program, the activities you plan, and the changes or results you hope to achieve" (WKKF, 2004, p. 1). Simply put, a logic model is a road map (Goldman & Schmalz, 2006). More specifically: "logic models increase the likelihood that program efforts will be successful because they

- Communicate the purpose of the program and expected results.
- Describe the actions expected to lead to the desired results.
- Become a reference point for everyone involved in the program.
- Improve program staff expertise in planning, implementation, and evaluation.
- Involve stakeholders, enhancing the likelihood of resource commitment.

Box 12.1   RESPONSIBILITIES AND COMPETENCIES FOR HEALTH EDUCATION SPECIALISTS

This chapter focuses on program implementation. Because implementation is a culmination of all the preparation and planning that has come before it, several of the responsibilities and competencies for health education specialists apply. The responsibilities and competencies related to these tasks that are associated with implementation include:

Responsibility II: Plan Health Education

Competency 2.4: Develop a Scope and Sequence for the Delivery of Health Education

Competency 2.5: Address factors That Affect Implementation

Responsibility III: Implement Health Education

Competency 3.1: Implement a Plan of Action

Competency 3.2: Monitor Implementation of Health Education

Competency 3.3: Train Individuals Involved in Implementation of Health Education

Responsibility V: Administer and Manage Health Education

Competency 5.1: Manage Fiscal Resources

Competency 5.4: Manage Human Resources

Competency 5.5: Facilitate Partnerships in Support of Health Education

Responsibility VI: Serve as a Health Education Resource Person

Competency 6.2: Provide Training

Competency 6.3: Serve as a Health Education Consultant

Responsibility VII: Communicate and Advocate for Health and Health Education

Competency 7.4: Engage in Health Education Advocacy

Source: NCHEC, SOPHE, & AAHE (2010).

- Incorporate findings from other research and demonstration projects.
- Identify potential obstacles to program operation so that staff can address them early on" (CDC, n.d., para. 3).

Logic models can take many different shapes (linear, circular, lists) and be presented in various levels of detail (simple, complex) but all depict the relationship and linkages of various components in a graphic display of boxes and arrows. "Program-level logic models are often meta-summaries of complex processes; as a result, additional logic models may be needed to 'unpack' each component in the original model so that more details can be articulated" (Helitzer et al., 2009, p. 64). In its most basic form a logic model includes three components: *inputs* (or resources), *outputs* (or activities), and *outcomes*

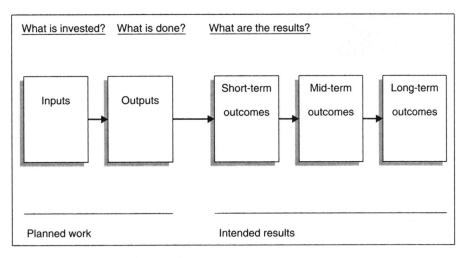

Figure 12.1 Basic Logic Model

(or results or effects). (See **Figure 12.1** for the basic logic model.) The **inputs** in a logic model are the resources that are used to plan, implement, and evaluate a program. They often include human resources (and related items like training, technical assistance, volunteers), partnerships, funding sources, equipment, supplies, materials, and community resources (e.g., space, gifts). The **outputs** in a logic model are the activities or interventions in a program. They often include products (e.g., curricula, educational DVDs, new software), services (e.g., in-service trainings, screenings, counseling), and infrastructure (e.g., structure, capacity, process, and relationships). Some logic model experts have a step in between input and outputs called activities (e.g., weekly sessions or newsletters); the outputs are then things like number of sessions and number participating, or number of newsletters. Others have included processes, tools, technology, events, and actions as activities.

The **outcomes** in a logic model are the intended results and are broken into *short-term* (or immediate) (e.g., changes in awareness, attitudes, knowledge, skills), *mid-term* (or medium) (e.g., changes in behavior or the environment), and *long-term* (e.g., risk reduction, change in health status, or quality of life). Some logic model experts have a step after outcomes called impact, which they define as the fundamental intended or unintended change occurring in organizations, communities, or systems as a result of program.

Basic logic models are good, but the more detailed a logic model the more useful it is to those interested in the program being planned. Thus, others (CDC, n.d.; CDC, 2010e; Goldman & Schmaltz, 2006; University of Kansas, 2011; WKKF, 2004) have suggested that logic models can also include (1) the purpose or mission of the program; (2) the context, conditions, or situations under which the program will be offered; (3) assumptions associated with the planned program; (4) external factors that could influence the success of the program; and (5) a description of the evaluation of the proposed program. **Box 12.2** provides an example of a logic model that was used as part of the planning process for a program aimed at reducing the incidence of colon cancer.

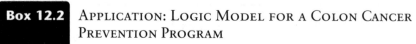

Box 12.2 APPLICATION: LOGIC MODEL FOR A COLON CANCER
PREVENTION PROGRAM

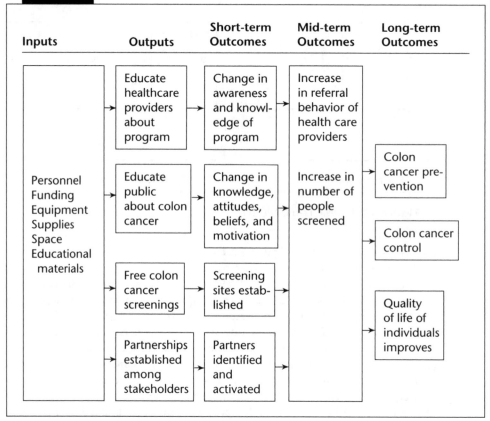

Defining Implementation

In the simplest terms, implementation means to carry out. Timmreck (1997) defined
implementation as the "the act of converting planning, goals, and objectives into action
through administrative structure, management activities, policies, procedures, regulations, and organizational actions of new programs" (p. 328). Keyser and colleagues
(1997) summarized implementation as the setting up, managing, and executing of a
project. Whereas Bartholomew and colleagues (2011) indicated that implementation is
one of the three stages of program diffusion, with the other two being *adoption* and
sustainability. Let's look now at the phases in the implementation process.

Phases of Program Implementation

The phases of implementation that we present here are a combination of some of our
own ideas with those of Parkinson and Associates (1982), Bartholomew and colleagues
(2011), and Johnson and Breckon (2007). It should be noted that the resulting generic

phases presented are flexible in nature and can be modified to meet the many different situations and circumstances faced by planners.

Phase 1: Adoption of the Program

Because the adoption process was presented at length earlier (in Chapter 11), we will not repeat it here. However, we do want to remind planners that great care must go into the marketing process to ensure that a relevant product (i.e., the health promotion program) is planned so that those in the priority population will want to participate in it.

Phase 2: Identifying and Prioritizing the Tasks to Be Completed

In order for a program to be implemented, planners will need to identify and prioritize a number of smaller tasks. Even though many of these tasks are small in nature, they cannot be overlooked if planners want a smooth implementation. Reserving space where the program is to be held, making sure audiovisual equipment is available when requested, ordering the correct number of participant education packets or manuals, and arranging for interpreters when working with a diverse population are examples of tasks that are important to the success of a program. Other implementation tasks are presented later in this chapter in the section titled "Concerns Associated with Implementation."

To assist with identifying and prioritizing these tasks, it is recommended that planners use some form of a planning timetable or time line. Planning timetables and time lines can graphically represent the dates, time span, and sequence of events involved in a program (Issel, 2009). They can also aid in monitoring program progress "so that midcourse corrections can be made, if needed" (McDermott & Sarvela, 1999, p. 72). Planning timetables that are commonly used include basic time lines, task development time lines (TDTLs) (Anspaugh, Dignan, & Anspaugh, 2000), Gantt charts, PERT charts, and the critical path method (CPM). A basic time line is the simplest of the tools. It places the key activities or tasks on a line in the order that they will be completed. It may or may not include an estimate of the dates when the activities or tasks will take place, and the time allocated to complete them (see **Figure 12.2**).

Task development time lines and Gantt charts are very similar. They are both composed of rows and columns. The rows on the left-hand side of the chart represent the tasks or activities to be completed, while the columns represent periods of time. In the examples presented in **Figures 12.3** and **12.4**, the columns represent months, but they could just as easily represent weeks or for that matter days if the chart were being used for a short-term project. The major difference between a TDTL and a Gantt chart is in the detail presented. A **task development time line** identifies the tasks that need to be completed and the time frame in which the tasks will be completed (Anspaugh et al., 2000). A **Gantt chart**, developed in 1917 by Henry Gantt as a production control tool

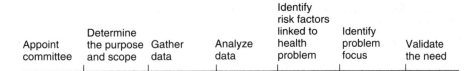

Figure 12.2 Sample Basic Time Line for a Needs Assessment

Tasks Year 1	Months											
	J	F	M	A	M	J	J	A	S	O	N	D
Develop program rationale	✔	✔										
Conduct needs assessment			✔									
Develop goals and objectives				✔								
Create intervention					✔							
Conduct formative evaluation						✔						
Assemble necessary resources						✔						
Market program						✔	✔					
Pilot test program								✔				
Refine program									✔			
Phase in intervention #1										✔		
Phase in intervention #2											✔	
Phase in intervention #3												✔

Tasks Year 2	Months											
	J	F	M	A	M	J	J	A	S	O	N	D
Phase in intervention #4	✔											
Total implementation		✔	✔	✔	✔	✔	✔	✔	✔	✔	✔	✔
Collect and analyze data for evaluation			✔									
Prepare evaluation report				✔								
Distribute report					✔							
Continue with follow-up for long-term evaluation						✔	✔	✔	✔	✔	✔	✔

Figure 12.3 Sample Task Development Time Line for Program Planning, Implementation, and Evaluation

Date
√

	Mar.	April	May	June	July	Aug.	Sept.	Oct.	Nov.	Dec.
Hire and train program facilitators	▬▬▬	▬▬▬								
Pilot test program			▬▬▬	▬▬▬						
Revise program based on pilot					▬▬					
Promote the program					▬▬▬	───				
Prepare for program "kick off"						▬▬ ─				
Phase in program							▬▬▬			
Full implementation								▬▬▬		
Evaluate program									▬▬▬	
Write final report										▬▬

▬▬▬ = planned time frame

─── = completed

Figure 12.4 Sample Gantt Chart for Program Implementation and Evaluation

(TechTarget, 2007a), does the same plus provides an indication of the progress made toward completing the task by using different size lines to distinguish between the projected time frame for a task and the progress toward completing the task. In addition, a Gantt chart uses a marker above the columns to indicate the current date (Timmreck, 2003). (See the check mark above the month of August in Figure 12.4.) Thus, when using a Gantt chart, planners would update their progress regularly on the chart.

PERT is an acronym for program evaluation and review technique. PERT charts are more complex than Gantt charts and have not been used as much with health promotion programs (Timmreck, 2003). PERT charts are composed of two components, a diagram and a timetable (Minelli & Breckon, 2009). The diagram presents a visual representation of the relationship between and among the tasks to be completed. The diagram also indicates the order of completion by sequentially numbering the tasks. This means that tasks identified with lower numbers must be completed prior to taking on tasks identified with higher numbers (TechTarget, 2007b). The timetable of a PERT chart is similar to the key activity chart but also includes three estimates of time for each task. Included in the estimates are an optimistic, pessimistic, and a probabilistic time frame. The complexity of PERT puts a detailed explanation beyond the scope of this textbook. If readers are interested in learning more about it, we recommend referring to business management textbooks.

The last planning timetable to be presented is the **critical path method** (CPM). CPM charts are similar to PERT charts and are sometimes referred to as PERT/CPM. Like all the other planning timetables presented here, the CPM provides a graphical view of the project and predicts the time required to complete the project. But what is unique to CPM is that it focuses on time by showing which tasks are critical to maintaining the planning schedule and which are not (NetMBA, 2002–2010). Thus, the critical path is indicated and consists of the set of dependent tasks (each dependent on the preceding one) that together take the longest time to complete. The tasks on the path are critical because any delay in their completion will lengthen program implementation unless appropriate action is taken (NetMBA, 2002–2010).

Phase 3: Establishing a System of Management

Once all the tasks have been identified and the timetable for completing them has been developed, planners can turn their attention to how the program will be managed. **Management** has been defined as "the process of assembling and using sets of resources in a goal-directed manner to accomplish tasks in an organizational setting" (Hitt, Black, & Porter, 2012, p. 483). Typically, the sets of resources include human, financial, and technical resources (Johnson & Breckon, 2007). Management is an important part of the program implementation process. "The efficient, satisfactory management of a health promotion program is vital to its long-term success" (Anspaugh et al., 2000, p. 124). Yet, management is both challenging and necessary (Hitt et al., 2012). It is challenging because the large number of responsibilities (e.g., planning, organization, coordination, and control) associated with the task of managing and because of change, both expected and unexpected, throughout the life of a program. Thus, good management is needed to ensure that programs are both *effective* and *efficient* (Gomez-Mejia & Balkin, 2012). Effective programs are ones that meet stated goals and objectives. They are efficient when the best possible use is made of program resources. Good managers can go a long way in making this happen. Hitt and colleagues (2012) have identified three types of skills needed by managers—technical, interpersonal, and conceptual. "Technical skills involve having specialized knowledge about procedures, processes, and equipment, and include knowing how and when to use that knowledge" (p. 19). Interpersonal skills include such qualities as sensitivity, persuasiveness, and empathy, while conceptual skills, sometimes called cognitive ability or cognitive complexity, include such skills as logical reasoning, judgment, and analytical abilities.

Depending on the type of program being planned, the management process could range from consuming a small portion of a single planner's time and resources, such as when a smoking cessation program is being planned for 10 people, to needing several people working full-time to manage a large community-wide program. Many of the tasks associated with the management phase of implementation are presented later in this chapter. In the space below we will provide an overview of the management of the three major resources.

Human Resources Management (HRM)   There are four fundamental functions associated with HRM. "These functions, designated by the acronym PADS, are planning, acquisition, development, and sanction" (Klingner, Nalbandian, & Llorens, 2010, p. 4). Personnel planning refers to the work that must be completed in order to be able to determine what positions are needed to carry out a program and how to fill them (Dessler, 2012), whether they are filled with employees or volunteers. (See Chapter 10 for more information on volunteers.) Thus knowing: (1) what tasks that must be completed by the personnel of a program, (2) what knowledge and skills the personnel need to complete the tasks, (3) how many people will be needed to complete the tasks, (4) how to describe the jobs (see Box 10.4 for a sample job description), and (5) how much compensation (pay and benefits) is appropriate for the jobs are all part of planning.

Once the planning for personnel is complete and job descriptions are in place, program managers can then focus on acquisition (the *A* of PADS) of personnel; that is, the recruitment and selection of the personnel. This process begins by generating a pool of candidates for the jobs through recruitment. This is typically handled through advertising via the *job posting* at various sites (e.g., newspapers; online on home pages or recruiting job boards; at employment agencies or career centers) where viable candidates will find the information (Dessler, 2012). Job postings not only describe the positions that need to be filled but also include information about the application process. It is not unusual to have applicants provide a letter of application, complete an application form, submit a résumé, and provide either letters of recommendation or the names of references to be contacted later. With the formal applications in hand, candidates must be screened (which in addition to looking for the appropriate qualifications may include testing, background checks, physical exams, and drug testing), decisions must be made on how and when to interview them, and finally the best candidates must be selected, and their services secured.

The *D* in PADS stands for development. Development includes the orientation, training, performance appraisal, and professional growth opportunities to increase the personnel's willingness and competencies to perform well (Dessler, 2012; Klingner et al., 2010). Orientation (often called *onboarding*) has two major purposes: (1) to provide background information to perform the job satisfactorily, and (2) to socialize new personnel to the work environment by instilling the attitudes, standards, values, and patterns of behavior that are expected (Dessler, 2012). Training involves providing personnel with the knowledge and skills needed to be successful in the position. Much training today revolves around building capacity and teamwork. (See Chapter 10 for more on these topics.) Performance appraisal and professional growth opportunities frequently go hand in hand. Performance appraisal often includes some informal appraisal in which feedback is provided as needed and a more formal evaluation that is conducted on either a semi-annual or annual basis. The results of these appraisals can be used to plan additional training to deal with deficiencies or plan professional growth opportunities to expand staff abilities and competencies.

The final fundamental function in HRM is sanction. Sanction (the *S* of PADS) deals with maintaining the expectations and obligations program personnel and their program manager have to one another through appropriate compensation, discipline/grievances, health and safety, and personnel rights (Klingner et al., 2010).

Much of the work of program managers as related to HRM is guided by laws and legal decisions. **Box 12.3** includes a list of a number of the important pieces of federal legislation that impact the management of human resources. Note that most of the legislation presented in Box 12.3 applies to all employees and most employers but not all. In certain situations specific requirements must be met for the legislation to apply. For example, the Family and Medical Leave Act (FMLA) only applies in work settings with 50 or more employees. Also note that in addition to the federal legislation individual states may also have laws that impact human resources. An example is the "state-by-state laws that establish insurance plans to compensate employees injured on the job" (Gomez-Mejia & Balkin, 2012, p. 286).

Box 12.3   IMPORTANT PIECES OF FEDERAL LEGISLATION
IMPACTING HUMAN RESOURCES

Year	Legislation	Topic
1935*	Social Security Act	Retirement system for workers
1938	Fair Labor Standards Act	Prescribes standards for wages and overtime pay
1959	Labor-Management Reporting and Disclosure Act (LMRDA)	Deals with the relationship between a union and its members
1963	Equal Pay Act	Prohibits discrimination in pay based on gender
1964**	Civil Rights Act	Prohibits discrimination based on race, color, religion, gender, or national origin
1967	Age Discrimination Employment Act	Prohibits discrimination against a person 40 or older because of age
1970	Occupational Safety and Health (OSH) Act	Workplace Safety
1973	Vocational Rehabilitation Act	Prohibits discrimination against qualified individuals with handicaps
1974	Vietnam Era Veterans' Readjustment Assistance Act	Requires affirmative action in employment for veterans of the Vietnam War era
1974	Employee Retirement Income Security Act	Regulates employers who offer pension or welfare benefit programs for their employees
1978	Pregnancy Discrimination Act	Prohibits discrimination in employment against pregnant women, or related conditions
1985	Consolidated Omnibus Budget Reconciliation Act (COBRA)	Provides opportunity to allow employee pay for continued health insurance coverage after termination
1988	Drug-Free Workplace Act	Employers must implement certain policies to restrict employee drug use
1990***	Americans with Disability Act (ADA)	Prohibits employment discrimination based on ability
1993***	Family and Medical Leave Act (FMLA)	Time off for medical issues for self and family
1996	Health Insurance Portability and Accountability Act (HIPAA)	Health insurance and privacy
2008	Genetic Information Nondiscrimination Act (GINA)	Prohibits discrimination in health coverage and employment based on genetic information

* Amended numerous times
**Amended in 1991
***Amended in 2008
Source: Created from Dessler (2012); Fallon & Zgodzinski (2012); Gomez-Mejia & Balkin (2012); Grudzien (2009); Johnson & Breckon (2007); Klingner et al. (2010); and USDL (n.d.).

Financial Management   Financial management "is the process of developing and using systems to ensure that funds are spent for the purposes for which they have been appropriated" (Klingner et al., 2010, p. 88). Financial management begins after funds have been obtained and the program budget has been created. (See Chapter 10 for more information on sources of funding and budgets.) Thus, it is the program manager who is responsible for ensuring that program funds are spent on the things for which they were appropriated. This process begins with a system to record the transactions that take place over the life of a program. These transactions include funds coming into, the income (e.g., grant money, gifts, participant fees), and going out, the expenditures (e.g., paying for salaries and wages, and the purchase of materials, supplies, and equipment) of the program. The process of recording and summarizing these transactions and interpreting their effects on the program budget is referred to as **accounting** (Fallon & Zgodzinski, 2012). Each organization has an accounting process and depending on the size of the organization responsibility for the accounting process may fall on the program manager or if the organization is large enough it may fall to an accounting department.

The accounting process generates financial statements. "Financial statements can be prepared at any point in time and can cover any period of time" (Fallon & Zgodzinski, 2012, p. 60). Most organizations work on a **fiscal year** (or funding year) running from either January 1st to December 31st or July 1st to June 30th. However, it is common for financial statements to be created at regular intervals (i.e., weekly, monthly, quarterly, semiannually, or annually) during the fiscal year. (See Figure 10.3.) Each "organization selects a reporting period and prepares financial statements at the end of the designated reporting period" (Fallon & Zgodzinski, 2012, p. 61). The statements usually include "actual revenue and expenses for the period, year-to-date actual, and year-to-date variance (Johnson & Breckon, 2007, p. 180). It is then the responsibility of the person in charge of program finance to determine the status of the budget and compare the financial statement to the program budget. Armed with such information, the program manager can make the necessary financial decisions. "The extent to which resources are managed according to the budget" (Issel, 2009, p. 323) is referred to as **fiscal accountability**.

Audits are conducted to ensure that the accounting process within an organization is being handled properly. An **audit** is a "review and confirmation that financial reports are accurate and that standard accounting procedures were used to prepare the reports" (Johnson & Breckon, 2007, p. 288). The main purpose of an audit "is to determine if fraud or other undesirable practices are occurring" (Johnson & Breckon, 2007, p. 292). Further, audits can be either external or internal. An **external audit** is one that is conducted by an qualified independent accountant usually just once a year, whereas an **internal audit** is a frequent and ongoing audit conducted by an employee of the organization not responsible for the accounting practices (BusinessDictionary.com, 2011a).

Technical Resources Management   Technical resources (also referred to as *other resources*) includes all other resources besides human or financial. Included in this category of resources are communication (both internal and external to the organization), equipment (e.g., computers), expertise, information, materials, partnerships, relationships, space, and supplies. This may be the most difficult category of resources to manage because sometimes it is difficult to quantify the amount of a technical resource like personnel and funding needed for a program. For example, how are external communication and relationships quantified?

Phase 4: Putting the Plans into Action

Parkinson and Associates (1982) suggested three major ways of putting plans into action: by using a piloting process; by phasing them in, in small segments; and by initiating the total program all at once. These three strategies are best explained by using an inverted triangle, as shown in **Figure 12.5**. The triangle represents the number of people from the priority population who would be involved in the program based on the implementation strategy chosen. The wider portion of the triangle at the top would indicate offering the program to a larger number of people than is represented by the point of the triangle at the bottom.

These three different implementation strategies exist in a hierarchy. It is recommended that all programs go through all three of the strategies, starting with piloting, then phasing in, and finally implementing the total program. However, keep in mind that limited time and resources may not always allow planners to work through all three strategies. In addition, if the priority population is relatively small it may not make sense to use all three strategies. In such cases the phasing in strategy would probably not be used.

Pilot Testing   Pilot testing (or *piloting* or *field testing*) a program is a crucial step. Even though planners work hard to bring a program to the point of putting it into action, it is important to try to identify any problems with the program that might exist. Pilot testing allows planners to work out any bugs before the program is offered to a larger segment of the priority population, and also to validate the work that has been completed

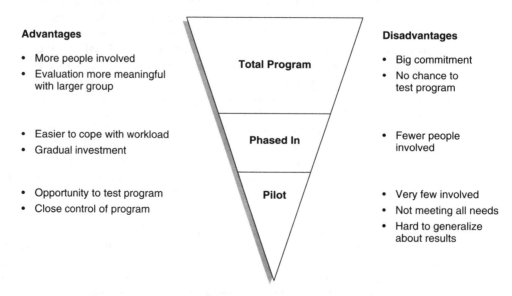

Figure 12.5 Putting Plans Into Action

up to this point. For the most meaningful results, a newly developed program should be piloted in a similar setting and with people as much like those who will eventually use the program as possible. Use of any other group may fail to identify problems or concerns that would be specific to the priority population. As an example of the piloting process, take the case of a hospital developing a worksite health promotion program that will be marketed to outside companies. It would be best if the program were piloted on a worksite group before it was marketed to worksites in the community. The hospital could look for a company that might want to serve as a pilot group, or it might use its own employees.

As part of piloting the program, planners should check on the following four areas:

1. The intervention strategies were implemented as planned.

2. The intervention strategies worked as planned.

3. Adequate resources were available to carry out the program.

4. Participants in the pilot group had an opportunity to evaluate the program.

It is important to have the program participants critique such aspects of the program as content, approaches used, facilitator's effectiveness, space, accommodations, and other resources used. Such feedback will help planners determine if they need to revise the program, and if so how to revise it. If many changes are made in the program as a result of piloting, planners may want to pilot it again before moving ahead. (This evaluation process during the piloting phase is part of formative evaluation and will be discussed further in Chapter 13.)

Phasing In   Once a program has been piloted and revised, the program should, if applicable, be **phased in** rather than implemented in its entirety. This is especially true when there is a very large priority population. Phasing in allows the planners to have more control over the program and helps to protect planners and facilitators from getting in over their heads. There are four ways in which to phase in a program:

1. By different program offerings

2. By a limit on the number of participants

3. By choice of location

4. By participant ability

Say a comprehensive health promotion program was being planned for Blue Earth County, Minnesota. To phase in the program by different offerings, planners might offer stress-management classes the first six months. During the next six-month period, they could again offer stress management but also add smoking cessation programs. This process would continue until all offerings are included.

If the program were to be phased in by limiting the number of participants, planners might limit the first month's enrollment to 25 participants, expand it to 35 the second month, to 45 the third month, and so on, until all who wanted to participate were included. To phase in the program by location, it might initially be offered only to those living in the southwest portion of the county. The second year, it might expand to include those in the southeast, and continue in the same manner until all were included. A program planned for a college town might be offered first on campus, then off campus to the general public. A program phased in by participant ability might start with a beginning group of exercisers, then add an intermediate group, and finally include an advanced group.

Total Implementation   Implementing the total program all at once, in most situations, would be a mistake. Rather, planners should work toward total implementation through the piloting and phasing in processes. The only exceptions to this might be "one-shot" programs, such as programs designed around a single lecture, and possibly screening programs, but even then piloting would probably help.

First Day of Implementation   No matter what program is being planned, there will be a "first day" for the program. The first day of the program, also referred to as the **program launch, program rollout,** or **program kickoff,** is just an extension of the fourth P of marketing: promotion (see Chapter 11). The focus of promotion is on creating and sustaining demand for a product (Weinreich, 1999). The creation of the demand for the product leads to the initiation of the program. As such, some special planning needs to take place for the first day of implementation. First, decide on a day when the program is to be rolled out. Consider launching the program to coincide with other already-occurring events or special days that can help promote the program. Examples include starting a weight loss program at the beginning of the calendar year to coincide with New Year's resolutions, beginning a smoking cessation program on the third Thursday of November (the day each year for the American Cancer Society's Great American Smokeout), having immunization programs and physical examinations for children prior to the beginning of a new school year, launching a skin cancer prevention program on a college campus prior to the annual spring break, or rolling out the community-wide exercise program at the beginning of February, Heart Health month.

Second, kick off the program in style. This is important to bring attention to the program, and to create momentum and enthusiasm for the program (Chapman, 2006). Planners should consider having a first day that includes some special event such as a ribbon cutting, health screening, health fair, contest, appearance by a celebrity, or some other event that starts the program on a positive note. Celebrities need not be individuals with national or international recognition, but may be individuals such as an executive or supervisor of the organization for which the program is being planned (e.g., chief executive officer [CEO] or executive director), a visible or well-known person from the community (e.g., the mayor or a coach), or a common person who has been affected by the health problem on which the program will focus.

Third, consideration should be given to obtaining news coverage (print and/or broadcast) for the first day to further publicize the program. If it is decided to seek such coverage, you should (CDC, 2003):

- Inform appropriate media representatives of your plans
- Make arrangements to meet the media representatives at the designated time and place

- Prepare the following and have them ready for the day:
  - ◆ Press releases
  - ◆ Video news releases
  - ◆ Spokespersons trained to respond to inquires from media representatives

To get news coverage it might be useful to use a **news hook** to interest the media in the program being launched. By news hook, we mean something that will make the media want to cover the launch. The planners' organization may have newsworthy data or information related to the health problem being targeted by the program, or there may be a related news event that is receiving media attention that would help bring attention to the new program (CDC, 2003). For example, if a new program is aimed at reducing teen pregnancy and new state legislation has been proposed to assist in such efforts or an event related to teen pregnancy is currently an important news item, then linking the new program with those timely events can make it more newsworthy (CDC, 2003). Human interest stories also make for good news hooks. For example, if you are starting a smoking cessation program, getting former quitters to talk about how quitting changed their lives can be of interest to others. Or, if your program is aimed at teaching children what to do in an emergency situation, and you know of a child who has completed a similar program and was able to put the education to use in helping someone, many people would like to know about that. Planners should even consider linking the launch of the program with some important date in history to make it newsworthy. Linking the influenza epidemic of 1918–19 to launch the countywide flu shot program may make it more newsworthy.

Phase 5: Ending or Sustaining a Program

The final phase of the implementation process is to determine how long to run a program. For some programs the answer will be simple: If the program met its goals and objectives and the priority population has been served to the fullest extent necessary, then the program can be ended. For example, a worksite health promotion program may have a goal to certify 50% of the workforce in CPR. If that goal is reached, then the program's resources could be used on other health promotion programming. However, a greater concern facing most planners is how to sustain a needed program for a longer period of time when the goals and objectives have not been met (e.g., only half of those who were expected to get flu shots got them), or goals and objectives of the program are long-term in nature (e.g., providing food and shelter for the homeless). This is especially difficult when original program funding and other types of resources and support may end or be withdrawn. Earlier (in Chapter 11), we presented information on how to maintain interest in program participants, but here we are referring to the maintenance and institutionalization of a program or its outcomes. Techniques that have been used by planners to sustain programs include: (1) working to institutionalize the program (see Chapter 2; Goodman & Steckler, 1989; and Goodman et al., 1993), (2) seeking feedback from program participants and evaluating the program in order to generate evidence to show its worth (Sleet & Cole, 2010), (3) advocating for the program (see Chapter 8 for a discussion of advocacy), (4) partnering with other organizations/agencies with similar missions to share resources, expenses, and responsibilities, and (5) by revisiting and revising the rationale used to create the program initially (see Chapter 2).

Concerns Associated with Implementation

Many matters of detail must be considered before and during the implementation process. Although we believe all the topics presented in this section are important, we feel that the topics of safety and medical concerns and ethical issues are the most important. That is why these topics are presented first.

Safety and Medical Concerns

The ultimate goal of most health promotion programs is to improve the health of its participants. As such, planners in no way want to put the health of participants in danger. Therefore, planners must give attention to the safety and medical concerns associated with health promotion programs. To ensure the safety of participants, planners need to inform participants about the program they are considering joining. Only after they understand what the program is all about should they agree to participate. This concept is referred to as informed consent. More formally, valid **informed consent** requires: "(1) Disclosure of relevant information to prospective subjects about the research [program]; (2) their comprehension of the information; and (3) their voluntary agreement, free of coercion and undue influence, to research [program] participation" (NIH, 2006, para. 1).

As a part of the process of obtaining informed consent from participants, program facilitators should take five steps:

1. Explain the nature and purpose(s) of the program.

2. Inform program participants of any inherent risks or dangers associated with participation and any possible discomfort they may experience.

3. Explain the expected benefits of participation.

4. Inform participants of alternative programs (procedures) that will accomplish the same thing.

5. Indicate to the participants that they are free to discontinue participation at any time.

In addition, planners must ask if the participants "have any questions, answer any such questions, and make it clear they should ask any questions they may have at any time during the program. Informed consent forms should be signed by participants before they enter the program" (Patton et al., 1986, p. 236).

Program planners must be aware that informed consent forms (sometimes called *waiver of liability* or *release of liability*) do not protect them from being sued. There is no such thing as a waiver of liability. If you are negligent, you can be found liable. However, informed consent forms do make participants aware of special concerns. Further, because people must sign the forms, they may not consider legal action even if they have a case, feeling that they were duly warned. **Box 12.4** presents a sample consent form.

Box 12.4	APPLICATION—EXAMPLE INFORMED CONSENT FORM

Consent to Perform Cholesterol Screening

I hereby grant permission to the Institute for Health Promotion personnel to perform a cholesterol screening on me. I am engaging in this screening voluntarily. I have been told this screening will provide an analysis of total blood cholesterol and that a trained employee will take my blood from a finger stick sample. This finger stick may be uncomfortable. I understand that the results of this screening are considered to be preliminary in nature and in no way conclusive. Results of a blood cholesterol screening like this can be affected by a number of factors including, but not limited to, smoking, stress level, amount of exercise, hormone levels, food eaten, heredity, and pregnancy. I also understand that my physician can perform a more complete blood lipid (fat) analysis for me, if I so desire.

Further, I have been told that all the information related to this screening is considered confidential.

I have read the above statement and understand what it means. I have also had an opportunity to ask questions about the screening, and all my questions have been answered to my satisfaction.

_____   _____   _____
Participant's Signature   Date   Signature of Witness

NOTE TO PROGRAM PLANNERS: To ensure this form meets all related organizational policies and local and state laws, this form should be submitted to legal counsel before use.

Once participants have agreed to participate in a program, if the act of participating in the program puts anyone at medical risk (e.g., cardiovascular exercise programs), then these individuals need to obtain medical clearance before participating. Some organizations that conduct such programs on a regular basis will have a medical clearance form that will need to be completed. Typically, a physician who is familiar with the person's health history must sign the form. If such a form is not available, then steps need to be taken to create one and have it reviewed by a lawyer to make sure it includes all the necessary information.

After participants have medical clearance and are enrolled in a program, steps must be taken to ensure the safety and health of all associated with the program (i.e., participants and staff members). Providing a safe program includes: finding a safe program location (e.g., low-crime area), providing appropriate security at the location; ensuring that all building codes are met at the location, and ensuring that the classroom, locker rooms, laboratories, and any other facilities used are free of hazards. In addition to a safe environment, programs need qualified instructors (i.e., appropriately trained and certified), and planners need to be prepared for emergency situations by supplying the appropriate first-aid supplies and equipment, and developing an emergency care plan. **Box 12.5** provides a checklist of items that should be considered when creating an appropriate emergency care plan.

Box 12.5	CHECKLIST OF ITEMS TO CONSIDER WHEN DEVELOPING AN EMERGENCY CARE PLAN

1. Duties of program staff in an emergency situation are defined.
2. Program staff is trained (CPR and first aid) to handle emergencies.
3. Program participants are instructed what to do in an emergency situation (e.g., medical, natural disaster).
4. Participants with high-risk health problems are known to program staff.
5. Emergency care supplies and equipment are available.
6. Program staff has access to a telephone.
7. Standing orders are available for common emergency problems.
8. There is a plan for notifying those needed in emergency situations.
9. Responsibility for transportation of ill/injured is defined.
10. Injury (incident) report form procedures are defined.
11. Universal precautions are outlined and followed.
12. Responsibility for financial charges incurred in the emergency care process are defined.
13. The emergency care plan has been approved by the appropriate personnel.
14. The emergency care plan is reviewed and updated on a regular basis.

Ethical Issues

"Ethical issues permeate almost every decision and action undertaken in health education" (Goldsmith, 2006, p. 33), including many of the decisions associated with program planning. By **ethical issues** we mean situations in which competing values are at play and program planners need to make a judgment about what is the most appropriate course of action. For example, planners may want to create an intervention that includes an economic incentive for a priority population that, for the most part, is composed of individuals with a low socioeconomic status. Because of the socioeconomic status of those in the priority population, the ethical issue that faces the planners is deciding at what dollar value does the incentive cross over from encouraging people to participate in a program to manipulating their participation in the program?

What guides ethical decision making? Most often, these decisions are compared to a standard of practice that has been defined by other professionals in the same field. For health promotion planners, the standard of practice is outlined in the *Code of Ethics for the Health Education Profession* developed by the Coalition of National Health Education Organizations (CNHEO, 2011a) (see the Appendix for a copy of the Code). The preamble of the *Code* states: "Health Educators are responsible for upholding the integrity and ethics of the profession as they face the daily challenges of making decisions. Health Educators value diversity in society and embrace a multiplicity of approaches in their work to support the worth, dignity, potential, and uniqueness of all people" (CNHEO, 2011a, p. 1). For program planners this means having integrity, and being honest, loyal, and accountable. Unethical practice leads to professional suicide; planners who act unethically damage their professional reputation and integrity (Bensley, 2009).

Many of the ethical issues that program planners will face revolve around the three fundamental principles of *The Belmont Report: Ethical Principles and Guidelines for the Protection of Human Subject Research* (National Commission, 1979). These principles include: (1) respect for persons, (2) beneficence, and (3) justice. Here are some examples of the application of these principles to program planning. The principle of *respect for persons* acknowledges the dignity and autonomy (i.e., freedom) of individuals, and requires that people with diminished autonomy (e.g., children, mentally disabled, and people with severe illnesses) be provided special protection (NIH, 2004). It is not unusual for health education specialists to be working with program participants who have values, behavior, including health behavior, and goals that are different than their own. Even though they are different, it is important to respect them. For example, health education specialists working in a family planning clinic may see clients choose a course of action that may be different than what they personally would select, but clients have the right to choose a course of action and it must be respected.

The principle of *beneficence* requires program planners to protect participants by maximizing anticipated benefits and minimizing harms (NIH, 2004). This principle dates back to the Hippocratic Oath written by the famous Greek physician Hippocrates who lived from about 460 B.C.E. until 377 B.C.E. (Cottrell et al., 2012). The principle embodies two concepts: doing good, **beneficence**, and not causing harm, **nonmaleficence**. The Hippocratic maxim "do no harm" has long been a fundamental principle of medical ethics, but also applies to the work of health education specialists. The concepts associated with this principle seem to be common sense, but well-intending health education specialists who may not be as well informed on best practices (see Chapter 8 for a discussion of best practices) could put participants at risk without knowing they are doing so. For example, much attention has been given to the public health issue of youth violence. Evidence shows that a number of well-meaning approaches to dealing with youth violence at all three levels of prevention—primary (e.g., holding youth back a grade in school), secondary (e.g., redirecting youth behavior or shifting peer group norm programs), and tertiary (e.g., "boot camps" for delinquent youths)—can bring harm to the youth (USDHHS, 2001).

When dealing with the principle of beneficence, health education specialists may need to make ethical decisions revolving around the "benefit-harm ratio." For example, should a health education specialist be barred from releasing information about a person without his or her consent, even if it will benefit that person? Consider a high school sophomore who approaches the health teacher with confidential information that she is pregnant. Should the health teacher tell anyone else, such as the girl's parents?

The principle of *justice* requires that program planners treat participants fairly (NIH, 2004). For example, the question of fairness may have ethical implications when it comes to charging a registration fee for a program. Because of the policies of the organization conducting the program, the program may need to turn a profit, but those in need of the program may not be able to afford the cost of registration. Other ethical issues of justice and fairness can arise from issues of sexism, racism, and other cultural biases.

The opportunities for dealing with ethical issues are many, and planners need to be prepared to handle them.

Legal Concerns

Legal liability is on the mind of many professionals today because of the concern over lawsuits. With this in mind, all personnel connected with the planned health promotion program, no matter how small the risk of injury to the participants (physical or mental), should make sure that they are adequately covered by liability insurance. In addition, program personnel should have an understanding of negligence and how to reduce one's risk of liability.

Negligence Negligence is failing to act in a **prudent** (reasonable) manner. If there is a question whether someone should or should not do something, it is generally best to err on the side of caution. Negligence can arise from two types of **acts: omission** and **commission**. An act of omission is not doing something when you should, such as failing to warn program participants of the inherent danger in participation. An act of commission is doing something you should not be doing, such as leading an aerobic dance program when you are not trained to do so.

Reducing the Risk of Liability The real key to avoiding liability is to reduce risk by planning ahead. Patton and colleagues (1986, p. 236) offer the following eight tips for reducing legal problems in exercise programs; however, similar advice would apply to all types of health promotion programs:

1. Be aware of legal liabilities (things you are legally responsible for).
2. Select certified instructors (in the activity and emergency care procedures) to lead classes and supervise exercise equipment (and for that matter all types of equipment).
3. Use good judgment in setting up programs and provide written guidelines for medical emergency procedures.
4. Inform participants about the risks and danger of exercise (or other activities) and require written informed consent.
5. Require that participants obtain medical clearance before entering an exercise program (or other strenuous programs).
6. Instruct staff members not to "practice medicine," but instead to limit their advice to their own area of expertise.
7. Provide a safe environment by following building codes and regular maintenance schedule for equipment.
8. Purchase adequate liability insurance for all staff.

With regard to item 8 in the preceding list, planners should check on the availability of liability insurance through their employer or special coverage from a professional organization. Liability insurance may also be available through one's homeowner's or renter's insurance.

Program Registration and Fee Collection

If the program you are planning requires people to sign up and/or pay fees, you will need to establish registration procedures. Program registration and fee collection may take place before the program (preregistration), by mail, in person, via an indirect method like payroll deduction, or at the first session. Planners should also give thought to the type of payment that will be accepted (cash, credit card, or check) and plan accordingly. Though it may seem obvious, some thought also must be given to the security of the money received. That is, how it will be handled, transported, and deposited or otherwise secured.

Procedures for Record Keeping

Almost every program requires that some records be kept. Items such as information collected at registration, medical information, data on participant progress, and evaluations must be accounted for. The importance of privacy for those planners working in health-care settings was further emphasized in 2003 with the enactment of the *Standards for Privacy of Individually Identifiable Health Information* section (the Privacy Rule) of the Health Insurance Portability and Accountability Act of 1996, officially known as Public Law 104–191 and referred to as **HIPAA**. The Rule sets national standards that health plans, health care clearinghouses, and health care providers who conduct certain health care transactions electronically must implement to protect and guard against the misuse of individually identifiable health information. Failure to implement the standards can lead to civil and criminal penalties (USDHHS, n.d.).

The two techniques that are used to protect the privacy of participants are anonymity and confidentiality. **Anonymity** exists when no one, including the planners, can relate a participant's identity to any information pertaining to the program. Thus information associated with a participant may be considered anonymous when such information cannot be linked to the participant who provided it. In applying this concept, planners need to ensure that collected data had no identifying information attached to them such as the participant's name, social security number, or any other less common information.

Confidentiality exists when planners are aware of the participants' identities and have promised not to reveal those identities to others. When handling confidential data, planners need to take every precaution to protect the participants' information. Often this means keeping the information "under lock and key" while participants are active in a program, then destroying (e.g., shredding) the information when it is no longer needed.

Procedural Manual and/or Participants' Manual

Depending on the type and complexity of a program, there may be a need to develop a *program procedural manual* and/or *participants' manual*. If a program is very involved (e.g., has several interventions or a very detailed curriculum) and/or may have a number of different people facilitating the program (i.e., one that will be used in a number of locations like an educational program of a voluntary health agency), there is probably a need to create a program procedural manual. The purposes of a program procedural manual (also sometimes referred to as a *training manual*) are to: (1) ensure that all who are associated with the program understand the program and its parameters, (2) standardize the intervention so it can be replicated and to avoid what Basch and colleagues (1985) referred to as **Type III errors**—failure to implement the health education intervention properly (see Chapter 15 for a discussion of Type I and II errors), (3) provide ideas for facilitation, (4) provide additional background information on the topic, and (5) provide citations for additional resources.

Participants' manuals may also be needed and/or useful for several reasons. First, they may be a good way of getting all program information into participants' hands at one time, including the educational materials and program procedures and guidelines. Second, they can help participants organize information they receive and keep it all in one place, especially if they are set up as loose-leaf notebooks or folders. Third, they can serve as a reference or resource for the participants. And fourth, if participants frequently use their manual as part of the program and become familiar with it, they may be more inclined to refer to it outside of the program sessions.

If a program is being developed in-house and manuals are needed, they will more than likely need to be developed in-house as well. Developing either type of manual—procedural or participant—in-house is a major task; therefore, adequate resources and time need to be given to developing the manuals. If a canned program is obtained from another organization (e.g., a voluntary health agency) or is being purchased from a vendor, it should more than likely include manuals.

Program Participants with Disabilities

A special situation for program planners during not only the implementation phase, but in all phases of program planning is ensuring that the programs being planned meet the needs of program participants with disabilities. From a legal, benefit, and social program perspective, **disability** is "often defined on the basis of specific activities of daily living, work and other functions essential to full participation in community-based living" (USDHHS, 2005, p. 4). Disability can range from sensory problems (e.g., seeing and hearing) to problems resulting from cognitive impairment, neuromuscular disorders, serious injury, and intellectual and developmental disabilities. However, "disability is not an illness. The concept of health means the same for persons with or without disabilities: achieving and sustaining an optimal level of wellness—both physical and mental—that promotes a fullness of life" (Krahn, 2003, as stated in USDHHS, 2005, p. 3). The number of people with disabilities in the United States range from an estimated 12% (~36+ million) (Erickson Lee, & von Schrader, 2010) to approximately 19% (~54+ million) (USDHHS, 2005) depending on how disability is defined. Regardless of the exact number of people, program planners must be prepared to work with individuals who have disabilities. Because most program planners have not received training developing programs for people with disabilities, Drum and colleagues (2009) have put forth useful guidelines and criteria. We have presented a list of their guidelines, criteria, and key questions (see **Box 12.6**) that need to be answered to ensure programs meet the needs of these individuals.

Training for Facilitators

An important part of the implementation process is to make sure that the program intervention is implemented as planned. There are a couple reasons for this. First, as you are now aware, a great deal of effort goes into creating an intervention for the specific priority population, possibly even tailoring the intervention; that effort should not be wasted. And second, appropriate implementation is necessary to be able to evaluate and document the effectiveness of an intervention. To ensure that a program is implemented as planned, the program facilitators need to be familiar with the intervention. This familiarity may come about by participating in the planning of the intervention or through a training session. If those who implement the intervention are also the ones who planned the intervention, then a brief review of the steps in the intervention may be all that is needed. If those who

Box 12.6	GUIDELINES, CRITERIA, AND ISSUES TO CONSIDER WHEN IMPLEMENTING PROGRAMS FOR INDIVIDUALS WITH DISABILITIES

Operational Guidelines for Health Promotion Programs for People with Disabilities

Criterion 1. Health promotion programs for people with disabilities should have an underlying conceptual or theoretical framework.

Issues:

1. Does the program use theories and concepts drawn from a wide variety of disciplines such as health promotion, disability studies, and/or education?
2. Does the program integrate appropriate theories and concepts into all aspects of the health promotion program (i.e., in planning, implementation, and evaluation)?

Criterion 2. Health promotion programs should implement process evaluation.

Issues:

1. Does the program include process evaluation measures for people with disabilities and their families or caregivers, including rating their satisfaction with the program?
2. Does the program make changes based on participant feedback?
3. Does the program have mechanisms for obtaining process feedback using appropriate methods such as the use of readers or interpreters?
4. Does the program record intervention-related expenses such as cost of materials, recruitment, equipment, space, and personnel?

Criterion 3. Health promotion programs should collect outcomes data using disability-appropriate outcomes measures.

Issues:

1. Does the program collect data on outcomes of health promotion activities?
2. Are the outcomes measures appropriate for people with disabilities (e.g., not penalizing for functional limitations)?

Participation Guidelines for Health Promotion Programs for People with Disabilities

Criterion 4. People with disabilities and their families or caregivers should be involved in the development and implementation of health promotion programs for people with disabilities.

Issues:

1. Did people with disabilities and their families or caregivers participate in the development of the program by identifying program outcomes or reviewing program content before implementation?
2. Are people with disabilities and their families or caregivers involved in implementing the program?

Criterion 5. Health promotion programs for people with disabilities should consider the beliefs, practices, and values of its target groups, including support for personal choice.

(Box 12.6 continues)

Box 12.6 (CONTINUED)

Issues:

1. Are the beliefs, practices, and values of people with disabilities reflected in the program's mode of delivery, training materials, and written materials?

2. Does the program support participants in identifying and achieving personal health goals?

Accessibility Guidelines for Health Promotion Programs for People with Disabilities

Criterion 6. Health promotion programs should be socially, behaviorally, programmatically, and environmentally accessible.

Issues:

1. Does the program consider social and behavioral and programmatic barriers that reduce participation among people with disabilities?

2. Does the program consider environmental barriers that reduce participation among people with disabilities, including environmental accessibility of the program site (e.g., physical and signage)?

3. Is the program site available via accessible public transportation?

4. Do the program materials (training materials and handouts) lend themselves to being translated into alternative formats?

5. Are process and outcomes measures produced in a variety of other formats, including but not limited to Braille, large print, and computer disk?

6. Are such accommodations provided when requested?

Criterion 7. Health promotion programs should be affordable to people with disabilities and their families or caregivers.

Issues:

1. Does the program maintain reasonable participant fees?

2. Does the program ensure low-cost transportation for participants?

Source: "Guidelines and Criteria for the Implementation of Community-Based Health Promotion Programs for Individuals With Disabilities" by C. E. Drum, J. J. Peterson, C. Culley, G. Krahn, T. Heller, T. Kimptron, J. McCubbin, J. Rimmer, T. Seekins, R. Suzuki, and G. W. White from *American Journal of Health Promotion.* Copyright © 2009 by the *American Journal of Health Promotion.* Reprinted with permission.

will be facilitating the intervention are brought in specifically for that task and are not familiar with the intervention more in-depth training will be needed. Also, regardless of how familiar the intended facilitators are with an intervention, if multiple facilitators are going to be used for implementation (e.g., the same program being implemented at different sites at the same time) then an implementation training would be useful to ensure there is a standardized delivery of the program. Without standardization of the intervention through training, the actual intervention delivered can deviate from what was intended depending on the personal preferences of the individuals facilitating the intervention (Issel, 2009). "This has serious implications for achieving the desired outcomes and, subsequently, for ensuring the long-term sustainability of the program" (Issel, 2009, p. 251).

A qualified instructor should conduct the actual training sessions. That instructor may be internal to the organization offering the program or it may be necessary to hire a vendor or consultant to conduct the training. It may also mean sending the people to be trained to other training classes outside the organization to become qualified facilitators. Finally, if the intervention being implemented needs a specially qualified person (e.g., certified or licensed) to facilitate it, such a person must be used. Do not assume some knowledgeable person who is not formally qualified to facilitate a program can do it because that places those who appoint/hire the facilitators in a high-liability situation. For example, if you are planning an exercise program for a group of people and someone comes to you and indicates he wants to lead the classes because he has been a participant in such a program for two years and knows just as much as past instructors but is not certified or licensed to facilitate the program, he should not be permitted to do so.

Dealing with Problems

With the program up and running, the task of the planners is to anticipate and deal with problems that might arise and to do so in a constructive manner. Even if a program has been piloted, problems can still arise. Astute and effective planners must anticipate the possibility of things going wrong (Timmreck, 2003). "If problems are anticipated, they can be resolved more easily should they occur in the implementation process" (Timmreck, 2003, pp. 182–183). The problems that could be encountered can range from petty concerns to matters of life and death. Problems might involve logistics (room size, meeting time, or room temperature), participant dissatisfaction, or a personal or medical emergency. Whatever the problem, it should be worked out as much as possible to the satisfaction of all concerned. If there is a question of whether to accommodate a program participant or the program personnel, 99% of the time the participants should be satisfied. They are the lifeblood of all programs. As a part of this implementation concern, it might be a good idea to conduct an early evaluation, say after one month, asking questions similar to the ones asked in the piloting evaluation.

Reporting and Documenting

Planners need to give attention to reporting or documenting the ongoing progress of the program to interested others (Ross & Mico, 1980). Planners should keep others informed about the progress of the program for several different reasons, including: (1) accountability, (2) public relations, (3) motivation of present participants, and (4) recruitment of new participants. The exact nature of the reporting or documenting will vary, but it is important for planners to keep all stakeholders informed.

SUMMARY

A great deal of work goes into developing a program before it is ready for implementation. The process used to implement a program may have much to say about its success. This chapter presents five phases planners can follow in implementing a program: (1) adoption of the program, (2) identifying and prioritizing the tasks to be completed: (3) establishing a system of management, (4) putting the plans into action, and (5) ending or sustaining a program. Also presented in this chapter are matters that need to be considered and planned for prior to and during implementation.

REVIEW QUESTIONS

1. What are logic models? Why are they used? What are the major components of logic models?

2. What is meant by the term *implementation*?

3. Name and briefly describe the five phases of implementation presented in this chapter.

4. Briefly describe how each of the following planning timetables can be used:
   a. Basic time line
   b. Task development time line
   c. Gantt chart
   d. PERT chart
   e. Critical path method

5. What is meant by *management*?

6. What are the three major categories of resources that need to be managed during implementation?

7. What are three strategies from the modified model of Parkinson and Associates (1982) for implementing health promotion programs?

8. What are some techniques planners can use to enhance the first day of implementation? What does it mean to kick off a program?

9. What is meant by the term *informed consent*?

10. What can program planners do to ensure the health and safety of program participants?

11. What is an ethical issue? What are the three ethical principles associated with the *Belmont Report*?

12. Where can you find the *Code of Ethics for the Health Education Profession*?

13. What is negligence? What is the difference between an act of omission and an act of commission?

14. How can program planners reduce their risk of liability?

15. What implications does HIPAA have for planners?

16. What is the difference between anonymity and confidentiality?

17. What are procedural and participant manuals? When should they be used?

18. Why is it important that those who implement planned interventions be trained well to do so?

ACTIVITIES

1. Using the guidelines presented in this chapter, create a logic model for a program you are planning.

2. Explain how you would implement a program you are planning, using a pilot study, phasing in, and total implementation. Also explain what you plan to do to kick off the program.

3. Develop an informed consent form that outlines the risks inherent in a program you are planning. Make sure the form includes a place for signatures of the participant and a witness and the date.

4. In a one-page paper, identify what you see as the biggest ethical concern of health promotion programming, and explain your choice.

5. Select one of the pieces of legislation listed in Box 12.3 to learn more about. Once selected, locate a U.S. government Website that includes information about the legislation and then write a one-page paper that describes why the legislation is important to human resources management.

WEBLINKS

1. http://www.hhs.gov/ocr/privacy

   U.S. Department of Health and Human Services (USDHHS)

   At the USDHHS Website you can get more information about the National Standards to Protect the Privacy of Personal Health Information.

2. http://www.history.com/this-day-in-history

   This Day in History

   This commercial Webpage allows you to input a specific date to find out what historical events took place that day. It can be of use to planners when trying to make the kick off of the program newsworthy by linking it to a historical event.

3. http://www.cnheo.org

   Coalition for National Health Education Organizations (CNHEO)

   You can find both the short and long versions of the *Code of Ethics for the Health Education Profession* at the CNHEO Website.

4. **http://asq.org/learn-about-quality/project-planning-tools/overview/gantt-chart.html**

   American Society for Quality (ASQ)

   The ASQ Webpage provides information on how to create a Gantt chart.

5. **http://www.cancer.gov/clinicaltrials/patientsafety/simplification-of-informed-consent-docs**

   National Cancer Institute (NCI)

   The NCI Website provides information on informed consent forms. It includes a consent form template that was created to include all of the federally required elements for such a form for a research project.

6. **http://www2a.cdc.gov/phlp/?source=govdelivery**

   Centers for Disease Control and Prevention (CDC)

   This page at the CDC Website presents the Public Health Law Program. The site was created in 2000 and has as its goals to: (1) improve the understanding and use of law as a public health tool, (2) develop CDC's capacity to apply law to achievement of its Health Protection Goals, and (3) develop the legal preparedness of the public health system to address all public health priorities.

7. **http://www.dol.gov/opa/aboutdol/lawsprog.htm**

   United States Department of Labor (USDOL)

   The USDOL Website presents a summary of the major laws associated with labor. You'll find brief descriptions of many of the principal statutes most commonly applicable to businesses, job seekers, workers, retirees, contractors, and grantees.

PART III

EVALUATING A HEALTH PROMOTION PROGRAM

The chapters in this section present an overview of the evaluation process, including how to plan an evaluation, how to analyze and interpret data, and how to report evaluation results. The chapters and topics presented in this section are:

CHAPTER 13

Evaluation:

An Overview

After reading this chapter and answering the questions at the end, you should be able to:

- Explain the two basic purposes of evaluation.
- Distinguish between formative and summative evaluation as well as between formative and process evaluation.
- Compare and contrast the various types of evaluation.
- Describe the process of conducting an evaluation.
- Identify some of the problems that may obstruct an effective evaluation.
- List reasons why evaluation should be included in all programs.
- Explain the difference between internal and external evaluations.
- Describe several considerations in planning and conducting an evaluation.

KEY TERMS

baseline data	formative evaluation	process evaluation
effectiveness	impact evaluation	quality
evaluation	internal evaluation	standards of acceptability
evaluation consultant	institutional review boards	standards of evaluation
external evaluation	outcome evaluation	summative evaluation

Performing adequate and appropriate evaluation is necessary for any program regardless of size, type, or duration. While it is true that program resources, namely the proportion of the budget that can be devoted to evaluation, as well as the evaluation expertise of program staff and partners, will influence the type and quality of the evaluation performed, every effort should be made to address the two most critical and basic

Box 13.1	Responsibilities and Competencies for Health Education Specialists

Responsibilities and competencies that are connected with the content in this chapter include:

Responsibility IV: Conduct Evaluation and Research Related to Health Education
Competency 4.1: Develop Evaluation/Research Plan
Competency 4.3: Collect and Analyze Evaluation/Research Data
Competency 4.5: Apply Findings from Evaluation/Research

Source: NCHEC, SOPHE, & AAHE (2010).

purposes of program evaluation: (1) assessing and improving **quality**, and (2) determining **effectiveness**.

As displayed in **Box 13.1**, conducting evaluation and research is a major area of responsibility for health education specialists who must demonstrate both knowledge of and the capacity to develop evaluation/research plans and collect and analyze related data (NCHEC, SOPHE, & AAHE, 2010). Your credibility as a planner and health professional will often be directly linked to your ability to perform these important tasks. Those who neglect evaluation do so at the peril of losing all or part of their program funding.

This chapter presents an overview of evaluation and introduces evaluation terminology; the basic purposes of evaluation, including distinctions between formative and process evaluation as well as summative, impact, and outcome evaluation; the process of conducting an evaluation; problems or barriers in program evaluation; and other issues to consider when conducting an evaluation.

Basic Terminology

In general, **evaluation** can be defined as the process of determining the value or worth of a health promotion program or any of its components based on predetermined criteria or standards of acceptability identified by stakeholders. **Standards of acceptability** are the minimum levels of performance, effectiveness, or benefits used to judge value (Green & Lewis, 1986). **Box 13.2** lists examples of standards of acceptability.

Two broad *categories* of evaluation correspond to the two basic *purposes* of evaluation, that is, assessing and improving quality and determining effectiveness. **Formative evaluation** relates to quality assessment and program improvement, whereas **summative evaluation** pertains to determining effectiveness.

Formative evaluation begins when programs are conceived and developed (or are forming). Though it continues through the implementation phase and usually ends when the program is concluded, it is particularly important and most relevant during the early

Box 13.2 STANDARDS OF ACCEPTABILITY

Standard of Acceptability	Examples
Appropriate response to mandates (policies, statutes, laws) of regulating agencies	Percent of children immunized; percent of priority population wearing safety belts; degree to which tobacco retailer laws are enforced
Enhanced health status among the priority population	Decreasing rates of mortality and morbidity compared with state or national data
Decreased risk factors among the priority population	Lowered rates of smoking, obesity, excessive alcohol use, etc.
Values expressed in the local community	Degree to which programs are developed in response to local values
Standards advocated by professional organizations	Passing scores on certification or registration examinations
Norms established by research	Treadmill tests or body mass index values
Norms established by evaluation of previous programs	Similar data that compare a program's results to benchmarks established by other programs (e.g., smoking cessation or weight loss programs, etc.)
Program implementation protocols	Degree to which programs implement protocols as per guidelines established previously by successful programs

stages of program development and implementation. The purpose of formative evaluation is to improve the overall *quality* of a program or any of its components before it is too late (i.e., the program concludes).

Another type of evaluation closely associated with formative evaluation is **process evaluation,** which assesses the implementation process in general, and tracks and measures what went well and what went poorly and how these factors contributed to the success or failure of a particular program. For example, when a protocol has been created for the implementation of a program, process evaluation will determine how closely the protocol was followed. Process evaluation also measures how many products were distributed or how many services were offered as well as how many people participated in the program (i.e., the extent of a program's reach). An occasional criticism leveled at health promotion is that programs sometimes limit their assessment to process evaluation (e.g., the number of program participants, etc.) and do not adequately address summative evaluation (the degree to which actual changes occurred as a result of the program). While process evaluation is important, it should not be performed in isolation of formative or summative evaluation.

In professional practice, formative and process evaluations are often used interchangeably and have become somewhat synonymous. However, commonly accepted features serve to distinguish the two, at least in theory. For example, formative evaluation attempts to enhance program components before and during implementation so that the very best products and services are offered to the priority population. Formative evaluation includes pretesting program components (e.g., curriculum, video clips, public service announcements, language for potential policy change, etc.) as well as pilot testing (testing the complete program with a small segment of the priority population before full-blown implementation). Though both formative and process evaluations are related to implementation, formative evaluation focuses on improving the quality of the program and its components while they are being implemented, whereas process evaluation measures the degree to which the program was successfully implemented and generally applies lessons learned in subsequent versions or implementations of the program. (Specific examples of both formative and process evaluation, which will more clearly distinguish the two, are presented in Chapter 14.)

The purpose of summative evaluation on the other hand, is to assess the *effectiveness* of the intervention and the extent to which awareness, attitudes, knowledge, behavior, the environment, or health status changed as a result of a particular program. Summative evaluation requires the measurement and establishment of a baseline value (the starting point or status of a health indicator prior to the implementation of an intervention) as well as measurement of the same health indicator after the program is concluded (i.e., a posttest).

Closely associated with summative evaluation are both **impact and outcome evaluations.** While summative evaluation is more generally an umbrella term associated with effectiveness, impact evaluation tends to focus on intermediary measures such as behavior change or changes in attitudes, knowledge, and awareness; whereas outcome evaluation tends to measure the degree to which end points such as diseases or injuries actually decreased. Collectively speaking, at least in health promotion practice, impact and outcome evaluations together constitute summative evaluation.

To summarize, in formative evaluation the quality of program components is measured and improved prior to or during program implementation. In process evaluation the mechanics of program implementation are assessed. In summative evaluation program outcomes are measured including impact evaluation (e.g., behavior change) and outcome evaluation (e.g., disease). Without evaluation, claims related to program quality and effectiveness can rarely, if ever, be made.

Supporting definitions for *formative, summative, process, impact, and outcome evaluation* are presented below.

- **Formative evaluation:** "Any combination of measurements obtained and judgments made before or during the implementation of materials, methods, activities or programs to control, assure or improve the quality of performance or delivery" (Green & Lewis, 1986, p. 362). Examples include, but are not limited to, pretesting, or pilot-testing a program. Data derived from formative evaluation help revise intervention components (content, methods, and materials) as well as instruments and data collection procedures (Windsor et al., 2004).

- **Summative evaluation:** "Any combination of measurements and judgments that permit conclusions to be drawn about impact, outcome, or benefits of a program or method" (Green & Lewis, 1986, p. 366). "Summative evaluations in the strictest sense are done at the conclusion of a program to provide a conclusive statement regarding program effects" (Issel, 2009, p. 21).

- **Process evaluation:** "Is used to monitor and document program implementation and can aid in understanding the relationship between specific program elements and program outcomes" (Saunders, Evans, & Joshi, 2005, p. 134). The central purposes for process evaluation are to "identify the key components of an intervention that are effective, to identify for whom the intervention is effective, and to identify under what conditions the intervention is effective" (Steckler & Linnan, 2002, p. 1). It also evaluates the "extent to which a program is being implemented as planned" (Harris, 2010, p.207).

- **Impact evaluation:** Focuses on "the immediate observable effects of a program, leading to the intended outcomes of a program; intermediate outcomes" (Green & Lewis, 1986, p. 363). Measures of awareness, knowledge, attitudes, skills, and behaviors yield impact evaluation data. Most notably, impact evaluation is associated with behavioral impact or change (Windsor et al., 2004).

- **Outcome evaluation:** Focuses on "an ultimate goal or product of a program or treatment, generally measured in the health field by mortality or morbidity data in a population, vital measures, symptoms, signs, or physiological indicators on individuals" (Green & Lewis, 1986, p. 364). Outcome evaluation is long-term in nature and generally takes more time and resources to conduct than impact evaluation. Ultimately, it makes a determination of the effect of a program or policy on its beneficiaries (Harris, 2010).

Purpose of Evaluation

Beyond improving the quality of programs and their components and measuring effectiveness, stakeholders will determine which factors will be measured to determine the worth or value of the program. While the outcome of any health promotion program should relate in some way to improved health, a myriad of factors leading to this outcome can be measured in the evaluation process. These include how broadly and successfully a program was implemented and the degree to which the program influenced knowledge, attitudes, confidence, abilities, and behaviors.

An evaluation can also assess less tangible benefits deemed important by stakeholders. These benefits may include outcomes such as the degree of good will or organizational presence produced by a program, the amount of social capital or community cohesiveness created, or the extent to which consumers are satisfied with a program for reasons other than improved health status. Ultimately, stakeholders will determine the worth of a program based on criteria unique and important to them.

In the most basic sense, programs are evaluated to gain information and make decisions. The information gained through evaluation may be used by planners during the implementation of a program to make immediate improvements (i.e., formative evaluation) as well as improvements to the implementation process in subsequent versions of the program (i.e., process evaluation). In other words, you do not want to continue indefinitely with a bad program. Evaluation may also be used to see if certain immediate outcomes—such as knowledge, attitude, skills, environment, and behavior change—have occurred (i.e., impact evaluation). It may also be used over time to determine whether long-term program goals and objectives associated with disease outcomes and improved health status have been met (i.e., outcome evaluation). Capwell, Butterfoss, and Francisco (2000) identified six general reasons why stakeholders may want programs evaluated:

1. *To determine achievement of objectives related to improved health status:* Probably the most common reason for program evaluation is to determine the degree to which program objectives related to improved health conditions were met. In this sense, evaluation may also be used to determine which of several programs was most effective in achieving a given objective. You should always attempt to link and limit the scope of evaluation (and the degree to which your personal or program performance is assessed) to program goals and objectives. For this reason, it is important to ensure that goals and objectives are specific, measurable, attainable, realistic and time-phased.

2. *To improve program implementation:* Planners should always be interested in improving a program. Program evaluation can help planners understand why a particular intervention worked (Valente, 2002) or did not work, and thus, weak elements can be identified, removed, and replaced (Green & Lewis, 1986). This is most closely associated with process evaluation.

3. *To provide accountability to funders, the community, and other stakeholders:* Many stakeholders are interested in the value of a program to a community, or if the program is worth its cost. Thus, an evaluation may provide decision makers with the information to determine if program funding should continue, discontinue, or increase.

4. *To increase community support for initiatives:* The results of an evaluation can increase community awareness of a program. Positive evaluation data channeled through proper communication channels can generate backing for a program, which in turn may lead to additional funding.

5. *To contribute to the scientific base for community public health interventions:* Program evaluation can provide findings that can lead to new hypotheses about human behavior and individual or community change, which in turn may lead to new and better programs.

6. *To inform policy decisions:* Program evaluation data can be used to impact policy within the community. For example, studies on passive or secondhand smoke have been the impetus for many states and local communities to pass laws or ordinances prohibiting indoor smoking.

Framework for Program Evaluation

In 1999, the Centers for Disease Control and Prevention (CDC, 1999a) published an evaluation framework for public health programs. The framework was developed by a working group that included evaluation experts, public health program managers and directors, state and local public health officials, teachers, researchers, U.S. Public Health Service agency representatives, and CDC staff members. This framework has stood the test of time and is still very robust.

The framework (see **Figure 13.1**) comprises six steps that should be completed for any evaluation, regardless of type (formative, summative, etc.) or setting. These steps are not a prescription; rather, they are starting points for tailoring the evaluation. The early steps provide the foundation, and all steps should be finalized before moving to the next step:

• *Step 1—Engaging stakeholders:* This step begins the evaluation cycle. Stakeholders must be engaged to ensure that their perspectives are understood. The three primary groups of stakeholders are (1) those involved in the program operations, (2) those served or affected by the program, and (3) the primary users of the evaluation results. Because stakeholders will decide the fate of the program based on the evaluation results, it is important to understand their expectations up front. The scope and level of stakeholder involvement will vary with each program being evaluated.

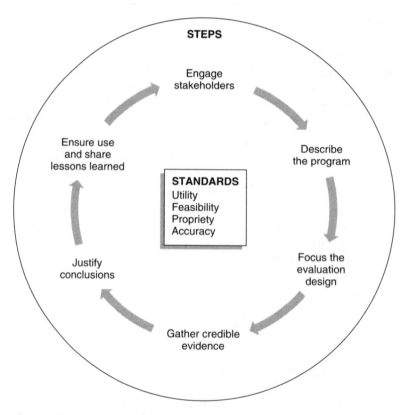

Figure 13.1 Framework for Program Evaluation
Source: CDC (1999c), p. 4.

- *Step 2—Describing the program:* This step sets the frame of reference for all subsequent decisions in the evaluation process. At a minimum, the program should be described in enough detail that the mission, goals, and objectives are understood. Also, the program's capacity to effect change, its stage of development, and how it fits into the larger organization and community should be known. Usually, a logic model is used in this step to display a sequence of program events (see Chapter 12 for a discussion of logic models) and the relationship among inputs, activities, and outputs or outcomes.

- *Step 3—Focusing the evaluation design:* This step involves making sure that the interests of the stakeholders are addressed while using time and resources efficiently. Among the items to consider in this step are: stating the reason for the evaluation (e.g., gain insight, change practice, assess effects, affect participants' behavior, etc.), determining the uses and users of the evaluation results, formulating research questions and/or hypotheses, determining the specific type of evaluation design that will be used, deciding on the types of statistical analyses that will be used, and finalizing any agreements about the process.

- *Step 4—Gathering credible evidence:* During this step, evaluators decide on measurement indicators, sources of evidence, quality and quantity of evidence, and logistics for collecting the evidence. This step also involves organizing data including specific processes related to coding, filing, and cleaning.

- *Step 5—Justifying conclusions:* This step includes the comparison of the evidence against the standards of acceptability (i.e., analyzing and synthesizing data); interpreting those comparisons; judging the worth, merit, or significance of the program; and creating recommendations for actions based on the results of the evaluation.

- *Step 6—Ensuring use and sharing lessons learned:* This step focuses on the use and dissemination of the evaluation results. When carrying out this final step, the needs of each group of stakeholders must be addressed. This is sometimes referred to as the evaluation feedback loop. And in order for evaluation data to be useful it must be processed by stakeholders who can approve the continuation of improved programs or stop the perpetuation of ineffective programs.

In addition to these six steps, the framework uses four **standards of evaluation**, which are displayed in the box at the center of Figure 13.1. These standards provide practical guidelines for the evaluators to follow when having to decide among evaluation options. For example, these standards help evaluators avoid evaluations that may be accurate and feasible but not useful or those that would be useful and accurate but not feasible (CDC, 1999a). The four standards are:

1. "Utility standards ensure that information needs of evaluation users are satisfied" (CDC, 1999a, p. 27).

2. "Feasibility standards ensure that the evaluation is viable and pragmatic" (CDC, 1999a, p. 27). In other words, the evaluation is realistic and affordable.

3. "Propriety standards ensure that the evaluation is ethical (i.e., conducted with regard for the rights and interests of those involved and effected)" (CDC, 1999a, p. 27).

4. "Accuracy standards ensure that the evaluation produces findings that are considered correct" (CDC, 1999a, p. 29). This means findings are both valid and reliable.

Practical Problems or Barriers in Evaluation

Several authors (Glasgow, 2002; Glasgow et al., 1999; NCI, 2002; Solomon, 1987; Timmreck, 2003; Valente, 2002) have identified practical problems or barriers to effective evaluation. Some of the more common problems or barriers which remain consistent over time are presented below.

1. Planners either fail to build evaluation in the program planning process or do so too late (Solomon, 1987; Timmreck, 2003; Valente, 2002).

2. Adequate resources (e.g., personnel, time, money) may not be available to conduct an appropriate evaluation (NCI, 2002; Solomon, 1987; Valente, 2002).

3. Organizational restrictions on hiring consultants and contractors may prohibit evaluation efforts (NCI, 2002).

4. Effects are often hard to detect because changes are sometimes small, come slowly, or do not last (Glasgow, 2002; Solomon, 1987; Valente, 2002).

5. Length of time allotted for the program and its evaluation is not realistic given the nature of behavior change or the interval that is necessary to measure mortality or morbidity (NCI, 2002).

6. Restrictions (i.e., policies, ethics, lack of trust in the evaluators) that limit the collection of data among the priority population (NCI, 2002).

7. It is difficult to make an association between cause and effect (Solomon, 1987).

8. It is difficult to separate the effects of multiple interventions within a program (Glasgow et al., 1999), or multiple programs within a community, or to isolate program effects on the priority population since evaluators/researchers cannot control all the influences of real-world phenomena (NCI, 2002).

9. Discrepancies arise between professional standards and actual practice (Solomon, 1987) with regard to appropriate evaluation design, particularly among novice evaluators.

10. Sometimes evaluators' motives to demonstrate success introduce bias (Solomon, 1987; Valente, 2002).

11. Stakeholders' perceptions of the evaluation's value may vary too drastically (NCI, 2002).

12. Intervention strategies are sometimes not delivered as intended (i.e., Type III error) (Glasgow, 2002), or are not culturally specific (NCI, 2002; Valente, 2002).

Examples of these problems in health promotion programs may occur by not collecting initial information from participants because evaluation plans were not in place, failing to budget for the cost of the evaluation (e.g., printing questionnaires, additional staff, postage), or conducting the evaluation prematurely before a change can occur (e.g., changes in cholesterol level) or too long after program completion (e.g., posttest effects of a smoking cessation program). Those without evaluation expertise may conduct an evaluation without a sound design, such as not using appropriate sampling techniques or comparison groups. Program managers who are motivated to make their programs cost effective may minimize costs and unwittingly jeopardize the integrity of an evaluation.

Awareness of these problems and development of strategies to deal with them will likely improve the accuracy of program evaluation. The remainder of this chapter discusses strategies that can help minimize problems with evaluation, such as including evaluation in the early stages of program planning, accounting for ethical considerations, determining who will conduct the evaluation, carefully considering the evaluation design, increasing objectivity, and developing a plan to use the evaluation results.

Evaluation in the Program Planning Stages

Evaluation design must reflect the goals and objectives of the program (see Chapter 6). In turn, the results of the evaluation will determine whether the goals and objectives were met. To be most effective, the evaluation must be planned in the early stages of program development and should be in place before the program begins. Results from evaluations conducted early in the program planning process can assist in improving the program (i.e., formative evaluation). Having a plan in place to conduct an evaluation before the end of a program will make collecting data related to program outcomes much easier and more reliable.

Discussion on how evaluation plans can be included in program planning will focus on examples of formative and summative evaluations. The formative evaluation should provide feedback to the program administrator, with program monitoring beginning in the early stages. Collecting information and communicating it to the administrator quickly allows for the program to be modified and improved.

Data reflecting the initial status or interests of the participants—**baseline data**— or something like qualitative data from focus groups can be used to assess participant satisfaction. Additional information from the formative evaluation may indicate that the necessary number of staff members has been hired, the program sites are available, brochures have been printed, participants are satisfied with the times the programs are offered, and classes are offered with the needs of the prospective participants in mind.

Initial data regarding the program should be analyzed promptly to make any necessary adjustments to the program. This type of evaluation can improve both new and existing programs. Information from the formative evaluation can also be useful in answering questions such as whether the programs are provided at convenient locations for the community members, whether the necessary materials arrived on time, and whether people are attending the workshops at all the various times they are offered. If the answer to these questions is no, specific program attributes needing quality improvement can be identified and addressed.

By developing the summative evaluation plan at the beginning of the program, planners can ensure that the results will be less biased. Early development of the summative evaluation plan ensures that the questions answered relate to the original objectives and goals of the program. This type of evaluation can provide answers to many questions, such as whether the group approach or the individual approach was more effective in reducing tobacco use among the participants in a smoking cessation program, whether the participants in a weight loss program actually lost weight and/or maintained the weight loss, and how many people in the priority population increased their knowledge, changed their attitudes, or reduced their risks.

Ethical Considerations

Always remember that evaluation or research should never cause mental, emotional, or physical harm to those in the priority population. Nor should it cause a delay in products or services that could potentially improve health among those being evaluated/researched. Evaluation participants should always be informed of the purpose and potential risks of any evaluation and should always give their consent before participating. Generally, evaluators assure the confidentiality and anonymity of evaluation responses. Although evaluation data are reported in the aggregate, no individual should ever have his or her personal information revealed in any setting or circumstance.

Because evaluations may have ethical considerations for the individuals involved, most colleges, universities, school systems, and large health organizations have boards to review the evaluation design and potential risk to participants. These groups are most often referred to as **institutional review boards** (IRBs) or human subjects committees (Cottrell & McKenzie, 2011). These boards serve to safeguard the rights, privacy, health, and well-being of those involved in the evaluation/research. Before conducting any evaluation or research involving human subjects, make sure to get IRB approval.

Who Will Conduct the Evaluation?

At the beginning of the program, planners must determine who will conduct the evaluation. The program evaluator must be as objective as possible and should have nothing to gain from the results of the evaluation. The evaluator may be someone associated with the program or someone from outside.

If an individual trained in evaluation and personally involved with the program conducts the evaluation, it is called an **internal evaluation**. For example, a local health department may assign one of its own employees to evaluate its programs. An internal evaluator would have the advantage of: (1) being more familiar with the organization and the program history, (2) knowing the decision-making style of those in the organization, (3) being present to remind others of results now and in the future, and (4) being able to communicate technical results more frequently and clearly (Fitzpatrick, Saunders, & Worthen, 2004). Conducting an internal evaluation is also less expensive than hiring additional personnel to conduct the evaluation. The major drawback, however, is the possibility of evaluator bias or conflict of interest. Someone closely involved with the program has an investment in the outcome of the evaluation and may not be completely objective. After all, a positive evaluation of the program may result in future funding that would enhance the positions of the staff members.

An **external evaluation** is one conducted by someone who is not connected with the program. Often an external evaluator is referred to as an **evaluation consultant**. Having a researcher from a university or some other type of research institute conduct evaluations for the local health department would be an example of an external evaluator. External evaluators are somewhat isolated, often lacking knowledge of and experience with the program that the internal evaluator possesses. Evaluation of this nature is also more expensive, since an additional person must be hired to carry out the work. However, an external evaluator: (1) can often provide a more objective review and a fresh perspective, (2) can help to ensure an unbiased evaluation outcome, (3) brings a global knowledge of evaluation having worked in a variety of settings, and (4) "typically brings more breadth and depth of technical expertise" (Fitzpatrick et al., 2004, p. 23). **Box 13.3** presents a list of characteristics that program planners can use when selecting an external evaluator. In addition, when selecting an external evaluator, planners should look for someone with formal training in evaluation methods.

Whether an internal or external evaluator conducts the program evaluation, the main goal is to choose someone with credibility and objectivity. The evaluator must have a clear role in the evaluation design and accurately report the results regardless of the findings.

Box 13.3 CHARACTERISTICS OF A SUITABLE EVALUATION CONSULTANT

- Is not directly involved in the development or administration of the program being evaluated
- Is impartial about evaluation results (i.e., has nothing to gain by skewing the results in one direction or another)
- Will not succumb to any pressure by senior staff or program staff to produce particular findings
- Will give the staff the full findings (i.e., will not gloss over or fail to report certain findings for any reason)
- Has experience in the type of evaluation needed
- Communicates well with key personnel
- Considers programmatic realities (e.g., a small budget) when designing an evaluation
- Delivers reports and protocols on time
- Past professional experience relates to the program and its evaluation needs
- Sees beyond the evaluation to other programmatic activities
- Explains both the benefits and risks of evaluation
- Educates program personnel about conducting evaluation, thus allowing future evaluations to be done in house
- Explains material clearly and patiently
- Respects all levels of personnel

Source: Thompson & McClintock (1998), p. 13.

Evaluation Results

The question of who will receive the evaluation results is also an important consideration. The evaluation can be conducted from several vantage points, depending on whether the results will be presented to the program administrator, the funding source, the organization, or the public. These stakeholders may all have different sets of questions they would like answered. The evaluation results must be disseminated to groups interested in the program. Different aspects of the evaluation can be stressed, depending on the group's particular needs and interests. An administrator may be interested in which program approach was more successful, the funding source may want to know if all objectives were reached, and a community member may want to know if participants felt the program was beneficial.

The planning process associated with the evaluation should include a determination of how the results will be used. It is especially important in formative evaluation to implement the findings rapidly to improve the program. However, a feedback loop and action plan are needed in summative, impact, and outcome evaluation to ensure that results and lessons learned are not filed away, but are used to determine how to proceed with health promotion programs.

SUMMARY

Evaluation can be thought of as a way to make sound decisions regarding the value and effectiveness of health promotion programs, to compare different types of programs, to eliminate weak program components, to meet requirements of funding sources, or to provide information about programs. The evaluation process takes place before, during, and after program implementation. If the evaluation is well designed and conducted appropriately, the findings can be very beneficial to program stakeholders.

REVIEW QUESTIONS

1. What are the two basic purposes of program evaluation?

2. What are the two broad categories of evaluation and how do they relate to the two basic purposes of program evaluation?

3. List and describe the six steps in CDC's framework for program evaluation.

4. List and describe the four standards in CDC's framework for program evaluation.

5. Give an example of a question that could be answered in a process evaluation, impact evaluation, and outcome evaluation.

6. What are some of the more common problems associated with or barriers to effective evaluation?

7. What different types of information could an evaluation provide for the various stakeholders (planners, funding source, administrators, and participants)?

8. Why is it important to begin the evaluation process in the program planning stages?

9. Explain how feedback from an evaluation can be used in program planning.

10. In what type of situation would an internal evaluation be more appropriate than an external evaluation?

11. What are the desirable characteristics of an external evaluator (evaluation consultant)?

ACTIVITIES

1. Describe potential roles and results of formative and summative evaluations in a program related to an HIV needle-exchange program.

2. Describe how process, impact, and outcome evaluation could be used in a stress management program for college students.

3. Write a rationale to a funding source for hiring an external evaluator (evaluation consultant).

4. Review the evaluation component from a health promotion program in your community and/or discuss an evaluation plan with a planner or evaluator. Look for the planning process used, the rationale for the data collection method, and how the findings were reported. To what extent did the program follow CDC's framework for evaluation?

5. Assume you are responsible for selecting an evaluator for a health promotion program you are planning. Would you select an internal or an external evaluator? Explain your rationale. If you select an external evaluator (evaluation consultant), where do you think you could find such a person?

WEBLINKS

1. http://www.eval.org

   American Evaluation Association (AEA)

   The AEA is an international professional association of evaluators devoted to the application and exploration of program evaluation, personnel evaluation, technology, and many other forms of evaluation.

2. http://www.evaluationcanada.ca/site.cgi?s=1

   Canadian Evaluation Society (CES)

   The CES is a professional association of evaluators dedicated to the advancement of evaluation theory and practice. Information at this Website is available in both English and French.

3. http://ctb.ku.edu/en/default.aspx

   Community Tool Box

   This Website has long provided technical assistance to health professionals on a number of tasks related to planning and evaluation in health promotion. With respect to evaluation, a general search for evaluation will present a number of specific links including introduction to evaluation, developing an evaluation plan, and selecting appropriate designs.

4. http://www.cdc.gov/mmwr/preview/mmwrhtml/rr4811a1.htm

   CDC Framework for Program Evaluation in Public Health

   This is CDC's framework described earlier in this chapter published in *Morbidity and Mortality Weekly Report*. This document describes in detail the six steps related to the framework.

5. http://www.phac-aspc.gc.ca/php-psp/toolkit-eng.php

   Program Evaluation Tool Kit (Public Health Agency of Canada)

   According to this Website, "the Program Evaluation Tool Kit is a practical, step-by-step guide to evaluating programs. It is presented in a series of short modules with simple explanations and specific tools for planning, conducting and using evaluation." This tool is similar to CDC's framework for program evaluation in public health.

6. http://www.rand.org/pubs/technical_reports/TR101.html

   Getting to Outcomes: Promoting Accountability through Methods and Tools for Planning, Implementation, and Evaluation

   An excellent evaluation resource related to establishing and measuring evidence-based program outcomes.

7. http://whqlibdoc.who.int/hq/2000/WHO_MSD_MSB_00.2e.pdf

   Process Evaluations

   This is a document on process evaluations from the World Health Organization. It is good resource for designing and conducting process evaluations.

Evaluation Approaches and Designs

After reading this chapter and answering the questions at the end, you should be able to:

- Describe the difference between formative and summative evaluations as well as their relationship to process, impact, and outcome evaluations.
- Identify elements and strategies related to both formative and process evaluations.
- List important considerations in selecting an evaluation design.
- Compare and contrast quantitative and qualitative methods of evaluation.
- List the various qualitative methods that can be used in evaluation and research.
- Differentiate between experimental, control, and comparison groups.
- Compare and contrast the major types of evaluation designs.
- Identify the threats to internal and external validity and explain how evaluation design can increase control.

KEY TERMS

accountability	cost-identification analysis	inductive
adjustment	deductive	interaction
approaches	designs	internal validity
blind	dose	justification
capacity	double blind	multiplicity
comparison group	evidence	nonexperimental design
confounding variable	experimental design	pilot testing
consumer orientation	experimental group	posttest
context	external validity	pretest
control group	fidelity	pretesting
cost-benefit analysis	generalizability	qualitative method
cost-effectiveness analysis	inclusion	quantitative method

Key Terms, continued

quasi-experimental design	resources	support
reach	response	triple blind
recruitment	satisfaction	

This chapter focuses on evaluation approaches and designs. The term **approaches** refers to formative, process, and summative evaluation and suggests these types of evaluation are clearly distinct. **Designs** relates specifically to summative evaluation. Whereas formative and process evaluations are typically defined with descriptions of associated elements and strategies, summative evaluations are generally associated with experimental, quasi-experimental, and nonexperimental designs. **Box 14.1** identifies the responsibilities and competencies for health education specialists that pertain to the material presented in this chapter.

Formative Evaluation

At its core, formative evaluation focuses on the quality of program content and program implementation. Some elements of formative evaluation occur before the start of the implementation phase and help ensure that a program and its elements have been

---

Box 14.1 RESPONSIBILITIES AND COMPETENCIES FOR HEALTH EDUCATION SPECIALISTS

This chapter describes evaluation approaches including formative, process, and summative evaluations (including impact and outcome evaluations), elements of formative and process evaluations, and evaluation designs associated with summative evaluation. Responsibilities and competencies connected with this chapter include:

Responsibility IV: Conduct Evaluation and Research Related to Health Education

Competency 4.1: Develop Evaluation/Research Plan

Competency 4.3: Collect and Analyze Evaluation/Research Data

Source: NCHEC, SOPHE, & AAHE (2010).

conceptualized and developed appropriately. Formative evaluation collects data and informs stakeholders of important findings that could potentially improve a program or its delivery, and allows for appropriate changes before the program is fully implemented and completed. Although a formative evaluation can be used to improve a program between implementation cycles (i.e., an evaluator identifies various issues that need to be addressed before the program is implemented again), it is usually better to allow a formative evaluation to inform and guide the development and implementation of a program as it actually unfolds. In cases where a program implementation is ongoing, the distinction between formative and process evaluation is not as clear or relevant as long as programs are being improved based on feedback collected in the evaluation process.

Table 14.1 displays the elements of a comprehensive formative evaluation. The degree to which these elements are used will be determined by many factors including the preferences of stakeholders. However, all 15 elements are important and have a bearing on program quality which, in turn, leads to program effectiveness as measured in summative evaluation.

Formative evaluation occurs from the time of program inception through implementation. By nature, certain elements of formative evaluation are more applicable at the time of program inception. This is when planners either begin developing a new program or decide to use an existing program and adapt it for their priority population. For example, addressing the elements termed **justification** and **evidence** provides assurance that programs are supported by key stakeholders and are evidence based. It is easy to make assumptions about these issues during a planning process. But addressing these key matters initially will orient and influence planners to make careful assessments about other program and evaluation components. In this regard, formative evaluation can be beneficial before much, if any, time and effort are applied to the program.

Three additional elements displayed in Table 14.1 relate to issues that should be addressed early in the formative evaluation process. Assessing **capacity** requires evaluators to carefully examine the competency of those who are designing and implementing a program. This can be somewhat challenging if those performing the evaluation are the same professionals designing and implementing the program. Despite this potential challenge, planners and evaluators should identify the strengths and weaknesses of the internal staff and external partners and either invest in training or contract for external evaluation as necessary.

Resources relate to adequate internal or external funding and/or assistance from partner organizations. Although it is easy to underestimate program costs, evaluators performing a formative evaluation should match the projected costs with available resources to determine whether the program can be realistically implemented. Closely related to the concept of resources are three types of cost analyses that can help guide planners in the selection of specific interventions. **Cost-identification analysis** (or cost-feasibility analysis) is used to compare different interventions available for a program, often to determine which intervention would be the least expensive. With this type of

Table 14.1 Elements of a Comprehensive Formative Evaluation

Justification	Degree to which a program, service, or activity is mandated or approved by relevant stakeholders and justified by needs assessment data and analysis
Evidence	Degree to which the program, service, or activity is evidence based (i.e., documented evaluation results in the literature suggest the program is effective or at least promising)
Capacity	Extent to which professionals have adequate knowledge, skills, and abilities to design and implement a program, service, or activity or the degree to which they can access or contract with other organizations and professionals to provide the same program, service or activity
Resources	Adequacy of resources (e.g., budget, community resources or assistance, assets, time, etc.)
Consumer-Orientation	Degree to which the program, activity, or service is tailored to the priority population (i.e., culturally appropriate and based on consumer preferences)
Multiplicity	Degree to which multiple components (i.e., intervention strategies) are built into the program, service, or activity (e.g., education, communication, policy, environmental change, etc.)
Support	Degree to which a support component is built into a program, service, or activity (e.g., a hot line/quit line for a tobacco media campaign, development of walking paths for a community physical activity campaign)
Inclusion	Extent to which an adequate range and number of appropriate partners or organizations are involved with the program, service, or activity
Accountability	Extent to which internal staff and external partners are fulfilling their responsibilities as planned and are communicating needs appropriately
Adjustment	Degree to which programs, services, or activities are modified based on feedback received from participants, partners, or other stakeholders
Recruitment*	Degree to which members of the priority population are adequately recruited through appropriate channels and places consistent with cultural and other unique characteristics
Reach*	Proportion of the priority population given the opportunity to participate in the program, activity, or service
Response*	Proportion of the priority population actually participating in the program, activity, or service
Interaction	Quality of interactions (e.g., customer service; interpersonal, counseling, and presentation skills; clarity of instructions) between professionals (those providing programs, services, and activities) and participants
Satisfaction	Degree to which the needs of participants are being met, how satisfied they are with the program, service, or activity, and their belief that a positive impact is being made in their lives

*These items relate to formative evaluation as they help ensure that an adequate number of people are participating in the program. But they also relate to process evaluation as an evaluation of the implementation process itself would naturally measure not only how many people had the opportunity to participate in the program, but more importantly, how many people actually participated.

analysis, evaluators identify the different items (e.g., personnel, facilities, curriculum, etc.) associated with a given intervention, determine a cost for each item, total the costs for that intervention, and then compare the total costs associated with each of several interventions. For example, if a health department is interested in providing a tobacco prevention and control program for a school district, it could conduct a cost-identification analysis on three different interventions: (1) teacher led, (2) peer-to-peer, and (3) voluntary agency provided. Costs for each of these interventions—such as staff time, staff benefits, curriculum materials, and volunteer training—would be identified, compared, and analyzed.

Cost-benefit analysis looks at how resources can best be used. It will yield the dollar benefit received from the dollars invested in the program. **Cost-effectiveness analysis** is used to quantify the effects of a program in monetary terms. It is more appropriate for health promotion programs than cost-benefit analysis, because a dollar value does not have to be placed on the outcomes of the program. Instead, a cost-effectiveness analysis will indicate how much it costs to produce a certain effect. For example, based on the cost of a program, the effect of years of life saved, number of smokers who stop smoking, or morbidity or mortality rates can be determined.

Continuing with elements displayed in Table 14.1, evaluators must also ensure that **consumer orientation,** or the degree to which programs are adapted to the needs of the priority population, is adequately addressed. Professionals commonly assume that members of the priority population hold the same understanding and value for programs as those who design and implement the programs. Data from social marketing studies indicate this is not the case (Neiger & Thackeray, 2002). Assuring that programs are tailored to the values, wants, and needs of the priority population is an important component of a formative evaluation and helps ensure that programs are more readily accepted by the priority population and that intended outcomes occur.

Two elements displayed in Table 14.1 relate to the development and content of a program. The term **multiplicity** relates to a concept in health promotion where, compared with single-component programs (i.e., one intervention strategy), multiple-component programs cater more effectively to the varied needs of consumers and tend to be accepted more readily. For example, the Truth Campaign in Utah offers a multidimensional approach to preventing and controlling tobacco use among both youth and adults. Program components involve educational materials including a comprehensive guide for schools, media resources, models for policy and legislation, materials for healthcare professionals, and a quit line to assist current smokers in cessation efforts (Utah Department of Health, 2011). **Support,** a closely related concept to multiplicity, assures that programs have appropriate built-in reinforcement components to assist participants with the expected level of involvement and/or behavior change. For example, a well-baby program that promotes prenatal care through a media campaign cannot responsibly broadcast messages without an infrastructure that can actually support prenatal care. In addition, a well-baby program of this nature should also be prepared to make referrals based on a variety of demographic variables within the priority population, including the ability to pay for services.

Certain elements in formative evaluation relate to key components of program implementation and ensure that: the right people and organizations are participating in the delivery of the program; partners are doing what they're assigned to do; and necessary changes are being made based on feedback from both participants and partners.

Inclusion ensures that the right partners are involved with the program. The natural inclination of most professionals or organizations is to include as many partners as possible to bear the burden of a program's cost and implementation. Care should be taken, however, to ensure that only those organizations that share the same values and commitment are included as program partners. This is not to suggest that organizations should not seek diverse or nontraditional partners. However, ideally, all partners should bring a similar level of vision and energy to the program development and implementation process.

Accountability ensures that each partner organization performs its work as previously arranged. For this reason, it is important for partners to meet regularly, report on progress and identify ways to improve performance. **Adjustment**, perhaps the most critical element of formative evaluation, is the process whereby planners make necessary changes to the program or its implementation based on feedback from participants and partners. In this regard, those who develop and implement programs must collect data (or information) on what needs to change and then see to it that appropriate changes are made. **Recruitment, reach,** and **response** pertain to promoting a program and ensuring that people in the priority population are aware of the program, have the opportunity to engage in the program, and an adequate number actually participate in the program. Obviously, the budget, among other factors, influences the proportion of the priority population that has access to the program. Evaluators must develop projections for participation early and then match projections with actual participation. Furthermore, evaluators must determine whether methods for recruitment or promotion are appropriate based on communication capabilities and preferences of the priority population. For example, social media approaches will not work if members of the priority population do not subscribe to the right (matching) applications. Similarly, newspaper advertisements will do little good if word-of-mouth communication is a preferred channel within the priority population.

Interaction and **satisfaction** address the degree to which practitioners effectively work and communicate with program participants and how satisfied participants are with the program in general or with specific components. For example, an evidence-based curriculum for weight loss among adults may be appealing to participants, theoretically grounded and technically sound in every way but not resonate with participants because of an ineffective instructor. A formative evaluation can identify this problem and generate the necessary recommendations or adjustments (e.g., a new instructor). Likewise, data regarding participant satisfaction may produce important modifications during program implementation or in future applications of the program.

In contrast to formative evaluation, a process evaluation looks back on the implementation process and measures what went well and what went poorly. While data from process evaluation can certainly inform subsequent versions of a program, its main objectives are to describe how closely the program implementation followed protocols; how successful it was in recruiting and reaching members of the priority population; how many people participated or how many products or services were distributed; and what other factors may have competed with or confounded program results.

Elements of process evaluation are displayed in **Table 14.2**. Fidelity ensures that programs are implemented either as intended or as per protocol. Because the results of effective programs should be published in scientific journals or other reporting mechanisms, methods sections should provide a sequential order or step-by-step description of how the program was implemented. Other practitioners should then rely on this information to replicate the program. In addition, programs should routinely include some type of procedures outline or protocol that guides implementation. In this regard, process evaluation can assure that appropriate procedures are followed throughout implementation.

Dose is a measurement of how many products, services, or other program components were actually delivered to the priority population (e.g., number of educational sessions presented, number of nicotine devices distributed, number of car seats on loan, number of times a public service announcement was aired). Oftentimes, process evaluation is associated with dose. In other words, the practitioner tracks and reports how many products were distributed and equates this with the quality of a program. Although dose is an important element in process evaluation, it should not be the sole focus of any evaluation. As an independent measurement, it cannot fully represent process evaluation nor should it be used as a proxy measure to describe the quality, value or effectiveness of a program.

As described in formative evaluation, recruitment, reach, and response are also measured in process evaluation since an evaluation of the implementation process itself would naturally measure fairness and adequacy of recruiting practices, how many

Table 14.2 Elements of a Process Evaluation*

Fidelity	Extent to which the program, activity, or service was delivered as planned or as per protocol including the use of Gantt charts (i.e., time lines) and logic models
Dose	Number of program units delivered (e.g., presentations, products, services, messages)
Recruitment*	Degree to which members of the priority population are adequately recruited through appropriate channels and places consistent with cultural and other unique characteristics Proportion of the priority population given the opportunity to participate in the program, activity, or service
Reach*	Proportion of the priority population given the opportunity to participate in the program, activity, or service
Response*	Proportion of the priority population actually participating in the program, activity, or service
Context	External factors that may influence program results (e.g., competing programs, conflicting messages, other confounders)

*Adapted from Steckler & Linnan (2002); and Saunders, Evans, & Joshi (2005).

members of the priority population had the opportunity to participate in the program, and most importantly, how many people actually participated.

Finally, **context** assesses the presence of any confounding factors, or naturally occurring events in the same environment that may affect program participation and results. For example, participation in a school-based alcohol/drug-free graduation celebration may be diminished by alternative activities that appeal more directly to the intended participants. Negative aspects of the physical environment or location of a program may have a harmful effect on program participation or retention. A television program documenting disabling aspects of cancer aired at the same time a cancer screening program is initiated may scare potential program participants and impact their involvement.

Strategies for conducting formative evaluations, and to some extent process evaluations, are displayed and briefly described in **Table 14.3**. Although no single strategy is inherently superior to another, the element being evaluated (see Tables 14.1 and 14.2) will largely influence the selection of the appropriate strategy. For example, a key informant interview would generally be appropriate if an evaluator is measuring capacity or resources. In this scenario, the key informant would probably be an administrator with adequate information about the skill sets of his/her staff and the type of budget that would be dedicated to the program. On the other hand, assessing fidelity in a process evaluation can be accomplished with a protocol checklist. Certain elements can be addressed by one of many strategies or a combination of strategies. For example, assessing interaction or satisfaction can be accomplished by focus groups, in-depth interviews, or surveys.

Each of the strategies listed in Table 14.3 has a specific protocol to guide its use. Evaluators must ensure that these strategies are used appropriately and that data are not extrapolated or projected beyond their natural or appropriate function. (For further explanation on specific strategies, see Chapter 4 for information on focus groups, survey methods, interviews, use of forms (existing records), and observations, etc.)

Two additional strategies, pretesting and pilot testing, commonly associated with formative evaluation, are presented here as ways to assess the quality of distinct components associated with a program and to assess the overall quality of a program before full implementation occurs. Although the two terms are often used interchangeably, certain distinctions are important to make and understand.

Pretesting

Pretesting can be defined in at least two ways: (1) testing components of a program (e.g., strategies and materials), services, and products with the priority population prior to implementation (Grier & Bryan, 2005); and (2) collecting baseline data prior to program implementation that will be compared with posttest data to measure the effectiveness of programs. The type of pretesting that relates to formative evaluation pertains to the first definition—testing components of a program prior to program implementation. This type of pretesting is often associated with social marketing and health communication. When applied to health communication, pretesting has been defined as an evaluation that involves systematically collecting intended-audience reactions to messages and materials before the messages and materials are produced in final form (NCI, 2002).

Table 14.3 Procedures Used in Formative Evaluation

Focus Groups*	Qualitative research wherein a trained moderator uses an interview or moderator's guide to ask questions about new programs, products, services, ideas, or topics to determine the attitudes, opinions, and preferences of a group of 6–12 individuals from a subgroup of the priority population (see Chapter 4).
Surveys	The collection of data, generally through questionnaires, from a representative sample of the priority population that allows evaluators to draw general conclusions about the entire priority population. May involve face-to-face interviews or written questionnaires, mailed questionnaires, telephone interviews, electronic questionnaires, and so on. An intercept survey attempts to approach consumers in their natural environments (e.g., grocery stores, malls, community events) for a brief face-to-face interview (see Chapter 4).
In-Depth Interviews*	Formal interviews with program participants generally lasting a half hour or longer with the use of an interview guide and related probes. Allows evaluators to observe body language and facial expressions as prompts for additional questions and information.
Informal Interviews	Brief interviews with program participants that may take the form of a conversation rather than a formal interview.
Key Informant Interviews	Qualitative, in-depth interviews with individuals who understand the priority population and can represent their attitudes, values, and opinions to evaluators. Key informants are often people of influence within the priority population (see Chapter 4).
Direct Observation	A process wherein evaluators immerse themselves in the program and assess the interactions between professionals and other participants, the general reactions and behaviors of the participants, and any problems or issues associated with program content and delivery. Use of this procedure sometimes involves concealing the observer from the program participants (see Chapter 4).
Expert Panel Reviews	A process wherein a small group of professionals, not associated with the program but who have expertise related to the program, volunteer or are contracted to collect data, analyze the program, draw conclusions about its strengths and weaknesses, and make recommendations.
Quality Circles	A qualitative approach wherein internal staff from the same program or work area meet regularly to discuss the strengths and weaknesses of a product, program, service, or activity and make recommendations for improvement. As an alternative to quality circles, evaluators may choose to interview program staff directly.
Protocol Checklist	A linear or sequential list of tasks or procedures that allows evaluators to compare how a program is being implemented and compared with how it was originally intended to be implemented, or compared with what has been done elsewhere and reported in published studies or reports. Use of logic models may be used in lieu of the protocol checklist.
Gantt Chart	A type of bar or line chart that displays a program's time line or project schedule. Whereas protocol checklists or logic models are not usually time phased, Gantt charts display the start and finish dates of key program elements (e.g., program objectives or key activities and tasks) (see Chapter 12).
Program and Evaluation Forms	Program forms collected prior to program implementation may provide relevant information to evaluators (e.g., factors that have motivated participation, identification of goals, previous participation). Data from forms compiled during the program may reveal information helpful to program improvement (e.g., strengths, barriers, risks). Evaluation forms are generally administered at the conclusion of a program to measure the awareness, knowledge, attitudes, skills and behaviors, and general levels of satisfaction as well as feedback on specific program components.

*Responses are recorded, transcribed, coded, and analyzed to identify themes and draw conclusions. (Note: see Chapter 4 for types of data collection.)

Pretesting, however, can be applied to any component of a program (e.g., specific sessions of an educational curriculum, a participant manual, draft language for a legislative bill, the visual presence and structural layout of a booth that will be used in a health fair, a planned location and structure of a community exercise path, etc.).

Pretesting assumes that program components have already been reviewed for evidence. That is, the component is demonstrated to be evidence-based in the literature or through some other reporting mechanism. Pretesting also assumes that practitioners have done their best to prepare program components in final form. In other words, it is not appropriate for practitioners to take short cuts and present materials with the mindset that members of the priority population will correct any flaws.

Many of the same strategies displayed in Table 14.3 are used to pretest program components. The most common strategies involve focus groups, in-depth interviews, and surveys (NCI, 2002). Practitioners would be well advised to receive training in these strategies before attempting to conduct them. Otherwise, it is wise to contract for services with professionals who have appropriate experience and expertise.

Pilot Testing

Whereas pretesting focuses on specific program components, **pilot testing** (also referred to as field testing or alpha testing) generally assesses programs in limited areas and/or time periods (NCI, 2002). In other words, pilot testing generally presents the entire program to a limited and manageable number of members of the priority population so necessary modifications can be made before the program is implemented to a larger segment of the priority population.

Pilot testing allows for "dry runs" to assess and measure the overall quality of a program. Occasionally, pilot testing may be associated with shorter durations of time compared with actual implementation time, but this is generally not advisable. Implementing the entire program to a limited number of people in the actual time frame is helpful for evaluators to discover important issues related to timing, spacing, and duration of interventions. (See Chapter 12 for more information on this application.) Pilot testing offers evaluators a wide angle or broad view of the program to assess how the entire program impacts participants.

Conducting a pilot test generally involves collecting data from participants. It is advisable to use the same data collection instruments that will be used in the actual implementation of the program to make adjustments to the instruments and program components simultaneously. (The specific methodologies associated with summative evaluation are addressed later in this chapter and in Chapter 15. Chapter 5 also provides useful information on measurement, data collection, and sampling.)

Summative Evaluation

If a program accounts for the elements displayed in Table 14.1 and adequately monitors and improves quality through formative evaluation, practitioners can assume that the collective efforts of stakeholders in designing and implementing a high-quality program will result in the accomplishment of program goals and objectives related to changes in behaviors and disease indicators. These expected outcomes are the focus of **summative evaluation,** which is any combination of measurements that permit conclusions to be drawn about impact, outcome, or benefits of a program (Green & Lewis, 1986).

By way of review, summative evaluation includes both impact evaluation, which focuses on intermediate indicators such as awareness, knowledge, attitudes, skills, environment, and most importantly, behaviors, as well as outcome evaluation, which focuses on long-term program measures such as mortality, morbidity, or disability. Indicators used in summative evaluation might include years of potential life lost (or saved), prevalence of tobacco use, reductions in diabetes mortality, a decreased incidence of HIV/AIDS, reduced absenteeism, number of pounds lost, and health care costs saved due to health promotion programs. As in formative and process evaluations, the list of potential indicators in summative evaluation is nearly endless.

Although many types of indicators and outcomes may be related to summative evaluation, the process itself is usually associated with the development of designs. This is particularly true of impact evaluation which requires a thoughtful design, appropriate data collection procedures, valid and reliable questionnaires or other instruments, and proper analysis and data reporting. Outcome evaluation related to communities or large populations often involves analysis of vital statistics and trend data with the evaluator trying to account for confounding, when the relationship between a risk factor or some other determinant and an outcome is modified by an additional variable, called the **confounding variable** (Sullivan, 2008). In other words, community-wide programs often have great difficulty identifying with any precision the degree to which the programs themselves had an impact when the priority population was exposed to so many influences at the same time. As described earlier, confounding variables relate to the element of context as measured in process evaluation. In more controlled environments such as clinical or worksite settings, many of the same procedures related to designs used in impact evaluation can be applied to outcome evaluation.

An evaluation design is used to organize a summative evaluation and to provide for planned, systematic data collection, analysis, and reporting. A well-planned evaluation design helps ensure that the conclusions drawn about the program will be as accurate as possible. The design is developed during the early stages of program planning and has program goals and objectives as its focus. CDC's Framework for Program Evaluation (discussed in Chapter 13) suggests the study design should be addressed in Step 3, only after engaging stakeholders and describing the program. As designs are developed, evaluators must consider the audience and/or stakeholders who will read the results of the evaluation. In other words, the design must produce information that will answer the evaluation questions of stakeholders.

Selecting an Evaluation Design

There are no perfect evaluation designs, because no situation related to program design and implementation is ideal, and there are always restraining factors, such as limited resources. The challenge is to devise an *optimal* evaluation—as opposed to an *ideal* evaluation (CDC, 1999a). Planners should give much thought to selecting the best design for each situation. The following questions may be helpful in the selection of a design for summative evaluation:

- How much time do you have to conduct the evaluation?
- What financial resources are available?
- How many participants can be included in the evaluation?
- Are you more interested in qualitative or quantitative data?
- Do you have data analysis skills or access to statistical consultants?
- In what ways can validity be increased?
- Is it important to be able to generalize your findings to other populations?
- Are the stakeholders concerned with validity and reliability?
- Do you have the ability to randomize participants into experimental and control groups?
- Do you have access to a comparison group?

Dignan (1995) presents four steps in choosing an evaluation design. These four steps are outlined in **Figure 14.1**. The first step is to orient oneself to the situation.

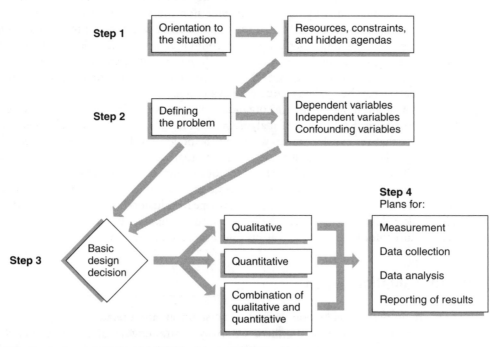

Figure 14.1 Steps in Selecting an Evaluation Design

Source: Measurement and Evaluation of Health Education. M. B. Dignan. Copyright © 1995 by Charles C. Thomas Publisher, Ltd. Reprinted with Permission.

The evaluator must identify resources (time, personnel), restraints, and hidden agendas (unspoken goals). During this step, the evaluator must determine what is to be expected from the program and what can be observed.

The second step involves defining the problem—determining what is to be evaluated. During this step, definitions are needed for independent variables (what the sponsors think makes the difference), dependent variables (what will indicate a difference, e.g., awareness, knowledge, attitudes, skills, environmental change, behaviors, disease prevalence), and confounding variables (what the evaluator thinks could be impacting the results in addition to or in place of the program under investigation).

The third step involves making a decision about the design—that is, whether to use qualitative or quantitative methods of data collection or both. The **quantitative method** is **deductive** in nature (applying a generally accepted principle to an individual case), so that the evaluation produces numeric (hard) data, such as counts, ratings, scores, or classifications. Examples of quantitative data include the posttest scores on a nutrition knowledge test, a decrease in percent of body weight from pretest to posttest, and reduction of mortality rates related to cancer. This method is suited to programs that are well defined and compares outcomes of programs with those of other groups or the general population. It is the method most often used in evaluation designs.

The **qualitative method** is an **inductive** method (individual cases are studied to formulate a general principle) and produces narrative data, such as words and descriptions. This is a good method to use for programs that emphasize individual outcomes or in cases where other descriptive information from participants is needed. That is, qualitative data provide depth of understanding, study motivation, enable discovery, are exploratory and interpretive, and allow insights into behavior and trends. Conversely, quantitative data measure levels of occurrence, provide proof, and measure levels of actions and trends (NCI, 2002). **Box 14.2** provides a summary of various qualitative methods.

Patton (1988) produced a checklist to determine whether qualitative data might be appropriate in a particular program evaluation. Collecting qualitative data may be a good strategy if there is a need to describe individual outcomes, to understand the dynamics and process of the programs, to obtain in-depth information on certain clients or sites, to focus on the diversity of program clients or sites, or to gather information to improve the program during process evaluation. Many of the strategies displayed in Table 14.2 use qualitative data.

Rather than choose one method, it may be advantageous to combine quantitative and qualitative methods. Steckler, McLeroy, and colleagues (1992) described the advantage of combining qualitative and quantitative methods, because, to a certain extent, the weaknesses of one method are compensated for by the strengths of the other. **Figure 14.2** illustrates four ways this can occur. In Model 1, qualitative methods are used to help develop quantitative methods and instruments. For example, evaluators could use a focus group with stakeholders to determine what type of questions should be included on a data collection instrument. With Model 2, qualitative results are used to help interpret and explain findings from a quantitative evaluation. For example, evaluators could collect quantitative data from a large sample of people and more in-depth qualitative data from a few in the sample. Supplementing the hard data with anecdotal information further describes the findings. Model 3 is the reverse of Model 2. In this model,

Box 14.2 QUALITATIVE METHODS USED IN EVALUATION

- *Case studies:* In-depth examinations of a social unit, such as an individual, family, household, worksite, community, or any type of institution as a whole.
- *Content analysis:* A systematic review identifying specific characteristics of messages.
- *Delphi techniques:* A process that generates consensus through a series of questionnaires. (See Chapter 4 for an in-depth discussion of the Delphi technique.)
- *Ethnographic studies:* A variety of techniques (participant-observer, observation, interviewing, and other interactions with people) used to study an individual or group.
- *Films, photographs, and videotape recording (film ethnography):* Includes the data collection and study of visual images.
- *Focus group interviewing:* Interviews used to obtain information about the feelings, opinions, perceptions, insights, beliefs, misconceptions, attitudes, and receptivity of a group of people concerning an idea or issue. (See Chapter 4 for an in-depth discussion of focus group interviewing.)
- *Historical analysis:* A review of historical accounts that may include an interpretation of the impact on current events.
- *In-depth interviewing:* Formal interviews with program participants. Allows evaluators to observe body language and facial expressions as prompts for additional questions and information. See also Table 14.3.
- *Nominal group process:* A highly structured process in which a few knowledgeable representatives of the priority population are asked to qualify and quantify specific needs. (See Chapter 4 for an in-depth discussion of the nominal group process).
- *Participant-observer studies:* Those in which the observers (evaluators) also participate in what they are observing.
- *Quality circle:* A group of internal program people who meet at regular intervals to discuss problems and to identify possible solutions. See also Table 14.3.
- *Unobtrusive techniques:* Data collection techniques that do not require the direct participation or cooperation of human subjects and include such things as unobtrusive observation, review of archival data, and study of physical traces.

Source: Health Education Evaluation and Measurement: A Practitioner's Perspective. Robert McDermott and Paul Sarvela. Copyright © 1999 by McGraw-Hill. Reprinted with permission.

quantitative results are used to help interpret predominately qualitative findings. For example, after observing a group of people for a period of time, evaluators may want to conduct a survey of the group. In the last model, Model 4, qualitative and quantitative data are used equally with cross-validation of findings.

The fourth step in selecting an evaluation design includes choosing how to measure the dependent variable, deciding how to collect the data (these components were discussed in Chapter 4) and how the data will be analyzed, and determining how the results will be reported. (These components are discussed in Chapter 15.)

Model 1
Qualitative methods are used to help develop
quantitative measures and instruments.

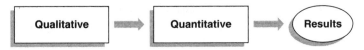

Model 2
Qualitative methods are used to help explain quantitative findings.

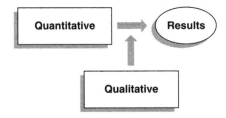

Model 3
Quantitative methods are used to embellish a primarily qualitative study.

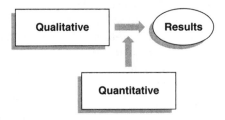

Model 4
Qualitative and quantitative methods are used equally and parallel.

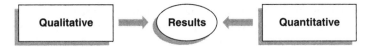

Figure 14.2 Four Possible Ways That Qualitative and Quantitative Methods Might
Be Integrated

Source: "Toward Integrating Qualitative and Quantitative Methods: An Introduction." Allan Steckler, Kenneth R. McLeroy, Robert M. Goodman, Sheryl T. Bird, Lauri McCormick, from *Health Education & Behavior*, 19(1). Copyright © 1992 by SAGE Publications. Reprinted with Permission.

Experimental, Control, and Comparison Groups

As in research studies, when evaluating a health promotion program, the group of individuals who receive the intervention is known as the **experimental group** (or treatment group). The evaluation is designed to determine what effects the program has on these individuals. To make sure that the effects are caused by the program and not by some other factor, a **control group** should be used. The control group should be as similar to the experimental group as possible, but the members of this group do not receive the program (intervention or treatment) that is to be evaluated.

Without the use of a properly selected control group, the apparent effect of the program could actually be due to a variety of factors (confounding variables), such as differences in participants' educational background, environment, or experience. By using a control group, an evaluator can show that the results or outcomes are due to the program and not to confounding variables. Ideally, participants should be randomly selected, then randomly assigned to one of two groups, and finally it should be randomly determined which group becomes the experimental group and which becomes the control group. Theoretically, this would evenly distribute the characteristics of the participants. This technique, called *randomizing* or *randomization*, increases the credibility of the evaluation by controlling for extraneous events and factors.

It is not always possible or ethical to assign participants to a control group, especially in population-based programs or if doing so would mean that they would be denied a necessary program or service. For example, a health promotion program could be designed for individuals with hypertension. Individuals diagnosed with hypertension could be referred by a physician into a health promotion class focused on reducing the risk factors associated with this disease. Denying some individuals access to the program in order to form a control group would clearly be unethical.

One way to deal with this problem is to provide the control group with an alternative program or to offer the regular program to the group at a later time (if a delay is not potentially harmful). Another alternative is to compare two programs: Offer an innovative program to some participants and continue the conventional program for others. Wagner and Guild (1989) described the advantage of this strategy as providing service to all participants (which fulfills a moral obligation) and still providing a comparison to assess the effectiveness of the innovative program.

Because the main purpose of social programs is to help individuals, the individuals' viewpoints should be the primary concern. It is important to keep this in mind when considering ethical issues in the use of control groups. Conner (1980) identifies four underlying premises for the use of control groups in social program evaluation:

1. All individuals have a right to status quo services.

2. All individuals involved in the evaluation are informed about the purpose of the study and the use of a control group.

3. Individuals have a right to new services, and random selection gives everyone a chance to participate.

4. Individuals should not be subjected to ineffective or harmful programs.

The ethical issues that must be considered involve the potential denial of a service and allocation of scarce resources. When randomization is not feasible, planners should consider an equitable process of providing services for individuals while maintaining control over the evaluation design.

When participants cannot be randomly assigned to an experimental or control group, a nonequivalent group may be selected. This is known as a **comparison group.**

It is important to find a group that is as similar as possible to the experimental group, such as two classrooms of students with similar characteristics or a group of residents in two comparable cities. Factors to consider include participants' age, gender, education, location, socioeconomic status, and experience, as well as any other variable that might impact program results. Comparison groups are not randomly selected or assigned.

Evaluation Designs

Measurements used in evaluation designs can be collected at three different times: after the program; both before and after the program; and several times before, during, and after the program. *Measurement* is defined as the process of applying numerical or narrative data from an instrument (i.e., questionnaire) or other data yielding tools to objects, events or people (Windsor et al., 2004).

Figure 14.3 presents evaluation designs commonly used in health promotion. In the figure, the letter O refers to measurement involving data derived from questionnaires, tests, interviews, observations, or other methods of gaining information. When multiple measurements are taken, the subscript number beside each O indicates the order in which the measurements are made. Measurement before the program begins is known as the **pretest**, and measurement after the completion of the program is known as the **posttest**. The letter X represents the program (intervention, or independent variable); the relative positions of the two letters in the table indicate when measurements are made in relation to when the program is provided. The figure also shows which groups receive the program and when participants are randomly assigned to groups [(R)].

Windsor and colleagues (2004) differentiate among three types of evaluation designs: experimental, quasi-experimental, and nonexperimental. **Experimental design** offers the greatest control over the various factors that may influence the results (confounding variables). It involves random assignment to experimental and control groups with measurement of both groups. This evaluation design produces the most interpretable and defensible evidence of effectiveness. **Quasi-experimental design** results in interpretable and supportive evidence of program effectiveness, but usually cannot control for all factors that affect the validity of the results. There is no random assignment to the groups, and comparisons are made on experimental and comparison groups. **Nonexperimental design**, without the use of a comparison or control group, has little control over the factors that affect the validity of the results.

The most powerful design is the experimental design, in which participants are randomly assigned to the experimental and control groups. The difference between designs I.1 and I.2 in Figure 14.3 is the use of a pretest to measure the participants before the program begins. Use of a pretest would help ensure that the groups are similar and provide baseline measurement. Random assignment should equally distribute any of the variables of the participants (such as age, gender, and race) between the different groups. Potential disadvantages of the experimental design are that it requires a relatively large group of participants and the intervention may be delayed for those in the control group.

A design more commonly found in evaluations of health promotion programs is the quasi-experimental pretest-posttest design using a comparison group (II.1 in Figure 14.3). This design is often used when a control group cannot be formed by random assignment. In such a case, a comparison group (a nonequivalent control group) is identified, and both

I. Experimental design

1. Pretest-posttest design
— Experimental group   (R) O_1 X O_2
— Control group   (R) O_1 O_2

2. Posttest-only design
— Experimental group   (R)   X   O
— Control group   (R)   O

3. Time series design
— Experimental group   (R) O_1 O_2 O_3 X O_4 O_5 O_6
— Control group   (R) O_1 O_2 O_3 O_4 O_5 O_6

II. Quasi-experimental design

1. Pretest-posttest design
— Experimental group O_1 X O_2
— Comparison group O_1 O_2

2. Time series design
— Experimental group O_1 O_2 O_3 X O_4 O_5 O_6
— Comparison group O_1 O_2 O_3 O_4 O_5 O_6

III. Nonexperimental design

1. Pretest-posttest design
— Experimental group O_1 X O_2

2. Time series design
— Experimental group O_1 O_2 O_3 X O_4 O_5 O_6

Key: (R) = Random assignment
      O = Measurement/Observation
      X = Program/Intervention

Figure 14.3 Evaluation Designs

groups are measured before and after the program. For example, a program on healthy eating for two ninth-grade classrooms could be evaluated by using pre- and post–food inventory instruments. Two other ninth-grade classrooms not receiving the program could serve as the comparison group. Similar pretest scores between the comparison and experimental groups would indicate that the groups were equal at the beginning of the program. However, without random assignment, it would be impossible to be sure that other variables (e.g., a unit on meal preparation in a family and consumer science course, a reality television show related to weight loss, changes made by the primary meal preparer at home, etc.) did not influence the results.

Sometimes participants cannot be assigned to a control group and no comparison group can be identified. In such cases, a nonexperimental pretest-posttest design (III.1 in Figure 14.3) can be used, but the results are of limited significance, because changes could be due to the program or to some other event. An example of this type of nonexperimental design would be the measurement of safety belt use after a community program on that topic. An increase in use might mean that the program successfully motivated individuals to use safety belts; however, it could also reveal the impact of increased enforcement of the mandatory safety belt law, of a traffic fatality in the community, or a safety article in the local newspaper.

Experimental group 1	(R)	X	O_1		O_2		O_3		O_4	
Experimental group 2	(R)		O_1	X	O_2		O_3		O_4	
Experimental group 3	(R)				O_1	X	O_2		O_3	
Experimental group 4	(R)							X	O_1	

Key: (R) = Random assignment
    O = Measurement/Observation
    X = Program/Intervention

Figure 14.4 Staggered Treatment Design

A time series evaluation design (I.3, II.2, III.2 in Figure 14.3) can be used to examine differences in program effects over time. Random assignment to groups (I.3) offers the most control over factors influencing the validity of the results. The use of a comparison group (II.2) offers some control; without a control group or comparison group (III.2), it is possible to determine changes in the participants over time, but one cannot be sure that the changes were due only to the program.

In the time series design, several measurements are taken over time both before and after a program is implemented. This process helps to identify other factors that may account for a change between the pretest and posttest measurements and is especially appropriate for measuring delayed effects of a program. A time series design could be used in a weight loss program to indicate the amount of participants' weight loss over time and their ability to maintain a desired weight.

Another design that may be used is the staggered treatment design (see **Figure 14.4**), which is used to determine the effects of a program over time by including several measurements after the end of the program. It also indicates the effects of testing, since not all groups in this design receive a pretest. The staggered treatment design can also be used in quasi-experimental and nonexperimental designs, although with the limitations of not using a control group or comparison group.

Internal Validity

The **internal validity** of evaluation is the degree to which change that was measured can be attributed to the program and allows evaluators to speak with more confidence that the program itself actually made a difference (Issel, 2009). Many factors can threaten internal validity, either singly or in combination, making it difficult to determine if the outcome was brought about by the program or some other cause. Cook and Campbell (1979) identified common threats to internal validity, summarized as follows:

- *History* occurs when an event happens between the pretest and posttest that is not part of the health promotion program. An example of history as a threat to internal validity is having a national antismoking campaign coincide with a local smoking cessation program.

- *Maturation* occurs when the participants in the program show pretest-to-posttest differences due to growing older, wiser, or stronger. For example, in tests of muscle strength in an exercise program for junior high students, an increase in strength could be the result of muscular development and not the effect of the program.

- *Testing* occurs when the participants become familiar with the test format due to repeated testing. This is why it is helpful to use a different form of the same test for pretest and posttest comparisons.

- *Instrumentation* occurs when there is a change in measurement between pretest and posttest, such as the observers becoming more familiar with or skilled in the use of the testing format over time.

- *Statistical regression* is when extremely high or low scores (which are not necessarily accurate) on the pretest are closer to the mean or average scores on the posttest.

- *Selection* reflects differences in the experimental and comparison groups, generally due to lack of randomization. Selection can also interact with other threats to validity, such as history, maturation, or instrumentation, which may appear to be program effects.

- *Mortality* refers to participants who drop out of the program between the pretest and posttest. For example, if most of the participants who drop out of a weight loss program are those with the least (or the most) weight to lose, the group composition is different at the posttest.

- *Diffusion or imitation of treatments* results when participants in the control or comparison group interact and learn from the experimental group. Students randomly assigned to an innovative drug prevention program in their school (experimental group) may discuss the program with students who are not in the program (control or comparison group), biasing the results.

- *Compensatory equalization of treatments* occurs when the program or services are not available to the control or comparison group and there is an unwillingness to tolerate the inequality. For instance, the control or comparison group from the previous example (students not enrolled in the innovative drug prevention program) may complain, since they are not able to participate.

- *Compensatory rivalry* is when the control or comparison group is seen as the underdog and is motivated to work harder.

- *Resentful demoralization of respondents receiving less desirable treatments* occurs among participants receiving the less desirable treatments compared to other groups, and the resentment may affect the outcome. For example, an evaluation to compare two different smoking cessation programs may assign one group (control) to the regular smoking cessation program and another group (experimental) to the regular program plus an exercise class. If the participants in the control group become aware that they are not receiving the additional exercise class, they may resent the omission, and this may be reflected in their smoking behavior and attitude toward the regular program.

The most significant way in which threats to internal validity can be controlled is through *randomization*. By random selection of participants, random assignment to groups, and random assignment of types of intervention or no intervention to groups, any differences between pretest and posttest can be interpreted as a result of the program. When random assignment to groups is not possible and quasi-experimental or nonexperimental designs are used, the evaluator must make all threats to internal validity explicit and then rule them out one by one.

External Validity

The other type of validity that should be considered is **external validity,** or the extent to which the program can be expected to produce similar effects in other populations. This is also known as **generalizability** which is most closely associated with program evaluations that involve large sample sizes and are found to be internally valid (Harris, 2010). However, the more a program is tailored to a particular population, the greater the threat to external validity, and the less likely it is that the program can be generalized to another group.

As with internal validity, several factors can threaten external validity. They are sometimes known as *reactive effects,* since they cause individuals to react in a certain way. The following are several types of threats to external validity:

- *Social desirability* occurs when individuals give a particular response to try to please or impress the evaluator. An example would be children who tell their teacher they brush their teeth every day, regardless of their actual behavior.

- *Expectancy effect* is when attitudes projected onto individuals cause them to act in a certain way. For example, in a drug abuse treatment program, the facilitator may feel that a certain individual will not benefit from the treatment; projecting this attitude may cause the individual to behave in self-defeating manners.

- *Hawthorne effect* refers to a behavior change because of the special status of those being tested. This effect was first identified in an evaluation of lighting conditions at an electric plant; workers increased their productivity when the level of lighting was raised as well as when it was lowered. The change in behavior seemed to be due to the attention given to them during the evaluation process.

- *Placebo effect* causes a change in behavior due to the participants' belief in the treatment.

Cook and Campbell (1979) discussed the threats to external validity in terms of statistical interaction effects. These include interaction of selection and treatment (the findings from a program requiring a large time commitment may not be generalizable to individuals who do not have much free time); interaction of setting and treatment (evaluation results from a program conducted on campus may not be generalizable to the worksite); and interaction of history and treatment (results from a program conducted on a historically significant day may not be generalizable to other days).

Conducting the program several times in a variety of settings, with a variety of participants can reduce the threats to external validity. Threats to external validity can also be counteracted by making a greater effort to treat all subjects identically. In a **blind** study, the participants do not know to what group (control or experimental) they have been assigned. In a **double blind** study, the type of group participants are in is not known by either the participants or the planners. In a **triple blind** study, this information is not available to the participants, planners, or evaluators.

It is important to select an evaluation design that provides both internal and external validity. This may be difficult, because lowering the threat to one type of validity may increase the threat to the other. For example, tighter evaluation controls make it more difficult to generalize the results to other situations. There must be enough control over the evaluation to allow evaluators to interpret the findings while sufficient flexibility in the program is maintained to permit the results to be generalized to similar settings.

SUMMARY

This chapter focused on evaluation approaches, design elements, and strategies for conducting a comprehensive evaluation. Distinctions between formative and process evaluation were made and key issues related to summative evaluation were outlined.

The steps for selecting an evaluation design were also presented with a discussion about quantitative and qualitative methods. Evaluation design should be considered early in the planning process. Evaluators need to identify what measurements will be taken as well as when and how. In doing so, a design should be selected that controls for both internal and external validity.

REVIEW QUESTIONS

1. List the elements of a comprehensive formative evaluation and describe when in the design and implementation process they are most appropriately applied.

2. What are the fundamental differences between formative and process evaluations?

3. What is the difference between cost-benefit analysis and cost-effectiveness analysis? Which is more appropriate for use in health promotion programs?

4. What is the difference between quantitative and qualitative evaluations? When would one method be more appropriate than the other? How could they be combined in an evaluation design?

5. Name at least five different qualitative methods of evaluation and describe each.

6. What are the advantages of using a control group? What types of evaluation design do not use control groups? What is the difference between a control group and a comparison group?

7. What is the difference between experimental, quasi-experimental, and nonexperimental designs? What are the strengths and weaknesses of each?

8. What is the difference between internal validity and external validity?

9. What are some considerations in the selection of an evaluation design presented in this chapter? What considerations can you add to this list?

ACTIVITIES

1. Interview the manager of a health promotion program of your choice about how he or she measures quality. How many elements of formative evaluation can you detect?

2. Look at an evaluation of a health promotion program that has been conducted in your community. Identify the evaluation approach that it most closely follows. Discuss your view with the program evaluator.

3. Develop an evaluation design for a program you are planning. Explain why you chose this design, and list the strengths and weaknesses of the design.

4. If you were hired to evaluate a weight loss program in a community, what evaluation design would you use and why? Assume you have all the resources you need to conduct the evaluation.

5. Explain what evaluation design you would use in evaluating the difference between two teaching techniques. Why would you choose this design?

WEBLINKS

1. http://www.wmich.edu/evalctr/checklists/

   Evaluation Center at Western Michigan University (WMU)

   The Evaluation Center at WMU Website provides evaluation specialists and users with refereed checklists. The site's purpose is to improve the quality and consistency of evaluations and enhance evaluation capacity through the promotion and use of high-quality checklists targeted to specific evaluation tasks and approaches. Visitors to this site can download a number of checklists and information on how to create them.

2. http://oerl.sri.com/

   Online Evaluation Resource Library (OERL)

   Funded by the National Science Foundation (NSF), OERL was developed for professionals seeking to design, conduct, document, or review project evaluations. OERL's resources include instruments, plans, and reports from evaluations that have proven to be sound and representative of current evaluation practices.

3. http://www.eric.ed.gov/

   Educational Resources Information Center (ERIC)

   The ERIC Clearinghouse on Assessment and Evaluation Website offers a variety of resources and seeks to provide balanced information concerning educational assessment, and resources to encourage responsible test use.

4. http://www.nationalserviceresources.org/filemanager/download/ProgramMgmt/ Outcome_Measurement_Showing_Results_Nonprofit_Sector.pdf

   United Way of America (UWA)

   UWA's Outcome Measurement Resource Network offers information, downloadable documents, and links to resources related to the identification and measurement of program- and community-level outcomes.

5. http://whqlibdoc.who.int/hq/2000/WHO_MSD_MSB_00.2e.pdf

   World Health Organization

   This is a link to WHO's helpful document on process evaluation that supplements material in this chapter. It describes why a process evaluation should be performed and how to do a process evaluation.

6. http://www.rand.org/pubs/technical_reports/TR101/

   Rand Organization—Getting to Outcomes

   This document, which focuses on substance abuse, provides an excellent explanation of promoting accountability through methods and tools for planning, implementation, and evaluation. One focus of the document is how to get to outcomes that justify prevention programs in general.

CHAPTER 15

Data Analysis and Reporting

CHAPTER OBJECTIVES

After reading this chapter and answering the questions at the end, you should be able to:

- Define *data management*.
- List examples of univariate, bivariate, and multivariate analyses and explain how they can be used in evaluation.
- Differentiate between descriptive and inferential statistics.
- Explain the difference between the null hypothesis and the alternative hypothesis in significance testing.
- Define *level of significance*, *Type I error*, and *Type II error*.
- Define *independent variable* and *dependent variable*.
- Describe the format for the evaluation report, guidelines for presenting data, and ways to enhance the report.
- Discuss ways to increase the utilization of the evaluation findings.

KEY TERMS

alpha level
alternative hypothesis
analysis of variance
   (ANOVA)
bivariate data analysis
chi-square
correlations
data management
dependent variables
descriptive statistics

independent variables
inferential statistics
level of significance
mean
measures of central tendency
measures of spread or
   variation
median
mode
multiple regression

multivariate data analysis
null hypothesis
program significance
range
statistical significance
t-tests
Type I error
Type II error
univariate data analysis
variable

Like all other aspects of evaluation, the types of data analysis used in an evaluation should be determined in the pre-planning stage. Basically, the analysis determines what if any impact was made by the program. The evaluator then draws conclusions and prepares reports and/or presentations. The types of analyses used and how the information is presented are determined by the evaluation questions as well as the needs and requests of the stakeholders.

This chapter describes different types of analyses commonly used in evaluating health promotion programs. To present them in detail or to include all possible techniques is beyond the scope of this text. If you need more information, refer to statistics textbooks, research methods and statistics courses, or statistical consultants. **Box 15.1** identifies the responsibilities and competencies for health education specialists that pertain to the material presented in this chapter.

Evaluations affected by major methodological problems are not likely to inspire confidence. A common problem in this regard is inadequate documentation of methods, results, and data analysis. The evaluation should be well designed and the report itself should contain a complete background and description of the program, a thorough explanation of methodology including information about the instrumentation, the program participants and their selection, evaluation design and statistical analysis, as well as an objective interpretation of facts, and a discussion of features of the study that may have influenced the findings. Attention to these details will help ensure a more accurate assessment of program effectiveness as well as enhance the credibility of planners/evaluators among stakeholders. In addition, this level of professionalism will also increase the likelihood that evaluation reports can be translated to peer reviewed publications and contribute to the research and knowledge base of health promotion in general.

Box 15.1 RESPONSIBILITIES AND COMPETENCIES FOR HEALTH EDUCATION SPECIALISTS

This chapter describes managing data collected in evaluations or other research; types of data analyses; applications of data analyses; interpreting data; reporting the results of evaluation, including designing written reports and how and when to present evaluation reports; and increasing the use of evaluation results. Responsibilities and competencies related to the content in this chapter include:

Responsibility IV: Conduct Evaluation and Research Related to Health Education

Competency 4.1: Develop Evaluation/Research Plan

Competency 4.2: Design Instruments to Collect Evaluation/Research Data

Competency 4.3: Collect and Analyze Evaluation/Research Data

Competency 4.4: Interpret Results of the Evaluation/Research

Competency 4.5: Apply Findings from Evaluation/Research

Source: NCHEC, SOPHE, & AAHE (2010).

Data Management

Once data have been collected (see Chapter 4 for data collection methods), they must be organized in such a manner that they can be analyzed in order to interpret the findings. To do this, the data, whether quantitative or qualitative, must be coded, cleaned, and organized into a usable format. These steps are collectively referred to as **data management**. By coded, we mean that the data are assigned labels so they can be read and processed by a computer. The coding system outlines the process "through which raw data become translated for various forms of analysis (such as frequency counts, descriptive statistics, cross tabulations and other statistical procedures)" (McDermott & Sarvela, 1999, p. 77). For example, if the answer to a question on an instrument is yes, yes answers may be coded as the number 1 when entered into the computer, while no answers may be coded as a number 2. In addition to creating the coding scheme for raw data, a coding system also establishes rules for dealing with coding problems such as when respondents circle both yes and no for their answer to a question, or when neither yes nor no is circled but rather the space between the yes and no is circled.

Once the data have been coded, they must be cleaned before being entered into a computer system. "Data cleaning entails checking that the values are valid and consistent; i.e., all values correspond to valid question responses" (Valente, 2002, p. 136). For example, if the possible range of answers for a particular question is 1 to 3 and the frequency distribution identifies some 4s, those response forms with the 4s must be identified and checked to determine if the person completing the instrument made an error or if there was an error made by the person coding the data. If it was a data coding error, it should be corrected. If the person completing the data collection instrument made an error, it would be treated as no response to that question or as missing data (Cottrell & McKenzie, 2011). Once data have been cleaned, the appropriate data analysis can begin.

Data Analysis

The goal of data analysis is to reduce, organize, synthesize, and summarize information in order to make sense of it and to be able to make inferences about the priority population (Fitzpatrick et al., 2004; McDermott & Sarvela, 1999). Regardless of the type of data analysis to be used, the analysis begins with the identification of the variables of interest. A **variable** is a characteristic or attribute that can be measured or observed (Creswell, 2002). In program evaluation, the variables are divided into independent and dependent variables. **Independent variables** are those that are either controlled by the evaluator or cause or exert some influence, whereas the **dependent variables** are the outcome variables being studied. In other words "independent variables influence dependent variables" (Valente, 2002, p. 165). Examples of independent variables include exposure to an intervention, gender, race, age, education, and income, and so on, while dependent variables may include awareness, knowledge, attitudes, skills, and behaviors.

Statistics are used to analyze variables. **Descriptive statistics** are used to organize, summarize, and describe characteristics of a group, while **inferential statistics** are concerned with relationships and causality in order to make generalizations (or inferences) about a population based upon findings from a sample. Statistical analyses also allow evaluators to measure the association and relationships between and among variables. When one variable is analyzed, it is called **univariate data analysis**. Analysis of two variables is called **bivariate data analysis** and analysis of more than two variables is referred to as **multivariate data analysis**.

The choice of a type of analysis is based on the evaluation questions, the type of data collected, and the audience that will receive the results (Newcomer & Wirtz, 2004). For some types of evaluation, descriptive data are all that are needed, and techniques are chosen to determine frequencies, counts, or other univariate procedures. Other evaluation questions focus on testing a hypothesis about relationships between variables; in such cases, more elaborate statistical techniques are needed. **Box 15.2** contains examples of the types of evaluation questions that can be answered by using different types of data analyses.

The level of measurement (i.e., nominal, ordinal, interval, or ratio) (discussed in Chapter 5) is an important factor in selecting the type of analysis to be used. For the most part, analytical techniques have been developed for use with selected levels of measurement. In other words, not all analytical techniques can be used with all levels of measurement. For example, multiple regression analysis is a technique that has been reserved for use with interval and ratio data. Newcomer and Wirtz (1994) created a particularly useful summary (see **Table 15.1**) to assist evaluators in selecting appropriate statistical techniques.

Box 15.2 EXAMPLES OF EVALUATION QUESTIONS ANSWERED USING UNIVARIATE, BIVARIATE, AND MULTIVARIATE DATA ANALYSIS

Univariate Analysis	Bivariate Analysis	Multivariate Analysis
What was the average score on the cholesterol knowledge test?	Is there a difference in smoking behavior between the individuals in the experimental and control groups after the healthy lifestyle program?	Can the risk of heart disease be predicted using smoking, exercise, diet, and heredity?
How many participants at the worksite attended the healthy lifestyle presentation?	Is peer education or classroom instruction more effective in increasing knowledge about the effects of drug abuse?	Can mortality risk among motorcycle riders be predicted from helmet use, time of day, weather conditions, and speed?
What percentage of the participants in the corporate fitness program met their target goal?	Do students' attitudes about bicycle helmets differ in rural and urban settings?	Which of the following most accurately predict successful management of stress among program participants: physical activity, diet, meditation, anger management, yoga, or deep breathing?

Table 15.1 Selecting Statistical Techniques

Purpose of the Analysis	How the Variables Are Measured	Appropriate Technique	Appropriate Test for Statistical Significance	Appropriate Measure of Magnitude
To compare a sample distribution to a population distribution	Nominal/ordinal	Frequency counts	Chi-square	NA
	Interval	Means and medians Standard deviations/interquartile range	Chi-square	NA
To analyze the relationship between two variables	Nominal/ordinal	Contingency tables	Chi-square	Difference in column percentages
	Interval	Contingency tables/test of differences of means or proportions	Chi-square or t-test	Difference in column percentages or in means
To reduce the number of variables by identifying factors that explain variation in a larger set of variables	Interval	Factor analysis	NA	Pearson's correlations; Eigenvalues
To sort units into similar clusters or groupings	Nominal/ordinal/ interval	Cluster analysis; discriminant functions analysis	F; Wilk's Lambda	Cannonical/correlation coefficient[2]
To predict or estimate program impact	Nominal/ordinal dependent variable	Log linear regression	t and F	Odds estimates
	Interval dependent variable	Regression	t and F	R^2, beta weights
To describe or predict a trend in a series of data collected over time	Nominal, ordinal, or interval independent variables but interval dependent variable	Regression	t and F	R^2, beta weights

Note: NA = not applicable.
Source: Handbook of Practical Program Evaluation. Joseph S. Wholey, Harry P. Hatry, and Kathryn E. Newcomer. Copyright © 1994 by John Wiley & Sons, Inc. Reproduced with permission.

The issue of who will receive the final evaluation report should also be considered when selecting the type of analysis. Evaluators want to be able to present the evaluation results in a form that can be understood by the stakeholders. With regard to this issue, it is probably best to err on the side of too simple an analysis rather than one that is too complex. Finally, regardless of the type of analysis selected for an evaluation, the method should be chosen early in the evaluation process and in place before the data are collected.

Univariate Data Analyses

Univariate data analyses examine one variable at a time. It is common for univariate analyses to be descriptive in nature. As noted earlier, descriptive statistics are used to describe, classify, and summarize data. Summary counts (frequencies) are totals, and they are the easiest type of data to collect and report. Summary counts can be used in process evaluation—for example, to count the number of participants in blood pressure screening programs at various sites. The information would assist the planners in publicizing sites with low attendance or adding additional personnel to busy sites. Other examples of frequencies, or summary counts, are the number of participants in a workshop, those who scored above 80% on a knowledge posttest, or the number of individuals wearing a safety belt.

Measures of central tendency are other forms of univariate data analyses. The **mean** is the arithmetic average of all the scores. The **median** is the midpoint of all the scores, dividing scores ranked by size into equal halves. The **mode** is the score that occurs most frequently. These are all useful in describing the results, and reporting all three measures of central tendency will be especially helpful if extreme scores are found.

Measures of spread or variation refer to how spread out the scores are in the data set. **Range** is the difference between the highest and lowest scores. For example, if the high score is 100 and the low score is 60, the range is 40. Measures of spread or variation— such as range, standard deviation, or variance—can be used to determine whether scores from groups are similar or spread apart.

Bivariate Data Analyses

Bivariate data analyses are used to study two variables simultaneously. Such analyses "are usually used to determine the presence of relationships or differences between groups" (McDermott & Sarvela, 1999, p. 300). When using bivariate analyses, it is common to state evaluation questions in the form of hypotheses. The **null hypothesis** holds that there is no observed difference between groups. The **alternative hypothesis** states there is a difference between groups. For example, a null hypothesis might state there is no difference between two groups, for example men and women, in knowledge about cancer risk factors, while the alternative hypothesis states there is a difference.

Statistical tests are used to determine if the relationships or differences between groups are statistically significant. **Statistical significance** "refers to whether the observed differences between the two or more groups are real or not or whether they are chance occurrences" (McDermott & Sarvela, 1999, p. 300). In other words, statistical tests are used to determine whether the null hypothesis is rejected (meaning a relationship between the groups probably does exist) or whether it fails to be rejected (indicating that any apparent relationship between groups is due to chance).

There is the possibility that the null hypothesis can be rejected when it is, in fact, true; this is known as **Type I error**. There is also the possibility of failing to reject the null hypothesis when it is, in fact, not true; this is a **Type II error**. The probability of making a Type I error is reflected in the alpha level. The **alpha level**, or **level of significance**, is established before the statistical tests are run and is generally set at .05 or .01. This indicates that the decision to reject the null hypothesis is incorrect 5% (or 1%) of the time; that is, there is a 5% probability (or 1% probability) that the outcome occurred by chance alone.

When a smaller alpha level is used (.01 or .001), the possibility of making a Type I error is reduced; at the same time, however, the possibility of a Type II error increases. An example of a Type I error is the adoption of a new program due to higher scores on a knowledge test, when, in reality, increases in knowledge occurred by chance and the new program is not more effective than the existing program. An example of a Type II error is not adopting the new program when it is, in reality, more effective.

Bivariate analyses that are commonly used in program evaluation include chi-square, *t*-tests, analysis of variance, and correlations. **Chi-square** is a statistical test "that measures the association between two nominal and/or ordinal variables" (Valente, 2002, p. 170). An example of this type of analysis would be measuring the association of grade levels (e.g., third and fifth grades) with the attitudes of children toward the use of bicycle helmets (i.e., strongly agree, agree, disagree, and strongly disagree).

While chi-square is used to study nominal and/or ordinal variables, *t*-tests and **analysis of variance (ANOVA)** are statistical tests used to study group differences when the dependent variables involve interval or ratio data (e.g., scores on a test). There are several situations in which a *t*-test could be used. The most common use of a *t*-test is to determine whether a variable changed significantly in one group at two different points in time, such as between baseline before the intervention (pretest) and at follow-up after the intervention (posttest). This type of *t*-test is called a dependent *t*-test. A second common use of a *t*-test is to study the differences between two groups at a single point in time. An example of such a situation is the comparison of scores on nutrition practices after two groups have been exposed to different nutrition education interventions. This type of *t*-test is called an independent *t*-test.

ANOVA is a statistical test that can be used to study differences between two groups just like a *t*-test, but is more commonly used to study differences between more than two groups. For example, an ANOVA could be used to determine if there was a difference in the test scores of three groups (i.e., different age groups like 15–24, 25–45, and 46–65 year olds) on a physical activity assessment following exposure to a single health promotion intervention.

While the bivariate analyses discussed so far are used to determine if differences exist between groups, **correlations** are used to study the strength and direction of relationships between two variables (McDermott & Sarvela, 1999). Correlations are expressed as values between +1 (a positive correlation) and -1 (a negative correlation), with a 0 indicating no relationship between the variables. "The higher the value of the correlation coefficient (regardless of direction) the stronger the relationship between the two variables" (McDermott & Sarvela, 1999, p. 304).

Correlation between variables indicates only a relationship; this technique does not establish cause and effect. An example of the use of correlation would be to determine the relationship between safety belt use and age of the driver. If older people were found to wear their safety belts more often than younger people, that would constitute a positive correlation between age and safety belt use. If younger people wore their safety belts more often, it would be a negative correlation. If age made no difference in who wore safety belts more frequently, the correlation would be 0.

Multivariate Data Analyses

Multivariate data analyses are used to study three or more variables simultaneously. Examples of multivariate analyses include multiple regression, discriminant analysis, and factor analysis. Of these, the one that tends to be used most commonly in health promotion evaluation is **multiple regression.** "There are many different types of multiple regression, including stepwise regression, logistic regression, and general linear regression" (McDermott & Sarvela, 1999, p. 305). Though the procedures and applications for various types of regression differ, they are "useful in exploring relationships among variables or in exploring the independent effects of many variables on one dependent variable" (Fitzpatrick et al., 2004, p. 359). An example of the latter would be trying to predict the risk of heart disease (the dependent variable) using the independent variables of smoking, exercise, diet, and family history.

Applications of Data Analyses

Many evaluation concepts have been presented. Therefore, a few examples here will help you see how to move from a program goal to an intervention to an evaluation design to data analysis. To illustrate these concepts, a few statistics have been selected that are commonly used with health promotion programs: chi-square and t-tests.

Case #1

Program goal: Reduce the prevalence of smoking in the priority population
Priority population: The 140 employees of Company X who smoke
Intervention (independent variable): Two different smoking cessation programs
Variable of interest (dependent variable): Smoking cessation after six months
Evaluation design:

| R | A | X_1 | O_1 |
| R | B | X_2 | O_1 |

where:

R	=	random assignment
A	=	group A
B	=	group B
X_1	=	method 1
X_2	=	method 2
O_1	=	self-reported smoking behavior

Data collected: Nominal data; quit yes or no

	Smoking Employees	
	Group A Method 1	Group B Method 2
Quit	24%	33%
Did not quit	76%	67%

Data analysis: A chi-square test of statistical significance can be used to test the null hypothesis that there is no difference in the success of the two groups.

Case #2

Program goal: Increase knowledge of HIV/AIDS within the priority population
Priority population: The 3,200 incoming freshmen at University X
Intervention (independent variable): A two-hour lecture-discussion program presented during the freshmen orientation program
Variable of interest (dependent variable): Knowledge of HIV/AIDS
Evaluation design: O_1 X O_2

where:

$$O_1 \; = \; \text{pretest scores}$$
$$X \; = \; \text{two-hour program at freshman orientation}$$
$$O_2 \; = \; \text{posttest scores}$$

Data collection: Ratio data; scores on 100-point-scale test

	Test Results	
	Pretest	**Posttest**
Number of students	3,200	3,200
Mean score	69.0	78.5

Data analysis: A dependent *t*-test of statistical significance can be used to test the null hypothesis that there is no difference between the pre- and posttest means on the knowledge test.

Case #3

Program goal: To improve the testicular self-examination skills of the priority population
Priority population: All boys enrolled in the eighth grade at Junior High School X
Intervention (independent variable): Two-week unit on testicular cancer
Variable of interest (dependent variable): Score on testicular self-exam skills test
Evaluation design: A O_1 X O_2
                          B O_1 O_2

where:

$$A \; = \; \text{eighth-grade boys at Junior High School X}$$
$$B \; = \; \text{eighth-grade boys at Junior High School Y}$$
$$O_1 \; = \; \text{pretest scores}$$
$$X \; = \; \text{two-week unit on testicular cancer}$$
$$O_2 \; = \; \text{posttest scores}$$

Data collected: Ratio data; scores on 100-point skills test

	Test Results	
	Junior High X (*n* = 142)	**Junior High Y** (*n* = 131)
Pre	62	63
Post	79	65

Data analysis: An independent *t*-test of statistical significance can be used to (1) test the null hypothesis that there is no difference in the pretest scores of the two groups because the groups were not randomly assigned, and (2) test the null hypothesis that there is no difference in the posttest scores of the two groups.

Interpreting the Data

With the data analyses completed, attention turns to interpreting the data. By interpretation we mean attaching meaning to the analyzed data and drawing conclusions. "Interpretation should be characterized by careful, fair, open methods of inquiry." (Fitzpatrick et al., 2004, p. 364.)

To ensure that the interpretation is fair and as objective as possible, it is recommended that the interpretation not be the sole responsibility of the evaluator or, for that matter, any other single person. Earlier, when we began our discussion of evaluation, we spoke of the importance of making sure that the evaluation process is a collaborative process that includes representation from all of the stakeholders (see Chapter 13). That principle applies not only to the planning of the evaluation but also to the interpretation of the data. Over time, several authors (Fitzpatrick et al., 2004; Patton, 1986; Solomon, 1987; Weiss, 1984) have recommended bringing the stakeholders and evaluator together in one or more meetings to systematically review the findings. Such meetings take advantage of the diverse perspectives of the stakeholders, as well as allowing for a discussion of the implications of various interpretative conclusions.

There is no single method used to interpret data. In fact, a number of different methods could be used. Fitzpatrick and colleagues (2004) have identified eight methods:

1. "Determining whether objectives have been achieved;

2. Determining whether laws, democratic ideals, regulations, or ethical principles have been violated;

3. Determining whether assessed needs have been reduced;

4. Determining the value of accomplishments;

5. Asking critical reference groups to review the data and to provide their judgments of successes and failures, strengths, and weaknesses;

6. Comparing results with those reported by similar entities or endeavors;

7. Comparing assessed performance levels on critical variables to expectations of performance or standards;

8. Interpreting results in light of evaluation procedures that generated them" (p. 364).

Given this list, it becomes clear that there is a difference between what is termed statistical significance and **program significance**. Program significance measures the meaningfulness of a program (based on stakeholder preferences) regardless of statistical significance. Statistical significance is determined by statistical testing. It is possible—especially when a large number of people are included in the data collection—to have statistically significant results that indicate gains in performance but are not meaningful in terms of program goals. For example, if the mean scores on a knowledge test of two groups are 70 and 69 (out of 100 points) and the groups are large enough, it would be possible that the difference in the scores (i.e., 1 point) could be statistically significant. But in practical terms, the group with a mean score of 70 compared with 69 will likely not have more knowledge that will translate to more informed consumers. Thus, spending extra dollars on the program that generated the mean score of 70 versus the less expensive program that generated a mean score of 69 would not be cost-effective. Statistical significance is similar to reliability in that they are both measures of precision. It is important to consider whether statistical significance justifies the development, implementation, and costs of a program (Fink & Kosecoff, 1978). On the other hand, while program results may not be considered statistically significant, stakeholders may feel the program should be continued for various reasons (e.g., goodwill is being developed in the community or the organization is receiving a lot of positive attention that is drawing more clients to other programs, etc.).

Evaluation Reporting

The results and interpretation of the data analyses, as well as a description of the evaluation process, are incorporated into a final report that is presented to stakeholders. The report itself generally follows the format of a research report, including an introduction, methodology, results, conclusions, and discussion.

Some may see the creation of an evaluation report as a nonessential step in the larger process of evaluation; however, an evaluation report is essential for several reasons (Wurzbach, 2002). An evaluation report can provide:

- The impetus "to help you critically analyze the results of the evaluation and think about any changes you should make as a result

- A tangible product for your agency

- Evidence that your program or materials have been carefully developed—to be used as a sales tool with gatekeepers (e.g., television station public service directors)

- A record of your activities for use in planning future programs

- Assistance to others who may be interested in developing similar programs or materials

- A foundation for evaluation activities in the future (e.g., it is easier to design a new questionnaire based on one you have previously used than to start anew)" (p. 590).

The number and type of reports required are determined at the beginning of the evaluation based on the needs of the stakeholders. For a formative evaluation, reports are needed early and may be provided on a weekly or monthly basis. Related feedback may be formal or informal, ranging from scheduled presentations to informal telephone calls but must be submitted in a timely manner in order to provide immediate feedback so that program modifications can be made before program implementation has progressed too far. For a summative evaluation, the report is generally more formal and may resemble a scientific paper that can be submitted to a journal for publication. In fact, it is advisable in many circumstances to recommend to stakeholders that the evaluation report take the form of such a paper so that publication is an option. In this regard, successful programs can be shared with the larger profession of health promotion. Ultimately, stakeholders will determine the format of the report (technical report, journal article, news release, meeting, presentation, press conference, letter, or workshop, etc.) as well as the criteria that will define program success. Often, an oral presentation will accompany the submission of a final evaluation report and at times, more than one method is selected in order to meet the needs of all stakeholders. For example, following an innovative worksite health promotion program, the evaluator might prepare a story for the worksite newsletter, a letter of findings to all staff who participated, a technical report for the funding source, and an executive summary for the administrators.

Evaluators must be able to communicate to all audiences when presenting the results of the evaluation. The reaction of each audience—participants, media, administrators, funding sources—must be anticipated in order to prepare the necessary information. In some cases, technical information must be included; in other cases, anecdotal information may be appropriate. The evaluator must fit the report to the audience as well as prepare for a negative response if the results of the evaluation are not favorable. This involves looking critically at the results and developing responses to anticipated reactions.

Designing the Written Report

As previously mentioned, the evaluation report follows a similar format to that used in a scientific or research report. The evaluation report generally includes the following sections:

- *Abstract or executive summary:* This is a summary of the total evaluation including goals and objectives, methods, results, conclusions, and recommendations. It is a concise presentation of the evaluation because it may be the only portion of the report that some of the stakeholders read. Most abstracts/executive summaries range in length from 200 to 500 words.

- *Introduction:* This section of the report contains a complete description of the program including background information as well as rationale or justification for the program and its evaluation. Goals and objectives of the program are listed, as well as the evaluation questions to be answered.

- *Methods/procedures:* This section includes information on the evaluation design, priority populations, instruments used, and how the data were collected and analyzed.

- *Results:* This section is the most critical component of the report. It includes the findings from the evaluation, summarizing and simplifying the data and presenting them in a clear, concise format. Data are presented for each evaluation or research question. If null and alternative hypotheses were developed as part of the evaluation or research, they are also explained and answered as part of this section.

- *Conclusions/recommendations:* This section interprets the results (presented in the previous section) to determine significance and provide explanations for what was found. Judgments and recommendations are included in this section and may be based on findings from other studies, other literature previously published, or related theories.

Box 15.3 summarizes what is included in the evaluation report.

Box 15.3	WHAT TO INCLUDE IN THE EVALUATION REPORT

Abstract/executive summary	Overview of the program and evaluation
	General results, conclusions, and recommendations
Introduction	Purpose of the evaluation
	Rationale or justification for the evaluation
	Program and participant description (including staff, materials, activities, procedures, etc.)
	Goals and objectives
	Evaluation questions
Methods/procedures	Design of the evaluation
	Priority population
	Instrumentation, including information on validity and reliability
	Sampling procedures
	Data collection procedures
	Pilot study results
	Data analyses procedures
Results	Description of findings from data analyses
	Answers to evaluation questions
	Addresses any special concerns
	Explanation of findings
	Charts and graphs of findings
Conclusions/ recommendations	Interpretation of results
	Conclusions about program effectiveness
	Limitations
	Program recommendations
	Determining if additional information is needed

Presenting Data

The data that have been collected and analyzed are presented in the evaluation report. Data presentation should be simple and straightforward. Graphic displays and tables may be used to illustrate certain findings; in fact, they are often a central part of the report. They also often make it easier for the readers of a written report or the audience of an oral report to understand the findings of the evaluation. Graphic displays should be self-explanatory. In fact, it is usually ill-advised to describe in the text too much of what is already displayed in a table or figure. When presenting the data in graphic form it is often helpful to include a frame of reference—such as a comparison with national, state, local, or other data—and explain any limitations of the data. If graphic displays are used in a report, it is recommended (USDHHS, CDC, n. d.) that such displays are appropriate for the results:

- Use horizontal bar charts to focus attention on how one category differs from another.

- Use vertical bar charts to focus attention on a change in a variable over time.

Box 15.4 GUIDELINES FOR PRESENTING DATA

1. Use graphic methods of presenting numerical data whenever possible.

2. Build the results and discussion section of the evaluation report—and perhaps other sections as well—around tables and figures. Prepare the tables and graphs first; then write text to explain them.

3. Make each table and figure self-explanatory. Use a clear, complete title, a key, labels, footnotes, and so forth.

4. Discuss in the text the major information to be found in each table and figure.

5. Experiment with, and consider using, as many graphs as you have the time and ingenuity to prepare. Not only do they communicate clearly to your audiences, they also help you see what is happening.

6. Because graphs tend to convey fewer details than numerical tables, consider providing both tables and graphs for the same data, where appropriate.

7. If you have used a mixed evaluation design with both quantitative and qualitative data collection procedures, use the direct quotations and descriptions from the qualitative results to add depth and clarity to information reported graphically.

8. When presenting complicated graphs to a live audience, give some instruction about how to read the graph and a few sample interpretations of simpler versions, then present the real data.

9. When a complete draft of the report has been completed, ask yourself the following questions:
   a. Do the figure titles give a comprehensive description of the figures? Could someone browsing through the report understand the graphs?
   b. Are both axes of every graph clearly labeled with a name?
   c. Is the interval size marked on all axes of graphs?
   d. Is the number of cases on which each summary statistic has been based indicated in each table or on each graph?
   e. Are the tables and figures labeled and numbered throughout the report?
   f. If the report is a lengthy one, does it include a list of tables and figures at the front following the table of contents?

Source: How to Communicate Evaluation Findings. Lynn Lyons Morris. Copyright © 1987 by Sage Publications Inc.. Reprinted with permission.

- Use cluster bar charts to contrast one variable among multiple subgroups.

- Use line graphs to plot data for several periods and show a trend over time.

- Use pie charts to show the distribution of a set of events or a total quantity.

If many tables or graphs are included, only the most relevant should be inserted in the text of the report with the remainder placed in an appendix. **Box 15.4** lists guidelines to follow when presenting data in the evaluation report and/or presentation.

How and When to Present the Report

Evaluators must carefully consider the logistics of presenting the evaluation findings and should discuss this with the stakeholders involved in the evaluation. An evaluator may be in the position of presenting negative results, encountering distrust among staff members, or submitting a report that will never be read. Following are several suggestions for enhancing the evaluation report:

- Give key stakeholders advance information on the findings; this increases the likelihood that the information will be processed most appropriately. Avoid releasing any information to media outlets until all stakeholders have had an opportunity to read and discuss findings.

- Maintain anonymity of individuals, institutions, and organizations; use sensitivity to avoid judging or labeling people in negative ways; maintain confidentiality of the final report according to the wishes of administrators; and maintain objectivity throughout the report (Windsor et al., 2004).

- Choose ways to report the evaluation findings so as to meet the needs of diverse stakeholders, and include information that is relevant to each group.

Increasing Utilization of the Results

Far too often an evaluation will be conducted and a report submitted to the stakeholders without the recommendations being implemented. This occurs for a variety of reasons. Evaluators may not use findings because they are conducting the evaluation only to fulfill the requirements of the funding source, to serve their own self-interest, or to gain recognition for a successful program. If decision makers do not press those responsible for the program to make improvements, those implementing the program may not feel inclined to go to the trouble of making the necessary changes. Those who are given the evaluation results for their program may find that they are unable to make sense of the report due to language and concepts that are unfamiliar to them. Weiss (1984) developed the following guidelines to increase the chances that evaluation results will actually be used:

1. Plan the study with program stakeholders in mind and involve them in the planning process.

2. Continue to gather information about the program after the planning stage; a change in the program should result in a change in the evaluation.

3. Focus the evaluation on conditions about the program that the decision makers can change.

4. Write reports in a clear, simple manner and submit them on time. Use graphs and charts within the text and include complicated statistical information in an appendix.

5. Base the decision on whether to make recommendations on how specific and clear the data are, how much is known about the program, and whether differences between programs are obvious. A joint interpretation between evaluator and stakeholders may be best.

6. Disseminate the results to all stakeholders, using a variety of methods.

7. Integrate evaluation findings with other research and evaluation as they relate to the program focus.

8. Provide high-quality research.

SUMMARY

Evaluation questions developed in the early program planning stages can be answered once the data have been analyzed. Descriptive statistics can be used to summarize or describe the data, and inferential statistics can be used to generate or test hypotheses and infer and transfer findings to the broader population. These statistics are generated by applying the appropriate univariate, bivariate, and/or multivariate analyses. Evaluators then interpret the data and present the results to the stakeholders via a formal or informal report.

REVIEW QUESTIONS

1. What are some common problems with evaluations, and how can these problems be reduced or overcome?

2. What is meant by the term *data management*?

3. What is the difference between descriptive statistics and inferential statistics?

4. What are some types of univariate data analyses used in evaluation? When would these be used?

5. How are bivariate and multivariate data analyses used in evaluation?

6. Explain the concepts of hypothesis testing, level of significance, Type I error, and Type II error.

7. What are the roles of evaluators and stakeholders in interpreting program results and making recommendations?

8. What is the difference between statistical significance and program significance?

9. What information is included in the written evaluation report? How is the information modified for various audiences?

10. What are some guidelines for presenting data in an evaluation report?

11. How can the evaluation report be enhanced?

12. How can the evaluator increase the likelihood of utilization of the evaluation findings?

ACTIVITIES

1. Obtain an actual report from a program evaluation (perhaps in a data-based article in a scientific journal pertaining to health promotion). Look for the type of statistical tests used, level of significance, independent and dependent variables, interpretation of the findings, recommendations, and format for the report.

2. Discuss evaluation with a decision maker from a health agency. Find out what types of evaluation the agency conducted, who has conducted them, what the findings have been, whether the findings were implemented, and how the information was reported.

3. Compare an evaluation report with a research report (e.g., perhaps a peer-reviewed journal article). What are the similarities and differences? How could you improve the report?

4. Using data that you have generated or data presented by your instructor, create one table and one graph.

WEBLINKS

1. http://www.astho.org/

   Association of State and Territorial Health Officials (ASTHO)

   ASTHO is the national nonprofit organization representing the state and territorial public health agencies of the United States, the U.S. territories, and the District of Columbia. ASTHO's members are the chief health officials of these jurisdictions. At this site you can link to all the state and territorial public health agencies where you can find various examples of the presentation of health data using charts, graphs, and tables.

2. http://www.cancercontrol.cancer.gov/index.html

   National Cancer Institute (NCI)

   NCI's Website provides information on cancer control and population sciences, including evaluation/research reports on a number of cancer-related programs.

3. http://www.adb.org/Evaluation/reports/

   Asian Development Bank (ADB)

   The ADB, established 1966, is a multilateral development finance institution dedicated to reducing poverty in Asia and the Pacific. At this Website you can find a number of the final evaluation reports created by the ADB related to health programs implemented outside the United States. These reports provide good examples of how final evaluation reports are formatted. Some of the reports deal with health-related topics.

4. http://www.cdc.gov/Learning/

   Centers for Disease Control and Prevention (CDC Learning Connection)

   This is a CDC Webpage where you can access information related to concepts described in this chapter.

5. http://www.cdc.gov/nchs/

   National Center for Health Statistics (NCHS)

   This Website is a rich source of information about America's health and provides many examples of the presentation of health data.

6. http://www.nhtsa.gov/

   State Traffic Safety Information (STSI)

   This is NHTSA's National Center for Statistical Analysis Website. STSI presents a state-by-state profile of traffic safety data and information including crash statistics, economic costs, legislation status, funding programs, and more. You'll find lots of examples of the presentation of health data using charts, graphs, and tables.

Code of Ethics for the Health Education Profession

Preamble

The Health Education profession is dedicated to excellence in the practice of promoting individual, family, group, organizational, and community health. Guided by common goals to improve the human condition, Health Educators are responsible for upholding the integrity and ethics of the profession as they face the daily challenges of making decisions. Health Educators value diversity in society and embrace a multiplicity of approaches in their work to support the worth, dignity, potential, and uniqueness of all people.

The Code of Ethics provides a framework of shared values within the professions in which Health Education is practiced. The Code of Ethics is grounded in fundamental ethical principles including: promoting justice, doing good, and avoidance of harm. The responsibility of each health educator is to aspire to the highest possible standards of conduct and to encourage the ethical behavior of all those with whom they work.

Regardless of job title, professional affiliation, work setting, or population served, Health Educators should promote and abide by these guidelines when making professional decisions.

Article I: Responsibility to the Public

A Health Educator's responsibilities are to educate, promote, maintain, and improve the health of individuals, families, groups and communities. When a conflict of issues arises among individuals, groups, organizations, agencies, or institutions, health educators must consider all issues and give priority to those that promote the health and well-being of individuals and the public while respecting both the principles of individual autonomy, human rights and equality.

Section 1

Health Educators support the right of individuals to make informed decisions regarding their health, as long as such decisions pose no risk to the health of others.

Section 2

Health Educators encourage actions and social policies that promote maximizing health benefits and eliminating or minimizing preventable risks and disparities for all affected parties.

Section 3

Health Educators accurately communicate the potential benefits, risks and/or consequences

Source: The Coalition of National Health Education Organizations, Ethics Task Force, February 8, 2011. www.cnheo.org/. Reprinted by permission.

associated with the services and programs that they provide.

Section 4

Health Educators accept the responsibility to act on issues that can affect the health of individuals, families, groups and communities.

Section 5

Health Educators are truthful about their qualifications and the limitations of their education, expertise and experience in providing services consistent with their respective level of professional competence.

Section 6

Health Educators are ethically bound to respect, assure, and protect the privacy, confidentiality, and dignity of individuals.

Section 7

Health Educators actively involve individuals, groups, and communities in the entire educational process in an effort to maximize the understanding and personal responsibilities of those who may be affected.

Section 8

Health Educators respect and acknowledge the rights of others to hold diverse values, attitudes, and opinions.

Article II: Responsibility to the Profession

Health Educators are responsible for their professional behavior, for the reputation of their profession, and for promoting ethical conduct among their colleagues.

Section 1

Health Educators maintain, improve, and expand their professional competence through continued study and education; membership, participation, and leadership in professional organizations; and involvement in issues related to the health of the public.

Section 2

Health Educators model and encourage nondiscriminatory standards of behavior in their interactions with others.

Section 3

Health Educators encourage and accept responsible critical discourse to protect and enhance the profession.

Section 4

Health Educators contribute to the profession by refining existing and developing new practices, and by sharing the outcomes of their work.

Section 5

Health Educators are aware of real and perceived professional conflicts of interest, and promote transparency of conflicts.

Section 6

Health Educators give appropriate recognition to others for their professional contributions and achievements.

Section 7

Health educators openly communicate to colleagues, employers and professional organizations when they suspect unethical practice that violates the profession's Code of Ethics.

Article III: Responsibility to Employers

Health Educators recognize the boundaries of their professional competence and are accountable for their professional activities and actions.

Section 1

Health Educators accurately represent their qualifications and the qualifications of others whom they recommend.

Section 2

Health Educators use and apply current evidence-based standards, theories, and guidelines as criteria when carrying out their professional responsibilities.

Section 3

Health Educators accurately represent potential and actual service and program outcomes to employers.

Section 4

Health Educators anticipate and disclose competing commitments, conflicts of interest, and endorsement of products.

Section 5

Health Educators acknowledge and openly communicate to employers, expectations of job-related assignments that conflict with their professional ethics.

Section 6

Health Educators maintain competence in their areas of professional practice.

Section 7

Health Educators exercise fiduciary responsibility and transparency in allocating resources associated with their work.

Article IV: Responsibility in the Delivery of Health Education

Health Educators deliver health education with integrity. They respect the rights, dignity, confidentiality, and worth of all people by adapting strategies and methods to the needs of diverse populations and communities.

Section 1

Health Educators are sensitive to social and cultural diversity and are in accord with the law, when planning and implementing programs.

Section 2

Health Educators remain informed of the latest advances in health education theory, research, and practice.

Section 3

Health educators use strategies and methods that are grounded in and contribute to the development of professional standards, theories, guidelines, data and experience.

Section 4

Health Educators are committed to rigorous evaluation of both program effectiveness and the methods used to achieve results.

Section 5

Health Educators promote the adoption of healthy lifestyles through informed choice rather than by coercion or intimidation.

Section 6

Health Educators communicate the potential outcomes of proposed services, strategies, and pending decisions to all individuals who will be affected.

Section 7

Health educators actively collaborate and communicate with professionals of various educational backgrounds and acknowledge and respect the skills and contributions of such groups.

Article V: Responsibility in Research and Evaluation

Health Educators contribute to the health of the population and to the profession through research and evaluation activities. When planning and conducting research or evaluation, health educators do so in accordance with federal and state laws and regulations, organizational and institutional policies, and professional standards.

Section 1

Health Educators adhere to principles and practices of research and evaluation that do no harm to individuals, groups, society, or the environment.

Section 2

Health Educators ensure that participation in research is voluntary and is based upon the informed consent of the participants.

Section 3

Health Educators respect and protect the privacy, rights, and dignity of research participants, and honor commitments made to those participants.

Section 4

Health Educators treat all information obtained from participants as confidential unless otherwise required by law. Participants are fully informed of the disclosure procedures.

Section 5

Health Educators take credit, including authorship, only for work they have actually performed and give appropriate credit to the contributions of others.

Section 6

Health Educators who serve as research or evaluation consultants maintain confidentiality of results unless permission is granted or in order to protect the health and safety of others.

Section 7

Health Educators report the results of their research and evaluation objectively, accurately, and in a timely fashion to effectively foster the translation of research into practice.

Section 8

Health Educators openly share conflicts of interest in the research, evaluation, and dissemination process.

Article VI: Responsibility in Professional Preparation

Those involved in the preparation and training of Health Educators have an obligation to accord learners the same respect and treatment given other groups by providing quality education that benefits the profession and the public.

Section 1

Health Educators select students for professional preparation programs based upon equal opportunity for all, and the individual's academic performance, abilities, and potential contribution to the profession and the public's health.

Section 2

Health Educators strive to make the educational environment and culture conducive to the health of all involved, and free from all forms of discrimination and harassment.

Section 3

Health Educators involved in professional preparation and development engage in careful planning; present material that is accurate, developmentally and culturally appropriate; provide reasonable and prompt feedback; state clear and reasonable expectations; and conduct fair assessments and prompt evaluations of learners.

Section 4

Health Educators provide objective, comprehensive, and accurate counseling to learners about career opportunities, development, and advancement, and assist learners in securing professional employment or further educational opportunities.

Section 5

Health Educators provide adequate supervision and meaningful opportunities for the professional development of learners.

Approved by the Coalition of National Health Education Organizations February 8, 2011

Task Force Members:
Michael Ballard
Brian Colwell
Suzanne Crouch
Stephen Gambescia
Mal Goldsmith, Chairperson
Marc Hiller
Adrian Lyde
Lori Phillips
Catherine Rasberry
Raymond Rodriquez
Terry Wessel

Glossary

accountability in a partnership arrangement, when each organization performs its work as previously arranged.

accounting the process of recording and summarizing transactions and interpreting their affects on the program budget (Fallon & Zgodzinski, 2012).

accuracy standards "ensure that the evaluation produces findings that are considered correct" (CDC, 1999c, p. 29); a standard of evaluation.

action research see *participatory research*.

action stage a stage of change in which a person has changed overt behavior for less than six months.

active participants those who take part in most group activities.

act of commission doing something you should not be doing.

act of omission not doing something you should be doing.

adjourning last stage of team development "in which teams complete their work and disband, if designed to do so" (Gomez-Mejia & Balkin, 2012, p. 391).

Administrative and Policy Assessment part of the fourth phase of PRECEDE-PROCEED, "an analysis of the policies, resources, and circumstances prevailing in an organizational situation to facilitate or hinder the development of the health program" (Green & Kreuter, 2005, p. G–1).

Advanced level 1 health educator "the level of a health educator with a baccalaureate or master's degree and five years' experience or more in the field of health education" (NCHEC, SOPHE, & AAHE, 2006, p. 56).

Advanced level 2 health educator "the level of a health educator with a doctoral degree and five years' experience or more in the field of health education" (NCHEC, SOPHE, & AAHE, 2006, p. 56).

advisory board see *planning committee*.

alpha level the level of statistical significance (usually set at .01 or .05).

alternative hypothesis the hypothesis that holds there is a difference between groups, treatments, or interventions.

analysis of variance (ANOVA) a statistical test used to study group differences when the dependent variables involved represent interval or ratio data.

anonymity exists when there is no link between personal information and the person's identity.

APEX-PH Assessment Protocol for Excellence in Public Health—a planning model developed by the National Association of County and City Health Officials in 1991 for city and county health departments.

approaches refers to formative, process, and summative evaluation and suggests these types of evaluation are clearly distinct.

attitude objective those that describe the desired attitude of those in the priority population.

attitude toward the behavior "the degree to which performance of the behavior is positively or negatively valued" (Ajzen, 2006).

audit "review and confirmation that financial reports are accurate and that standard accounting procedures were used to prepare the reports" (Johnson & Breckon, 2007, p. 288).

aversive stimulus unpleasant consequence of a behavior.

awareness objective those that describe of what those in the priority population will become aware.

barriers things that keep people from obtaining the product or adopting a behavior.

baseline data data collected prior to program implementation to serve as a comparison with data collected during the program, or more typically, with data collected at the completion of a program.

basic priority rating (BPR) a model used to prioritize needs assessment data.

behavior change theories "specify the relationships among causal processes operating both within and across levels of analysis" (McLeroy, Steckler et al., 1992, p. 3).

behavioral capability the knowledge and skills necessary to perform a behavior.

behavioral objective an impact objective that describes the action or behavior in which the priority population will engage.

beneficence doing good.

benefits value or outcome the priority population receives as a result of obtaining the product.

best experiences interventions from prior or existing programs of others that have not gone through the critical research and evaluation studies and thus fall short of best practice criteria but nonetheless show promise in being effective.

best practices "recommendations for an intervention, based on critical review of multiple research and evaluation studies that substantiate the efficacy of the intervention in the populations and circumstances in which the studies were done, if not its effectiveness in other populations and situations where it might be implemented" (Green & Kreuter, 2005, p. G–1).

best processes original intervention strategies that the planners create on their own based on their knowledge and skills of good planning processes.

bias a preference that inhibits impartiality.

bivariate data analysis analysis of two variables.

blind an evaluation wherein participants do not know if they belong to the experimental group or control group.

bottom up see *grassroots*.

BPR model 2.0 an updated version of the basic priority rating (see *basic priority rating*).

brand "name, term, design, symbol, or any other feature that identifies one seller's good or service as distinct from those of other sellers." (American Marketing Association, 2007)

budget a "formal statement of the estimated revenues and expenditures" (Johnson & Breckon, 2007, p. 170).

canned program one that has been developed by an outside group and includes the basic components and materials necessary to implement it.

capacity the individual, organizational, and community resources that enable a community to take action.

capacity building activities that enhance the resources of individuals, organizations, and communities to improve their effectiveness in taking action.

categorical funding funds that are earmarked or dedicated to support programs aimed at a specific health problem or determinant (i.e., risk factor).

census everyone in a population.

chi-square a statistical test that measures the association between two nominal and/or ordinal variables.

citizen initiated see *grassroots*.

cluster sampling a probability sample that selects participants from a sampling frame as groups not individuals.

coalition "a formal alliance of organizations that come together to work for a common goal" (Butterfoss, 2007, p. 30).

codes of practice guidelines or criteria for offering a certain type of program.

communication channel route through which a message is delivered to a priority population.

community a "group of people who have common characteristics" (Turnock, 2009, p. 502).

community advocacy a process in which the people of a community become involved in the institutions and decisions that will impact their lives.

community building an "orientation to community that is strength based rather than need based and stresses the identification, nurturing, and celebration of community assets" (Minkler, 2005b, p. 4).

community capacity the "characteristics of communities that affect their ability to identify, mobilize, and address social and public health problems" (Goodman et al., 1998, p. 259).

community development a "process designed to create conditions of economic and social progress for the whole community with its active participation and fullest possible reliance on the community's initiative" (United Nations, 1955, p. 6).

community empowerment when community members control decision making.

community forum a process that brings people from the priority population to discuss problems and needs.

community organization the "process by which community groups are helped to identify common problems or goals, mobilize resources, and in other ways develop and implement strategies for reaching the goals they have collectively set" (Minkler et al., 2008, p. 288).

community organizing the process of community organization.

comparison group as part of a summative evaluation or research study, a nonequivalent group (not randomly selected) that does not receive the treatment or program but is compared with the experimental group.

Competency Update Project (CUP) a six-year, multiphase process carried out by the health education profession in order to reverify the role of the entry-level health educator and to distinguish it from the role of the advanced-level health educator.

competition alternative choices for filling a need; programs or products that send messages that conflict with the behaviors program planners are promoting.

concepts primary elements or the building blocks of a theory (Glanz et al., 2008b).

concurrent validity a form of criterion validity in which a new instrument and an established valid instrument that measure the same characteristics are given to the same population and the new instrument correlates positively with the established instrument.

conditions a major component of an objective that describes when or how the outcome will be observed.

confidentiality exists when there is a link between personal information and the person's identity but that information is protected from others.

confounding variable "one that has an unpredictable or unexpected impact on the dependent variable" (Cottrell & McKenzie, 2011, p. 324).

construct a concept developed, created, or adopted for use with a specific theory (Kerlinger, 1986).

construct validity "the degree to which a measure correlates with other measures it is theoretically expected to correlate with" (Valente, 2002, p. 161).

consumer orientation a dedicated effort to understand a priority population prior to developing an intervention and then keeping this knowledge at the center of all program planning decisions.

consumer-based planning a planning process that incorporates the wants, needs, and preferences of the priority population directly into interventions and implementation.

contemplation stage a stage of change in which a person intends to take action in the next six months.

content validity the "assessment of the correspondence between the items composing the instrument and the content domain from which the items were selected" (DiIorio, 2005, p. 213).

contest a challenge between two individuals/groups in which the object is to try to outperform the competitor.

context assesses the presence of any confounding factors.

contingencies what happens if the objectives in a behavior change contract are either met or not met.

continuum theories those that identify variables that influence action and combine them into a prediction equation (Weinstein et al., 1998).

contract an agreement between two or more parties that outlines the future behavior of those parties.

control group as part of a summative evaluation or research study, a randomly selected group of individuals, similar to the experimental group that does not receive the treatment or program but is compared with the experimental group.

convergent validity "the extent to which two measures that purport to be measuring the same topic correlate (that is, converge)" (Bowling, 2005, p. 12).

correlation represents the strength and direction of relationships between two variables.

cost-benefit analysis (CBA) measures dollars spent on a program versus dollars saved or gained.

cost-effectiveness analysis (CEA) measures dollars spent on a program versus the impact achieved.

cost-identification analysis compares interventions to determine which is least expensive in the context of impact achieved.

criterion a major component of an objective that describes how much change will occur.

criterion-related validity the "extent to which data generated from a measurement instrument are correlated with the data generated from a measure (criterion) of the phenomenon being studied, usually an individual's behavior or performance" (Cottrell & McKenzie, 2011, p. 322).

critical path method (CPM) similar to PERT (see *PERT*) but focuses on total time to complete the tasks and the critical dependent tasks.

cultural audit an evaluation of the assumptions, values, normative philosophies, and cultural characteristics of an organization in order to determine whether they support or hinder that organization's central mission (Business Dictionary, 2011).

cultural competence "a developmental process defined as a set of values, principles, behaviors, attitudes, and policies that enable health professionals to work effectively across racial, ethnic and linguistically diverse populations" (Joint Committee, 2012).

culturally competent see *cultural competence*.

culturally sensitive relevant and acceptable within the cultural framework.

culture the "patterned ways of thought and behavior that characterize a social group, which are learned through socialization processes and persist through time" (Coreil, Bryant, & Henderson, 2001, p. 29).

curriculum "a planned set of lessons or courses designed to lead to competence in an area of study" (Gilbert et al., 2011, p. 412).

data management the process of organizing, coding, and cleaning data in a useable format for the purpose of analysis and reporting.

decision makers those who have the authority to approve a plan (e.g., administrator of an organization, governing board, chief executive officer).

decisional balance refers to the pros and cons of behavioral change.

deductive applying a generally accepted principle to an individual case.

Delphi technique a "group process that generates a consensus through a series of questionnaires" (Gilmore 2012, p. 82).

dependent variable an outcome variable or end result indicator in an evaluation or study.

descriptive statistics data used to organize, summarize, and describe characteristics of a group.

designs forms of different types of summative evaluation.

diffusion theory explains a pattern for how innovations (e.g., products) are adopted in a population.

direct reinforcement consequence given in a specific situation to increase a behavior.

disability "often defined on the basis of specific activities of daily living, work and other functions essential to full participation in community-based living" (USDHHS, 2005, p. 4).

discriminant validity "requires that the construct should not correlate with dissimilar (discriminant) variables" (Bowling, 2005, p. 12).

disincentive consequence for not acting in a certain way; also used as a means to discourage the consumer from purchasing a product or behaving in a certain way.

doers those who are willing to take on work to complete a task.

dose the number of program units delivered.

double blind study an evaluation wherein neither participants nor those implementing the program know which group is experimental and which group is the control.

early adopters in diffusion theory, the second group of people to adopt the innovation; often comprised of opinion leaders.

early majority in diffusion theory, the people who are interested in the innovation, but will need external motivation to become involved.

ecological framework see *socio-ecological approach*.

educational and ecological assessment the third phase of PRECEDE-PROCEED wherein planners identify predisposing, reinforcing, and enabling factors that contribute to problems identified in earlier phases of the model.

effectiveness in evaluation, a measure usually associated with the outcomes of a program—that is, did the program result in changes in awareness, knowledge, attitudes, skills, or especially behavior, and did the program result in improved health status (e.g., less mortality, morbidity, and disability).

efficacy expectations people's competency feelings.

elaboration amount of cognitive processing people put into receiving messages.

emotional-coping responses dealing with sources of anxiety that surround a behavior.

enabling factor "any characteristic of the environment that facilitates action and any skill or resource required to attain a specific behavior" (Green & Kreuter, 2005, p. G–3).

entry-level health educator those who are taking their first professional position in health education and possess a baccalaureate or master's degree and less than five years' experience.

environmental objective an impact objective that describes how the environments (e.g., economic, emotional, physical, political, service, social) around the priority population will change.

epidemiological assessment the second phase of PRECEDE-PROCEED, wherein planners identify specific health goals or problems that contribute to the social goals or problems identified in Phase 1; and "the identification of etiological factors, or determinants of health in the genetics, behavioral patterns, and environment of the population" (Green & Kreuter, 2005, pp. 11–12).

epidemiology "the study of the distribution and determinants of health-related states or events in specific populations, and the application of this study to control health problems" (Last, 2007, p. 111).

ethical issues situations where competing values are at play and program planners need to make a judgment about what is the most appropriate course of action.

evaluation the "comparison of an object of interest against a standard of acceptability" (Green & Lewis, 1986, p. 362)—may be formative (including process evaluation) or summative in nature.

evaluation approach refers to the use of process, formative, or summative evaluation and suggests these types of evaluation are clearly distinct.

evaluation consultant an external evaluator.

evaluation design used to organize the summative evaluation and to provide for planned, systematic data collection, analysis, and reporting.

evidence a body of data that can be used to make decisions about planning.

evidence-based practice process of systematically finding, appraising, and using evidence as the basis for decision making when planning a health promotion program (Cottrell & McKenzie, 2011).

exchange process of the marketer providing a product and its benefits to the consumer in trade for the consumer paying a price.

executive participants core group who are committed to resolution of the concern.

expectancies values people place on an expected outcome.

expenditure a cost incurred while planning, implementing, or evaluating a program.

expectations anticipation of certain outcomes from a certain behavior.

experimental design random assignment to experimental and control groups with measurement of both groups.

experimental group as part of a summative evaluation or research study, a group of individuals that receives the treatment or intervention.

external audit one conducted by an independent qualified accountant usually just once a year (Businessdictionary.com, 2011a).

external evaluation evaluation conducted by an individual or organization not affiliated with the organization conducting the program.

external personnel individuals from outside the planning agency/organization or people from within the priority population.

external validity extent to which the program can be expected to produce similar effects in other populations.

face validity if, on the face, a measure appears to measure what it is supposed to measure (McDermott & Sarvela, 1999).

fairness whether a measure is "appropriate for the individuals of various ethnic groups with different backgrounds, gender, educational levels, etc." (Torabi, 1994, p. 56).

feasibility standards "ensure that the evaluation is viable and pragmatic" (CDC, 1999c, p. 27); a standard of evaluation.

fidelity ensures that programs are implemented either as intended or as per protocol.

field study the most strenuous form of pilot testing in which people from the priority population assess the process being tested in a setting that is just like or closely represents the setting in which the program will be implemented.

financial management "the process of developing and using systems to ensure that funds are spent for the purposes for which they have been appropriated" (Klingner et al., 2010, p. 88).

fiscal accountability "the extent to which resources are managed according to the budget" (Issel, 2009, p. 323).

fiscal year (or funding year) 12 months of financial transactions typically running from either January 1st to December 31st or July 1st to June 30th.

flex time a system in which employees can vary their work schedule to meet their personal needs.

flexibility in terms of program planning, a process that is adapted to the needs of stakeholders.

fluidity in terms of program planning, a process that is sequential and logical in nature.

focus group an "exploratory process that is used for generating hypotheses, uncovering attitudes and opinions, and acquiring and testing new ideas" (Gilmore 2012, p. 118).

formative evaluation "any combination of measurements obtained and judgments made before or during the implementation of materials, methods, activities, or programs to control, assure or improve the quality of performance or delivery" (Green & Lewis, 1986, p. 362).

formative research a process that identifies differences among subgroups within a population, identifies a subgroup, determines the wants and needs of the subgroup, and identifies factors that influence its behavior, including benefits, barriers, and readiness to change (Bryant, 1998).

forming first stage of team development "which brings the team members together so they can get acquainted and discuss their expectations" (Gomez-Mejia & Balkin, 2012, p. 390).

Framework a shortened name for the *A Competency-Based Framework for Health Education Specialists—2010* (NCHEC, SOPHE, & AAHE, 2010).

full-time equivalent a unit of measurement that is calculated by dividing the average number of hours a person works by the average number of hours worked by a full-time employee.

functionality in terms of program planning, an assurance that the outcome of planning is improved health conditions, not just the production of a program plan.

Gantt chart a program management charting method that provides a graphical illustration of the time frame for tasks to be completed and what has been completed to date.

gatekeepers those who control, both formally and informally, the political climate of a community.

generalizability extent to which a program can be expected to produce similar effects in other populations.

Genetic Information Nondiscrimination Act of 2008 (GINA) (Public Law 110–233) amends portions of HIPAA by treating genetic information as protected health information, prohibits discrimination in health coverage and employment based on genetic information.

gifts sums of money or nonmonetary items that are given voluntarily without compensation.

goal general statement of intent (Neiger & Thackeray, 1998).

grant an award of financial assistance, the principal purpose of which is to transfer a thing of value from the grantor to a recipient to carry out a specific purpose (USDHHS, 2011a).

grantsmanship the ability to write grant proposals that are funded.

grassroots the creation of political "movement" in which those within the community are responsible for the organizing

Guide to Community Preventive Services (Community Guide) the "body of evidence and recommendations approved by the Task Force on Community Preventive Services" (Zara et al., 2005, p. 479).

hard money an ongoing source of funding that is part of the operating budget.

health advocacy "the processes by which the actions of individuals or groups attempt to bring about social and/or organizational change on behalf of a particular health goal, program, interest, or population" (Joint Committee on Terminology, 2012).

health assessments (HAs) include instruments known as health risk appraisals/assessments (HRAs), health status assessments (HSAs), various lifestyle-specific assessment instruments, and wellness and behavioral/habit inventories (SPMBoD, 1999).

health behavior behaviors that impact a person's health.

health communication the use of strategies to inform and influence individual and community decisions to enhance health (NCI, 2002).

health communication model a four-phase program planning model for health communication developed by the National Cancer Institute.

health education "any combination of planned learning experiences based on sound theories that provide individuals, groups, and communities the opportunity to acquire knowledge and the skills needed to make quality health decisions" (Joint Committee on Terminology, 2012).

health education specialist "someone having completed the education and/or training requirements currently associated with professionally prepared" (Hezel, 2007, p. 8).

health educator a "professionally prepared individual who serves in a variety of roles and is specifically trained to use appropriate educational strategies and methods to facilitate the development of policies, procedures, interventions, and systems conducive to the health of individuals, groups, and communities" (Joint Committee on Terminology, 2001, p. 100).

health impact assessment "a combination of procedures, methods, and tools by which a policy, program, or project may be judged as to its potential effects on the health of a population, and the distribution of those effects within the population" (ECHP,1999).

Health Insurance Portability and Accountability Act of 1996 (HIPAA) (Public Law 104–191) sets national standards that health plans, health care clearinghouses, and health care providers who conduct certain health care transactions electronically must implement to protect and guard against the misuse of individually identifiable health information.

health literacy the capacity to obtain, process, and understand basic health information and services to make appropriate health decisions (USD-HHS, 2000).

health numeracy "the degree to which individuals have the capacity to access, process, interpret, communicate, and act on numerical, quantitative, graphical, biostatistical, and probabilistic health information needed to make effective health decisions" (Golbeck et al., 2005, p. 375).

health promotion "any planned combination of educational, political, environmental, regulatory, or organizational mechanisms that support actions and conditions of living conducive to the health of individuals, groups, and communities" (Joint Committee on Terminology, 2012).

Healthy Communities a movement that began in the 1980s with assistance from the World Health Organization to mobilize and empower partnerships within cities and communities to enhance health and well-being.

Healthy People U.S. government publication that brought together much of what was known about the relationship of personal health behavior and health status.

Healthy Plan-It a six-phase planning model developed by the Centers for Disease Control and Prevention in 2000 to strengthen in-country management training capacity in the health sector of developing countries.

impact evaluation evaluation that focuses on the immediate observable effects of a program (e.g., awareness, knowledge, attitudes, skills, environment, and behaviors) leading to the intended outcomes of a program (Green & Lewis, 1986).

impact objectives a category of objectives comprised of learning (i.e., awareness, knowledge, attitudes, and skills), behavioral, and environmental objectives.

implementation the "act of converting planning, goals, and objectives into action through administrative structure, management activities, policies, procedures, regulations, and organizational actions of new programs" (Timmreck, 1997, p. 328).

incentives reward for achieving a goal; also used as a means to entice the consumer to purchase the product or adopt a behavior.

inclusion ensures that the right partners are involved with a program.

independent variable a variable that is manipulated, selected, or measured by the evaluator that causes or exerts some influence on the dependent variable.

inductive individual cases are studied to formulate a general principle.

inferential statistics data used to determine relationships and causality in order to make generalizations or inferences about a population based on findings from a sample.

influencers those who control resources to facilitate the planning and implementation of a program.

informed consent requires: "(1) Disclosure of relevant information to prospective subjects about the research [program]; (2) their comprehension of the information; and (3) their voluntary agreement, free of coercion and undue influence, to research [program] participation" (NIH, 2006, para. 1).

in-house materials educational materials developed by the program planners.

in-kind contributions nonmonetary gifts.

innovators in diffusion theory, the very first people to adopt the innovation.

inputs in a logic model, the resources that are used to plan, implement, and evaluate a program.

institutional review board (IRB) group of individuals with authority to grant or deny permission to conduct evaluation or research; it serves to safeguard the rights, privacy, health, and well-being of those involved in the research.

institutionalized imbedded in the organization so that it becomes sustained and durable.

instrumentation a "collective term that describes all measurement instruments used" (Cottrell & McKenzie, 2011, p. 326).

intention an "indication of a person's readiness to perform a given behavior, and it is considered to be the immediate antecedent of behavior" (Ajzen, 2006).

interactive contact methods data collection methods wherein those collecting the data interact with those from whom the data are being collected.

interaction the degree to which practitioners effectively work and communicate with program participants.

internal audit a frequent and ongoing audit conducted by an employee of the organization not responsible for the accounting practices (BusinessDictionary.com, 2011a).

internal consistency reliability the intercorrelations among individual items on the instrument, that is, whether all items on the instrument are measuring part of the total area.

internal evaluation evaluation conducted by one or more individuals employed by, or in some other way affiliated with, the organization conducting the program.

internal personnel individuals from within the planning agency/organization or from within the priority population.

internal validity degree to which change that was measured can be attributed to the program under investigation.

inter-rater reliability rater reliability using two or more raters.

interval level measures measurement form that puts data into categories that are mutually exclusive, exhaustive, and rank ordered; furthermore, the distance between categories can be measured and there is no absolute zero.

intervention "to come or occur between two things, events, or points in time; to come in or between so as to hinder or alter an action" (Anderson et al., 2002, p. 447).

intervention alignment part of the fourth phase of PRECEDE-PROCEDE wherein planners match appropriate strategies and interventions with projected changes and outcomes identified in earlier phases (Green & Kreuter, 2005).

intervention mapping a six-phase program planning model guided by diagrams and matrices that incorporate outputs of the assessment process with relevant theory to help develop appropriate interventions for priority populations.

intra-rater reliability rater reliability that is established by a single rater.

justification provides assurance that programs are supported by key stakeholders.

key informants strategically placed individuals in a community who have the knowledge and ability to report on the needs of those in the priority population.

knowledge objective an impact objective that describes the information those in the priority population will learn.

laggards in diffusion theory, people who are not very interested in innovation and would be the last to adopt it.

lapse a single slip back to an old behavior while attempting a behavior change.

late majority in diffusion theory, the people who are interested in the innovation but are more skeptical and need external motivation to become involved.

learning objectives a category of objectives composed of four levels: awareness, knowledge, attitudes, and skills.

lesson the amount of material that can be presented during a single educational encounter.

lesson plan the written outline of a lesson.

level of significance see *alpha level*.

levels of measurement a hierarchy of four measurement levels: nominal, ordinal, interval, and ratio.

likelihood of taking recommended preventive health action weighing the threat of disease against the difference between benefits and barriers.

literacy "the ability to use printed and written information to function in society, to achieve one's goals, and to develop one's knowledge and potential" (White & Dillow, 2005, p. 4).

literature the articles, books, and other documents that explain the past and current knowledge about a particular topic.

locality development a form of community organizing that is "heavily process oriented, stressing consensus, and cooperation and aimed at building group identity and a sense of community" (Minkler & Wallerstein, 2005, p. 30).

locus of control perception of the center of control over reinforcement.

logic model "a systematic and visual way to present and share your understanding of the relationships among the resources you have to operate your program, the activities you plan, and the changes or results you hope to achieve" (WKKF, 2004, p. 1).

macro practice methods of professional change that deal with issues beyond the individual, family, and small group level.

maintenance stage a stage of change in which a person has changed overt behavior for more than six months.

management "the process of assembling and using sets of resources in a goal-directed manner to accomplish tasks in an organizational setting" (Hitt, Black, & Porter, 2012, p. 483).

MAP-IT a planning guide or model used to assist communities in adapting *Healthy People 2020*.

MAPP Mobilizing for Action through Planning and Partnerships—a six-phase program planning model developed by the National Association of County and City Health Officials in 2001.

mapping the visual representation of data by geography or location, linking information to a place (Kirschenbaum & Russ, 2005).

mapping community capacity a process of identifying community assets.

market "the set of all people who have an actual or potential interest in a product or service" (Kotler & Clarke, 1987, p. 108).

marketing a "set of processes for creating, communicating, and delivering value to customers" (American Marketing Association, 2007).

marketing mix combination of the product, price, place, and promotion.

mean the arithmetic average of all scores in data analysis.

measurement the method or procedure of assigning numbers to objects, events, and people (Green & Lewis, 1986).

measurement instrument the item used to measure the variables.

measures of central tendency forms of univariate data analysis involving the mean, median, and mode.

measures of spread or variation how spread out the scores are in the data set.

median the midpoint of all scores in data analysis.

memorandum of understanding (MOU) (or memorandum of agreement [MOA]) "a document that describes the general principles of an agreement between parties, but does not amount to a substantive contract" (Dictionary.com, 2011).

mission statement a short narrative that describes the general focus or purpose of a program.

mode the score or response that occurs most frequently in data analysis.

model "is a composite, a mixture of ideas or concepts taken from any number of theories and used together" (Hayden, 2009, p. 1).

multiple regression a statistical test that explores the relationships between multiple independent variables and one dependent variable.

multiplicity refers to the number of components or activities that make up an intervention.

multivariate data analysis analysis of more than two variables.

need the "difference between the present situation and a more desirable one" (Gilmore 2012, p. 8).

needs assessment the process of identifying, analyzing, and prioritizing the needs of a priority population.

negative punishment removing a positive reinforcer to decrease a behavior.

negative reinforcement removing a negative reinforcer or aversive stimulus to increase a behavior.

negligence failing to act as a reasonable (prudent) person would.

networking interaction among professionals in order to share information.

news hook event that the media would want to cover.

no contact methods data collection methods wherein those collecting the data have no contact with those from whom the data are collected.

nominal group process a highly structured process in which a few knowledgeable representatives (five to seven) are asked to qualify and quantify specific needs.

nominal level measures measurement form that puts data into categories that are mutually exclusive and exhaustive.

nonexperimental design use of pretest and posttest comparisons, or posttest analysis only, without a control group or comparison group.

nonmaleficence not causing harm.

nonprobability sample a sample in which all members of a survey population do not have an equal and known probability of being selected.

nonproportional stratified random sample a stratified random sample in which the sampling units are selected so that there is equal representation from the strata.

norming third stage of team development "characterized by resolution of conflict and agreement over team goals and values" (Gomez-Mejia & Balkin, 2012, p. 390).

null hypothesis the hypothesis that holds there is no difference between two groups, treatments, or interventions.

numeracy the ability to understand and work with numbers; quantitative literacy.

objectives statements that specify intermediate accomplishments or benchmarks.

observation "notice taken of an indicator" (Green & Lewis, 1986, p. 363).

obtrusive observation when people are aware they are being measured, assessed, or tested.

occasional participants those who become involved on an irregular basis and usually only when major decisions are made.

opinion leaders those who are well respected in a community and can accurately represent the views of the priority population.

ordinal level measures measurement form that put data into categories that are mutually exclusive, exhaustive, and rank ordered.

organizational culture the formal and informal policies of an organization that express the organization's values.

outcome a major component of an objective that describes what will change as a result of the program; also the intended results in a logic model.

outcome evaluation evaluation that focuses on the end result of a program generally measured by improvements in mortality, morbidity, or vital measures of symptoms, signs, or physiological indicators (Green & Lewis, 1986).

outcome expectations value placed on expected outcomes.

outcome objective an objective that describes the change in health status, social benefits, risk factors, or quality of life of the priority population.

outputs the program activities or interventions in a logic model.

ownership a feeling that is derived from participating in the development of a program.

parallel (or equivalent or alternate) forms reliability focuses on whether different forms of the same instrument when measuring the same participants will produce similar results.

participation and relevance "community organizing that 'starts where the people are' and engages community members as equals" (Minkler & Wallerstein, 2005, p. 35).

participatory data collection members of the priority population participate in data collection.

participatory research has been "defined as systematic inquiry, with the collaboration of those affected by the issue being studied, for the purposes of education and of taking action or effecting change" (Mercer et al., 2008, p. 409).

PATCH an acronym for a planning process called Planned Approach to Community Health.

peer education a process wherein individuals are educated by others who have similar characteristics or standing as themselves.

penetration rate number in the priority population exposed or reached.

perceived barriers costs that must be overcome in order to follow a health recommendation.

perceived behavioral control perceived ease or difficulty of performing the behavior.

perceived benefits belief that a certain action could improve one's health.

perceived seriousness/severity belief that if a disease or condition were contracted it could be serious.

perceived susceptibility belief that one is vulnerable to a certain disease or condition.

perceived threat belief that one is vulnerable to a serious health problem or to the sequelae of that illness or condition.

performing fourth stage of team development "characterized by a focus on the performance of the tasks delegated to the team" (Gomez-Mejia & Balkin, 2012, p. 391).

PERT acronym for Program Evaluation and Review Technique; a program management charting method that provides a graphical illustration of the time frame for tasks to be completed that includes three estimates of time—optimistic, pessimistic, and probabilistic.

phased in implementation of a program by limiting the number of people able to start the program at any given time.

photovoice those in the priority population are provided with cameras and skills training, then use the cameras to convey their own images of the community's problems and strengths.

pilot testing a set of procedures used to try out various processes during program development using a small group of participants prior to implementation.

place where the priority population has access to the product or where they may engage in the desired behavior.

planning committee group of individuals who are responsible for creating a program and then overseeing its implementation and evaluation.

planning models those used for planning, implementing, and evaluating programs.

planning parameters the boundaries in which the planning committee must work when planning, implementing, and evaluating the program.

planning team see *planning committee.*

population as it relates to sampling, those in the universe specified by time or place.

population-based approach planning processes used with large populations.

positive punishment adding something to a situation that decreases a behavior.

positive reinforcement a consequence of a behavior that is enjoyable or makes a person feel good.

posttest testing components of a program, service, or product with the priority population after the completion of a program.

potential building blocks located resources originating outside the neighborhood and controlled by people outside.

practical significance refers to how those actually participating in a program will benefit from it.

PRECEDE-PROCEED (Predisposing, Reinforcing, Enabling Constructs in Ecological Diagnosis and Evaluation—Policy, Regulatory, and Organizational Constructs in Educational and Environmental Development) a widely known and robust eight-phase program planning model.

precontemplation stage a stage of change in which a person has no intentions to take action in the next six months.

predictive validity a form of criterion validity in which the measurement used will be correlated with another measurement of the same phenomenon at another time.

predisposing factor "any characteristic of a person or population that motivates behavior prior to the occurrence of the behavior" (Green & Kreuter, 2005, p. G–6).

preliminary review a form of pilot testing in which colleagues of planners review a process being tested.

preparation a stage of change in which a person intends to take action in the next 30 days and has taken some behavioral steps in this decision.

pre-pilot a form of pilot testing in which five or six people from the priority population assess the process being tested.

pre-planning a process carried out prior to the formal planning process that allows a core group of people to gather answers to key planning questions.

pretest testing components of a program, service, or product with the priority population prior to implementation.

pretesting can be defined in one of two ways: (1) getting feedback from the priority population on products, messages, and materials before launching a social marketing campaign, and (2) collecting baseline data prior to program implementation that will be compared with posttest data to measure the effectiveness of programs.

price what the priority population gives up to obtain the product and its associated benefits.

primary building blocks assets located in the neighborhood and largely under the control of those who live in the neighborhood.

primary data original data collected by the planners.

primary prevention measures that forestall the onset of illness or injury during the prepathogenesis period.

priority population the people for whom the program is intended.

probability sample a sample in which all in the survey population have an equal and known probability of being selected.

process evaluation "any combination of measurements obtained during the implementation of program activities to control, assure, or improve the quality of performance or delivery" (Green & Lewis, 1986, p. 364).

process objective an objective that expresses the tasks or activities to be carried out by the program planners.

processes of change a construct of the transtheoretical model that describes the covert and overt activities that people use to progress through the stages of change (Prochaska et al., 2008).

product something (e.g., goods, services, events, experiences, information, ideas, or behaviors) that fulfills a need customers have and provides a benefit they value; obtained for a price in the exchange.

profit margin the percent of financial gain after all the expenses are paid.

program kickoff see *program launch*.

program launch the first day of program implementation.

program ownership a feeling by those in the priority population that the program in part belongs to them.

program rollout see *program launch*.

program significance measures the meaningfulness of a program (based on stakeholder preferences) regardless of statistical significance.

promotion marketing communication strategy for letting a priority population know about a product and how to obtain or purchase it.

proportional stratified random sample a stratified random sample in which the sampling units are selected in the same proportion that the strata exist in the survey population.

proposal a formal written request for funding.

propriety standards "ensure that the evaluation is ethical" (CDC, 1999c, p. 27); a standard of evaluation.

proxy measure an outcome measure that provides evidence that a behavior has occurred.

prudent acting as a reasonable person would act in a given situation.

psychometric qualities an instrument's validity, reliability, and fairness.

public domain available for anyone to use without permission.

punishment any event that follows a behavior which decreases the probability that the same behavior will be repeated in the future.

qualitative data information presented in narrative form used in evaluation to provide detailed summaries or descriptions of observations, interactions, or verbal accounts (e.g., data from focus groups, in-depth interviews).

qualitative measure "tend to produce data in the language of the subjects, rarely with numerical values attached to observations" (Green & Lewis, 1986, p. 151).

qualitative method an inductive method that produces narrative data.

quality in evaluation, a measure usually associated with how a program is implemented and what can be done to improve program delivery.

quantitative data information expressed in numerical terms that can be compared on scales.

quantitative measure "rely on more standardized data collection and reduction techniques, using predetermined questions or observational indicators and established response items" (Green & Lewis, 1986, p. 151).

quantitative method a deductive method that produces numeric data.

quasi-experimental design use of a treatment group and a nonequivalent (nonrandomized) comparison group with measurement of both groups.

random selection a method of selecting participants in which all in the survey population have an equal chance or known probability of being selected.

random-digit dialing a method of selecting participants using random combinations of numbers to call telephone numbers.

randomized controlled trial research designs that include randomization, control groups, and experimental groups.

range the difference between the highest and lowest scores in data analysis.

rater (or observer) reliability associated with the consistent measurement (or rating) of an observed event by the same or different individuals (or judges or raters) (McDermott & Sarvela, 1999).

ratio level measure measurement form that puts data into categories that are mutually exclusive, exhaustive, and rank ordered; furthermore, the distance between categories can be measured and there is an absolute zero.

reach portion of the priority population that has an opportunity to participate in a program.

recidivism slipping back to an old behavior after attempting a behavior change.

reciprocal determinism behavior changes that result from the interaction between the person and the environment.

recruitment making those in the priority population aware of a program.

reforming a phase of team development when the team may continue on by refocusing its efforts on other tasks or problems.

reinforcement any event that follows a behavior which increases the probability that the same behavior will be repeated in the future (Skinner, 1953).

reinforcing factor "any reward or punishment following or anticipated as a consequence of a behavior, serving to strengthen the motivation for the behavior after it occurs" (Green & Kreuter, 2005, p. G–7).

relapse breakdown or failure in a person's attempt to change or modify a behavior (Marlatt & George, 1998).

relapse prevention a self-control program to help individuals to anticipate and cope with the problem of relapse in the behavior change process (Marlatt & George, 1998).

reliability "an empirical estimate of the extent to which an instrument produces the same result (measure or score), applied once or two or more times" (Windsor et al., 2004, p. 93).

request for application (**RFA**) a formal statement that invites grant or cooperative agreement applications for a specific task.

request for proposal (**RFP**) a call made by funding agencies to alert individuals and organizations that it will receive and review grant proposals.

resources the "human, fiscal, and technical assets available" (Johnson & Breckon, 2007, p. 296) to plan, implement, and evaluate a program.

response ensuring that an adequate number of people participate in a program.

return on investment (**ROI**) "measures the costs of a program (i.e., the investment) versus the financial return realized by that program" (Cavallo, 2006, p. 1).

Role Delineation Project a comprehensive process that led to the creation of the responsibilities and competencies of the entry-level health educator.

SAM (suitability assessment of materials) an instrument that can be used to determine the suitability of educational of materials.

sample a part of the whole.

sampling the process of selecting a sample.

sampling frame a list or quasi-list of all sampling units.

sampling unit an element or set of elements considered for selection as part of a sample (Babbie, 1992), for example, an individual, organization, or geographical area.

satisfaction approval after participation.

scope the breadth and depth of the material covered in a curriculum.

secondary building blocks assets located in the neighborhood but largely controlled by people outside.

secondary data those data that have been collected by someone else and are available for use by the planners.

secondary prevention measures that lead to early diagnosis and prompt treatment of a disease, illness, or injury to limit disability, impairment, or dependency and prevent more severe pathogenesis.

seed dollars funds designated to start up a new program or project.

segmentation process of identifying groups of consumers that share similar characteristics and will respond in a like way to a marketing strategy.

segmenting the act of segmentation.

self-assessments a process wherein an individual assesses him/herself.

self-control gaining control over one's own behavior through monitoring and adjusting it.

self-efficacy people's confidence in their ability to perform a certain behavior or task.

self-regulation see *self-control*.

self-reinforcement reinforcing oneself for a behavior performed in an appropriate manner.

self-report when individuals or groups answer questions about themselves.

sensitivity "the ability of the test to identify correctly all screened individuals who actually have the disease [problem]" (Friis & Sellers, 2009, p. 422).

sequence order in which the content of a curriculum is presented.

significant other one who has an important relationship (e.g., friend, family member, partner, spouse) with another.

simple random sample (SRS) most basic process for selecting a random sample.

single-step survey a means of gathering data in which collectors obtain the data from individuals or groups with a single contact.

skill development objective an impact objective that describes the skill those in a priority population will be able to perform.

sliding-scale fee a fee structure based on one's ability to pay.

SMART Social Marketing Assessment and Response Tool—a seven-phase social marketing planning model developed in 1998.

SMART objectives ones that are specific, measurable, achievable, realistic, and time-phased (CDC, 2003).

social action a form of community organizing that "is both task and process oriented" (Minkler & Wallerstein, 2005, p. 30) and deals with organizing a disadvantaged segment of the population.

social assessment the first phase of PRECEDE-PROCEED wherein planners seek to subjectively define the quality of life (problems and priorities) of those in the priority population.

social capital "the relationships and structures within a community, such as civic participation, networks, norms of reciprocity, and trust, that promote cooperation of mutual benefit" (Putnam, 1995, p. 66).

social context "is the sociocultural forces that shape people's day-to-day experiences and that directly and indirectly affect health and behavior (Burke et al., 2009, p. 56S).

social marketing "the application of commercial marketing technologies to the analysis, planning, execution, and evaluation of programs designed to influence the voluntary behavior of target audiences in order to improve their personal welfare and that of their society" (Andreasen, 1995, p. 7).

social math "the practice of translating statistics and other data so they become interesting to the journalist, and meaningful to the audience" (Dorfman et al., 2004, p. 112).

social media (or interactive media) any type media that uses the Internet and other technologies to allow for social interaction.

social network "web of social relationships that surround people" (Heaney & Israel, 2008, p. 190).

social planning a form of community organizing that is "heavily task oriented, stressing rational-empirical problem solving" (Minkler & Wallerstein, 2005, p. 30).

social support a network of individuals that provides assistance or encouragement to a person who is engaging in a new behavior.

socio-ecological approach recognizing that there are multiple levels of influence on behavior.

soft money a source of funding that is not an on-going part of an operating budget.

speakers bureau a service offered by various groups with experts who are willing to present information to others.

specificity "the ability of the test to identify only nondiseased individuals who actually do not have the disease" (Friis & Sellers, 2009, p. 424).

stage a step in the change process.

stage theory a theory composed of an ordered set of categories into which people can be classified, and for which factors could be identified that could induce movement from one category to the next (Weinstein & Sandman, 2002a).

stakeholders any person or organization with a vested interest in a health program, usually decision makers, program partners, or clients.

standard of acceptability the minimum levels of performance, effectiveness, or benefits used to judge value (Green & Lewis, 1986).

standards of evaluation utility, feasibility, propriety, and accuracy (*see* definitions for each term in other parts of the glossary).

statistical significance "refers to whether the observed differences between the two or more groups are real or not or whether they are chance occurrences" (McDermott & Sarvela, 1999, p. 300).

steering committee see *planning committee*.

storming second stage of team development "in which team members voice differences about team goals and procedures" (Gomez-Mejia & Balkin, 2012, p. 390).

strata in terms of sampling, subgroups of the survey population.

strategy a general plan of action for affecting a health problem; it may encompass several activities (CDC, 2003).

stratified random sample a probability sample that first divides the survey population into strata and then randomly selects participants from each strata.

subjective norm "the perceived social pressure to engage or not to engage in a behavior" (Ajzen, 2006).

summative evaluation "any combination of measurements and judgments that permit conclusions to be drawn about impact, outcome or benefits of a program or method" (Green & Lewis, 1986, p. 366).

support ensures that programs have appropriate built-in reinforcement components to assist participants with the expected level of involvement and/or behavior change.

supporting participants those who are seldom involved but help to swell the ranks of a program and may contribute in nonactive ways or through financial contributions.

survey population in terms of sampling, those in the universe specified by time or place, and who are accessible.

SWOT (Strengths, Weaknesses, Opportunities, and Threats) an approach to planning that minimizes planning time and moves quickly to action steps by assessing internal strengths and weaknesses as well as external opportunities and threats, usually displayed in a 2 × 2 matrix.

systematic sample a probability sample that selects participants from a sampling frame by taking every Nth person after a random start.

tailoring "any combination of information or change strategies intended to reach one specific person, based upon characteristics that are unique to that person, related to the outcome of interest, and have been derived from an individual assessment" (Kreuter & Skinner, 2000, p. 1).

task development time line a program management charting method that provides a graphical illustration of the time frame for tasks to be completed.

task force "a self-contained group of 'doers' that is not ongoing, but rather brought together due to strong interest in an issue and for a specific purpose" (Butterfoss, 2007, p. 30).

team "a small group of people with complementary skills who are committed to a common purpose, a set of performance goals, and an approach for which they hold themselves mutually accountable" (Gomez-Mejia & Balkin, 2012, p. 384.).

technical assistance (or *capacity building assistance*) a relationship in which individuals with specific knowledge and skills share them, via advice and training, with those who need them.

technical resources (or *other resources*) includes all other resources besides human or financial.

temptation "the intensity of urges to engage in a specific behavior when in difficult situations" (Prochaska et al., 2008, p. 102).

termination a stage of change in which a person who has changed a behavior has zero temptation to return to the old behavior.

tertiary prevention measure aimed at rehabilitation following significant pathogenesis.

test–retest (or *stability*) **reliability** "used to generate evidence of stability over time" (Torabi, 1994, p. 57).

theory "a set of interrelated concepts, definitions, and propositions that presents a *systematic* view of events or situations by specifying relations among variables in order to *explain* and *predict* the events of the situations" (Glanz et al., 2008b, p. 26).

three Fs of program planning fluidity, flexibility, and functionality (*see* definitions for each term in other parts of the glossary).

treatment see *intervention*.

triple blind study an evaluation wherein neither the participants, nor those implementing the program, nor the evaluators, know which group is experimental and which group is the control.

t-**test** a statistical test involving interval or ratio data that assesses whether the means of two groups are statistically different from each other.

Type I error rejecting the null hypothesis when it is actually true.

Type II error failing to reject the null hypothesis when it is, in fact, not true.

Type III error failure to implement the health education intervention properly (Basch et al., 1985).

units "an orderly, self-contained collection of activities educationally designed to meet a set of objectives" (Gilbert et al., 2011, p. 188).

univariate data analysis analysis of one variable.

universe as it relates to sampling, all those unspecific by time and place.

unobtrusive observation when people are not aware they are being measured, assessed, or tested.

utility standards "ensure that the information needs of evaluation users are satisfied" (CDC, 1999a, p. 27); a standard of evaluation.

validity whether an instrument correctly measures what it is intended to measure.

variable a construct, characteristic, or attribute that can be measured or observed.

vendors those who sell their products to program planners.

vicarious reinforcement observation of another being reinforced.

vision statement a description of where a program will be in the future.

volunteers those who serve an organization or cause without pay or compensation.

walk-through an observation completed by walking through an area at various times on different days looking for indicators of health.

windshield tour an observation completed by driving through an area at various times on different days looking for indicators of health.

References

Abroms, L. C., & Maibach, E. W. (2008). The effectiveness of mass communication to change public behavior. *Annual Review of Public Health, 28,* 219–234.

Adeyanju, M. (2008). Communication and cultural competence. In M. A. Pérez & R. R. Luquis, (Eds.), *Cultural competence in health education and health promotion* (pp. 147–162). San Francisco: Jossey-Bass.

Ad Hoc Work Group of the American Public Health Association. (1987). Criteria for the development of health promotion and education programs. *American Journal of Public Health, 77*(1), 89–92.

Agency for Healthcare Research and Quality (AHRQ). (2008). *Treating tobacco use and dependence.* Retrieved May 17, 2011, from http://www.ahrq.gov/path/tobacco.html

Airhihenbuwa, C. O., Cottrell, R. R., Adeyanju, M., Auld, M. E., Lysoby, L., & Smith, B. J. (2005). The national health educator competencies update project: Celebrating a milestone and recommending next steps for the profession. *American Journal of Health Education, 36*(6), 361–370.

Aitaoto, N., Tsark, J., & Braun, K. L. (2009). Sustainability of the pacific diabetes today coalitions. Preventing chronic disease, 6(4), 1–8. Retrieved May 29, 2011, from http://cdc.gov/pcd/issues/2009/oct/080181.htm

Ajzen, I. (1988). *Attitudes, personality, and behavior.* Chicago: Dorsey Press.

Ajzen, I. (2006). *Theory of planned behavior.* Retrieved April 27, 2011, from http://www.people.umass.edu/aizen/tpb.html

Aldana, S. G. (2001). Financial impact of health promotion programs: A comprehensive review of the literature. *American Journal of Health Promotion, 15*(5), 296–320.

Aldana, S. G. (2009). *The Top 5 strategies to enhance the ROI of worksite wellness programs (in economically challenging times).* Omaha, NE: Wellness Council of America. Retrieved March 22, 2011, from http://www.welcoa.org/freeresources/

Alexander, G. (1999). Health risk appraisal. In G. C. Hyner, K. W. Peterson, J. W. Travis, J. E. Dewey, J. J. Foerster, & E. M. Framer (Eds.), *SPM handbook of health assessment tools* (pp. 5–8). Pittsburgh, PA: Society of Prospective Medicine.

Alinsky, S. D. (1971). *Rules for radicals: A pragmatic primer for realistic radicals.* New York: Random House.

Allen, J., & Hunnicutt, D. (2007) A new way of thinking: Examining strategies for gaining leadership support for health promotion. *Absolute Advantage, 6*(2), 14–17. Retrieved March 19, 2011, from http://www.welcoa.org/freeresources/index.php?category=8

Allen, R. S., Phillips, M. A., Whitehead, D., Crowther, M. R., & Prentice-Dunn, S. (2009). Living well with living wills: Application of protection motivation theory to living will execution among older adults. *Clinical Gerontologist, 32,* 44–59.

Altschuld, J. W., & Witkin, B. R. (2000). *From needs assessment to action: Transforming needs into solution strategies.* Thousand Oaks, CA: Sage.

American Association for Health Education (AAHE), National Commission for Health Education Credentialing, Inc. (NCHEC), & Society for Public Health Education (SOPHE). (1999). *A competency-based framework for graduate-level health educators.* Reston, VA: Authors.

American Cancer Society (ACS). (2009). *Workplace Solutions: Building a Healthy Workforce.* Retrieved March 24, 2011, from http://www.acsworkplacesolutions.com/index.asp

American Cancer Society (ACS). (2011). *Learn about cancer.* Retrieved April 16, 2011, from http://www.cancer.org/Cancer/index.

American College of Sports Medicine (ACSM). (2010). *ACSM's guidelines for exercise testing and prescription* (8th ed.). Philadelphia: Lippincott, Williams, & Wilkins.

American Marketing Association. (2007). *Dictionary.* Retrieved August 13, 2011, from http://www.marketingpower.com/_layouts/Dictionary.aspx

American Psychological Association (APA). (2011). *PsycINFO.*®Retrieved April 2, 2011, from http://www.apa.org/pubs/databases/psycinfo/index.aspx

Ammary-Risch, N. J., Zambon, A., & Brown, K. M. (2010). Communicating health information effectively. In C. I. Fertman, & D. D. Allensworth (Eds.), *Health promotion programs: Theory to practice* (pp. 203–231). San Francisco: Jossey-Bass.

Anderson, B., Fortson, B. W., Kleindler, S. R., & Schonthal, H. (Eds.). (2002). *The American heritage dictionary.* New York, NY: Dell.

Anderson, G. (2004). *Chronic conditions: Making the case for ongoing care.* Baltimore: Johns Hopkins University.

Andreasen, A. R. (1995). *Marketing social change. Changing behavior to promote health, social development, and the environment.* San Francisco: Jossey-Bass.

Anspaugh, D. J., Dignan, M. B., & Anspaugh, S. L. (2000). *Developing health promotion programs.* Boston, MA: McGraw-Hill.

Arkin, E. B. (1990). Opportunities for improving the nation's health through collaboration with the mass media. *Public Health Reports, 105*(3), 219–223.

Association of State and Territorial Directors of Health and Public Health Education (ASTDHPHE). (2001). *Policy and environmental change: New directions for public research.* Atlanta: Centers for Disease Control and Prevention.

Auld, E. (1997). Practical tips for influencing public policy. *Health Education & Behavior, 24*(3), 272–274.

Auld, M. E., Radius, S. M., Galer-Unti, R., Hinman, J. M., Gotsch, A. R., & Mail, P. D. (2011). Distinguishing between health education and health information dissemination. *American Journal of Public Health, 101*(3), 390–391.

Backer, T. E., & Rogers, E. M. (1998). Diffusion of innovations theory and worksite AIDS programs. *Journal of Health Communication, 1,* 17–28.

Bagozzi, R. P. (1975). Marketing as exchange. *Journal of Marketing, 39,* 32–39.

Baker, E. A., Brownson, R. C., Dreisinger, M., McIntosh, L. D., & Karamehic-Muratovic, A. (2009). Examining the role of training in evidence-based public health: A qualitative study. *Health Promotion Practice, 10*(3), 342–348.

Bandura, A. (1977a). Self-efficacy: Toward a unifying theory of behavioral change. *Psychological Review, 84*(2), 191–215.

Bandura, A. (1977b). *Social learning theory.* Englewood Cliffs, NJ: Prentice Hall.

Bandura, A. (1986). *Social foundations of thought and action.* Englewood Cliffs, NJ: Prentice Hall.

Bandura, A. (2001). Social cognitive theory: An agentic perspective. *Annual review of psychology, 52,* 1–26.

Baranowski, T. (1985). Methodologic issues in self-report of health behavior. *Journal of School Health, 55*(5), 179–182.

Baranowski, T., Perry, C. L., & Parcel, G. S. (2002). How individuals, environments, and health behavior interact. In K. Glanz, B. K. Rimer, & F. M. Lewis (Eds.), *Health behavior and health education: Theory, research, and practice* (3rd ed., pp. 165–184). San Francisco, CA: Jossey-Bass.

Baric, L. (1993). The settings approach—Implications for policy and strategy. *Journal of the Institute of Health Education, 31,* 17–24.

Barnes, J. A. (1954). Class and committees in a Norwegian island parish. *Human Relations, 7,* 39–58.

Barnes, M. D., Neiger, B. L., & Thackeray, R. (2003). Health communication. In R. J. Bensley & J. Brookins-Fisher (Eds.), *Community health education methods* (2nd ed., pp. 51–82). Boston, MA: Jones & Bartlett.

Bartholomew, L. K., Parcel, G. S., Kok, G., & Gottlieb, N. H. (2006). *Planning health promotion programs: An intervention mapping approach* (2nd ed.). San Francisco, CA: Jossey-Bass.

Bartholomew, L. K., Parcel, G. S., Kok, G., Gottlieb, N. H., & Fernandez, M. E. (2011). *Planning health promotion programs: An intervention mapping approach* (3rd ed.). San Francisco, CA: Jossey-Bass.

Bartol, K. M., & Martin, D. C. (1991). *Management*. New York, NY: McGraw-Hill.

Basch, C. E., Sliepcevich, E. M., Gold, R. S., Duncan, D. F., & Kolbe, L. J. (1985). Avoiding Type III errors in health education program evaluations: A case study. *Health Education Quarterly, 12*(3), 315–331.

Bates, I. J., & Winder, A. E. (1984). *Introduction to health education*. Palo Alto, CA: Mayfield.

Becker, M. H. (Ed.). (1974). The health belief model and personal health behavior. *Health Education Monographs, 2* (entire issue).

Becker, M. H., Drachman, R. H., & Kirscht, J. P. (1974). A new approach to explaining sick-role behavior in low income populations. *American Journal of Public Health, 64*(March), 205–216.

Behrens, R. (1983). *Work-site health promotion: Some questions and answers to help you get started*. Washington, DC: Office of Disease Prevention and Health Promotion.

Belch, G. E., & Belch, M. A. (2007). *Advertising and promotion. An integrated marketing communications perspective*. New York: McGraw-Hill Irwin.

Bennett, G. G., & Glasgow, R. E. (2009). The delivery of public health interventions via the Internet: Actualizing their potential. *Annual Review of Public Health, 30*, 273–392.

Bensley, L. B. (2009). Using theory and ethics to guide method selection and application. In R. J. Bensley & J. Brookins-Fisher (Eds.) *Community health education methods: A practical guide* (3rd ed., pp. 3–30.). Sudbury, MA: Jones & Bartlett.

Bertrand, J. T. (2004). Diffusion of Innovations and HIV/AIDS. *Journal of Health Communication, 9*(S1), 113–121.

Berwick, D. M. (2003). Disseminating innovations in health care. *Journal of the American Medical Association, 15*, 1969–1975.

Bhatt, S. (2006, December 13). Taxi stand provides place for tipsy to get cabs. *Seattle Times*.

Block, L. E. (2008). Health policy: What it is and how it work. In C. Harrington, & C. L. Estes (Eds.), *Health policy: Crisis and reform in the U.S. health care delivery system* (5th ed., pp. 4–14). Sudbury, MA: Jones & Bartlett.

Bloom, B. S. (Ed.) (1956). *Taxonomy of educational objectives: The classification of educational goals. Handbook I: Cognitive domain*. New York, NY: David McKay.

Blumberg, S. J., & Luke, J. V. (2010). *Wireless substitution: Early release of estimates from the National Health Interview Survey, January–June 2010*. National Center for Health Statistics. Retrieved March 30, 2011, from: http://www.cdc.gov/nchs/nhis.htm.

Blumberg, S. J., Luke, J. V., Ganesh, N., Davern, M. E., Boudreaux, M. H., & Soderberg, K. (2011). Wireless substitution: State-level estimates from the National Health Interview Survey, January 2007–June 2010. *National Health Statistics Report, 39*, 1–28.

Boeka, A., Prentice-Dunn, S., & Lokken, K. (2010). Psychosocial predictors of weight loss and intentions to comply with post-surgical guidelines following bariatric surgery. *Psychology, Health, and Medicine, 15*, 188–197.

Borras, J. M., Fernandez, E., Schiaffino, A., Borrell, C., & LaVecchia, C. (2000). Pattern of smoking initiation in Catalonia, Spain, from 1948 to 1992. *American Journal of Public Health, 9*, 1459–1462.

Boslaugh, S. E., Kreuter, M. W., Nicholson, R. A., & Naleid, K. (2005). Comparing demographic, health status and psychosocial strategies of audience segmentation to promote physical activity. *Health Education Research 20*(4), 430–438.

Bowling, A. (2005). *Measuring health: A review of quality of life measurement scales* (3rd ed.). New York, NY: Open University Press.

Brager, G., Specht, H., & Torczyner, J. L. (1987). *Community organizing*. New York: Columbia University Press.

Braithwaite, R. L., Murphy, F., Lythcott, N., & Blumenthal, D. S. (1989). Community organization and development for health promotion within an urban black community: A conceptual model. *Health Education, 20*(5), 56–60.

Breen, M. (1999). Researching grants on the Internet. *Community Health Center Management*, March/April, 29.

Brennan Ramirez, L. K., Baker, E. A., & Metzler, M. (2008). *Promoting Health Equity: A Resource to Help Communities Address Social Determinants of Health*. Atlanta: Centers for Disease Control and Prevention. Retrieved March 29, 2011, from http://www.cdc.gov/nccdphp/dach/chaps

Breslow, L. (1999). From disease prevention to health promotion. *Journal of the American Medical Association, 281*(11), 1030–1033.

Brownson, R. C., Fielding, J. E., & Maylahn, C. M. (2009). Evidence-based public health: A fundamental concept for public health practice. *Annual Review of Public Health, 30*, 175–201.

Brownson, R. C., Haire-Joshu, D., & Luke, D. A. (2006). Shaping the context of health: A review of environmental and policy approaches in the prevention of chronic diseases. *Annual Review of Public Health, 27,* 341–370.

Bryan, R. L., Kreuter, M. W., & Brownson, R. C. (2009). Integrating adult learning principles into training for public health practice. *Health Promotion Practice, 10*(4), 557–563.

Burke, N. J., Joseph, G., Pasick, R. J., & Barker, J. C. (2009). Theorizing social context: Rethinking behavioral theory. *Health Education & Behavior, 36*(Suppl. 1), 55S–70S.

BusinessDictionary.com (2011a). *Audit, external audit, internal audit.* Retrieved June 20, 2011, from http://www.businessdictionary.com/definition/audit.html

BusinessDictionary.com (2011b). *Cultural audit.* Retrieved May 12, 2011, from http://www.businessdictionary.com/definition/cultural-audit.html

Butterfoss, F. D. (2006). Process evaluation for community participation. *Annual Review of Public Health, 27,* 323–340.

Butterfoss, F. D. (2007). *Coalitions and partnerships in community health.* San Francisco: Jossey-Bass.

Butterfoss, F. D. (2009). Building and sustaining coalitions. In R. J. Bensley & J. Brookins-Fisher (Eds.), *Community health education methods: A practical guide* (3rd ed., pp. 299–331). Sudbury, MA: Jones & Bartlett.

Capwell, E. M., Butterfoss, F., & Francisco, V. T. (2000). Why evaluate? *Health Promotion Practice, 1*(1), 15–20.

Catalani, C., & Minkler, M. (2010). Photovoice: A review of the literature in health and public health. *Health Education & Behavior, 37*(3) 424–451.

Cavallo, D. (2006). Using return on investment analysis to evaluate health promotion programs: Challenges and opportunities. *Health Promotion Economics, 1*(3), 1–4. Retrieved March 22, 2011, from http://www.rti.org/

Centers for Disease Control and Prevention. U.S. Department of Health and Human Services.

(n.d.). *Planned approach to community health: Guide for local coordinator.* Atlanta, GA: Author.

Centers for Disease Control and Prevention. (1999a). Framework for program evaluation in public health. *Morbidity and Mortality Weekly Report, 48*(RR-11), 1–40.

Centers for Disease Control and Prevention. (1999b). Ten great public health achievements— United States, 1900–1999. *Morbidity and Mortality Weekly Report, 48*(12), 241–243.

Centers for Disease Control and Prevention. (2000). *Healthy plan-it: A tool for planning and managing public health programs. Sustainable Management Development Program.* Atlanta, GA: Author.

Centers for Disease Control and Prevention. (2003). *CDCynergy 3.0: Your Guide Effective Health Communication* (CD ROM Version 3.0). Atlanta, GA: Author.

Centers for Disease Control and Prevention (CDC). (2008b). Smoking attributable mortality, years of potential life lost, and productivity losses— United States, 2000–2004. *Morbidity and Mortality Weekly Report, 57*(45), 1226–1228. Retrieved March 20, 2011, from http://www.cdc.gov/mmwr/preview/mmwrhtml/mm5745a3.htm

Centers for Disease Control and Prevention (CDC). (2009a). *Chronic disease and health promotion.* Retrieved March 15, 2011, from http://www.cdc.gov/chronicdisease/overview/index.htm.

Centers for Disease Control and Prevention (CDC). (2009b). *Health impact assessment.* Retrieved April 15, 2011, from http://www.cdc.gov/healthyplaces/hia.htm

Centers for Disease Control and Prevention (CDC). (2009c). *Social media at CDC: Data & metrics.* Retrieved May 8, 2011, from http://www.cdc.gov/SocialMedia/Data/index.html

Centers for Disease Control and Prevention (CDC). (2009d). *What we know about health literacy.* Retrieved May 7, 2011, from http://www.cdc.gov/healthmarketing/resources.htm

Centers for Disease Control and Prevention (CDC). (2010a). *Diabetes.* Retrieved March 15, 2011, from http://www.cdc.gov/chronicdisease/resources/publications/AAG/ddt.htm

Centers for Disease Control and Prevention (CDC). (2010b). Vital signs: Current cigarette smoking among adults aged ≥18 years—United States, 2009. *Morbidity and Mortality Weekly Report, 59*(35), 1135–1140. Retrieved March 20, 2011, from http://www.cdc.gov/mmwr/preview/mmwrhtml/mm5935a3.htm?s_cid=mm5935a3_w

Centers for Disease Control and Prevention (CDC). (2010c). *Workplace health promotion.* Retrieved March 20, 2011, from http://www.cdc.gov/workplacehealthpromotion/index.htm

Centers for Disease Control and Prevention (CDC). (2010d). *Recommendations and guidelines.* Retrieved May 19, 2011, from http://www.cdc.gov/hiv/resources/guidelines/index.htm

Centers for Disease Control and Prevention (CDC). (2010e). *Logic model.* Retrieved June 9, 2011, from http://www.cdc.gov/nccdphp/dnpao/hwi/programdesign/logic_model.htm

Centers for Disease Control and Prevention (CDC). (2011a). *Guide to community preventive services.* Retrieved March 25, 2011, from http://www.thecommunityguide.org/index.html

Centers for Disease Control and Prevention (CDC). (2011b). *Healthy Communities Program.* Retrieved July 31, 2011, from http://www.thecommunityguide.org/index.html

Centers for Disease Control and Prevention (CDC), Division of Heart Disease and Stroke Prevention. (n.d.). *Evaluation guide: Developing and using logic models.* Retrieved June 14, 2011, from http://www.cdc.gov/DHDSP/programs/nhdsp_program/evaluation_guides/logic_model.htm

Centers for Disease Control and Prevention (CDC), Division of Heart Disease and Stroke Prevention. (2008a). *Evaluation guide: Writing SMART objectives.* Retrieved April 19, 2011, from http://www.cdc.gov/dhdSP/programs/nhdsp_program/evaluation_guides/smart_objectives.htm

Central Intelligence Agency (CIA). (2011). *The world factbook.* Retrieved March 14, 2011, from https://www.cia.gov/library/publications/the-world-factbook/

Chaplin, J. P., & Krawiec, T. S. (1979). *Systems and theories of psychology* (4th ed.). New York: Holt, Rinehart & Winston.

Chapman, L. S. (1997). Securing support from top management. *The Art of Health Promotion, 1*(2), 1–7.

Chapman, L. S. (2003a). Meta-evaluation of worksite health promotion economic return studies. *The Art of Health Promotion, 6*(6), 1–14.

Chapman, L. S. (2003b). Biometric screening in health promotion: Is it really as important as we think? *The Art of Health Promotion, 7*(2), 1–12.

Chapman, L. S. (2005a). Incentives: An introduction and story–Part I. *Absolute Advantage, 4*(7), 1–46. Retrieved March 19, 2011, from http://www.welcoa.org/freesources/pdf/index.php?category=8

Chapman, L. S. (2005b). Meta-evaluation of worksite health promotion economic return studies: 2005 update. *The Art of Health Promotion, 19*(16), 1–11.

Chapman, L. S. (2006). Planning wellness: Getting off to a good start–Part I. *Absolute Advantage, 5*(4), 1–87. Retrieved March 19, 2011, from http://www.welcoa.org/freesources/pdf/index.php?category=8

Chapman, L. S. (2009). Building a sustainable administrative infrastructure for worksite wellness programs . *The Art of Health Promotion, 24*(12), 1–11.

Chapman, L. S., Whitehead, D., & Connors, M. C. (2008). The changing role of incentives in health promotion and wellness. *The Art of Health Promotion, 23*(11), 1–12.

Checkoway, B. (1989). Community participation for health promotion: Prescription for public policy. *Wellness Perspectives: Research, Theory and Practice, 6*(1), 18–26.

Chenoweth, D. H. (1987). *Planning health promotion at the worksite.* Indianapolis: Benchmark Press.

Clark, N. M., Friedman, A. R., & Lachance, L. L. (2006). *Summing it up: Collective lessons from the experience of seven coalitions, 7*(2), 149S–152S.

Clark, N. M., Janz, N. K., Dodge, J. A., & Sharpe, P. A. (1992). Self-regulation of health behavior: The "take PRIDE" program. *Health Education Quarterly, 19*(3), 341–354.

Cleary, M. J., & Neiger, B. L. (1998). *The certified health education specialist: A self-study guide for professional competency* (3rd ed.). Allentown, PA: National Commission for Health Education Credentialing.

Clow, K. E., & Baack, D. (2007). *Integrated advertising, promotion and marketing communications* (3rd ed.). Upper Saddle River, NJ: Pearson Prentice Hall.

Coalition of National Health Education Organizations (CNHEO). (2011a). *Code of ethics for the health education profession.* Retrieved June 21, 2011, from http://www.cnheo.org/

Coalition of National Health Education Organizations (CNHEO). (2011b). *Health education advocate.* Retrieved May 12, 2011, from http://www.healtheducationadvocate.org/

Cohen, J. (1960). A coefficient of agreement for nominal scales. *Educational and Psychological Measurement, 20*(1), 37–46.

Cohen, J. T., Neumann, P. J., & Weinstein, M. C. (2008). Does preventive care save money? Health economics and the presidential candidates. *The New England Journal of Medicine, 358*(7), 661–663.

Cook, T. D., & Campbell, D. T. (1979). *Quasi-experimentation: Design and analysis issues for field settings.* Boston: Houghton Mifflin.

Coreil, J., Bryant, C. A., & Henderson, J. N. (2001). *Social and behavioral foundations of public health.* Thousand Oaks, CA: Sage.

Cottrell, R. R., Girvan, J. T., & McKenzie, J. F. (2012). *Principles and foundations of Health promotion and education* (5th ed.). San Francisco: Benjamin Cummings.

Cottrell, R. R., & McKenzie, J. F. (2011). *Health promotion and education research methods: Using the five-chapter thesis/dissertation model* (2nd ed.). Sudbury, MA: Jones & Bartlett.

Courtney, A. (2004). Using community-based prevention marketing to promote physical activity among teens. *Social Marketing Quarterly, 10,* 3–4, 58–61.

Cowdery, J. E., Wang, M. Q., Eddy, J. M., & Trucks, J. K. (1995). A theory-driven health promotion program in a university setting. *Journal of Health Education, 26*(4), 248–250.

Creswell, J. W. (2002). Educational research: Planning, conducting and evaluating quantitative and qualitative research. Merrill Prentice Hall: Upper Saddle River, NJ.

Croker, K. S., Ryan, A., Morzenti, T., Cave, L., Maze-Gallman, T., & Ford, L. (2004). Delivering prostate cancer prevention messages to the public: How the National Cancer Institute (NCI) effectively spread the word about the Prostate Cancer Prevention Trial (PCPT) results. *Urologic Oncology, 22,* 369–376.

Crosby, R. A., Kegler, M. C., & DiClemente, R. J. (2009). Theory in health promotion practice and research. In R. J. DiClemente, R. A. Crosby, & M. C. Kegler (Eds.), *Emerging theories in health promotion practice and research* (2nd ed., pp. 4–17). San Francisco: Jossey-Bass.

Cummings, C., Gordon, J. R., & Marlatt, G. A. (1980). Relapse: Prevention and prediction. In W. R. Miller (Ed.), *Addictive behaviors* (pp. 291–322). Oxford, U.K.: Pergamon Press.

Dannenberg, A. L., Bhatia, R., Cole, B. L., Heaton, S. K., Feldman, J. D., & Rutt, C. D. (2008). Use of health impact assessment in the U.S.: 27 case studies, 1999–2007. *American Journal of Preventive Medicine, 34*(3), 241–256.

Davis, P. C., & Rankin, L. L. (2006). Guidelines for making existing health education programs more culturally appropriate. *American Journal of Health Education, 37*(4), 250–252.

Debus, M. (1988). *Handbook of excellence on focus group research.* Washington, DC: Academy for Educational Development.

Deeds, S. G. (1992). *The health education specialist: Self-study for professional competence.* Los Alamitos, CA: Loose Canon.

Della, L. J., DeJoy, D. M., Goetzel, R. Z., Ozminkowski, R. J., & Wilson, M. G. (2008). Assessing management support for worksite health promotion: Psychometric analysis of the leading by example (LBE) instrument. *American Journal of Health Promotion, 22*(5), 359–367.

Della, L. J., DeJoy, D. M., Mitchell, S. G., Goetzel, R. Z., Roemer, E. C., & Wilson, M. G. (2010). Management support of workplace health promotion. Field test of the leading by example tool. *American Journal of Health Promotion, 25*(2), 138–146.

Dessler, G. (2012). *Fundamentals of human resource management* (2nd ed.). Boston: Prentice Hall.

DiClemente, R. J., Crosby, R. A., & Kegler, M. (2009). *Emerging theories in health promotion practice and research* (2nd ed.). San Francisco: Jossey-Bass.

DiClemente, R. J., Salazar, L. E., & Crosby, R. A. (2013). *Health behavior theory for public health: Principles, foundations, and applications.* Burlington, MA: Jones & Bartlett Learning.

Dictionary.com. (2011). *Memorandum of understanding.* Retrieved June 5, 2011 from http://dictionary.reference.com/browse/memorandum+of+agreement?fromAsk=true&o=100074

Dignan, M. B. (1995). *Measurement and evaluation of health education* (3rd ed.). Springfield, IL: Charles C. Thomas.

DiIorio, C. K. (2005). *Measurement in health behavior.* San Francisco, CA: Jossey-Bass.

Dishman, R. K., Sallis, J. F., & Orenstein, D. R. (1985). The determinants of physical activity and exercise. *Public Health Reports, 100*(2), 158–171.

Doak, C. C., Doak, L. G., & Root, J. H. (1996). *Teaching patients with low literacy skills* (2nd ed.). Philadelphia, PA: J. B. Lippincott.

Dorfman, L., Woodruff, K., Herbert, K., & Ervice, J. (2004). *Making the case for early care and education: A message development guide for advocates.* Berkeley, CA: Berkeley Media Studies Group. Retrieved March 28, 2011, from http://www.bmsg.org/documents/YellowBookrev.pdf.

Downey, L. H., Ireson, C. L., & Scutchfield, F. D. (2009). The use of photovoice as a method of facilitating deliberation. *Health Promotion Practice, 10*(3), 419–427.

Drum, C. E., Peterson, J. J., Culley, C., Krahn, G., Heller, T., Kimpton, T., McCubbin, J., Rimmer, J., Seekins, T., Suzuki, R., & White, G. W. (2009). Guidelines and criteria for the implementation of community-based health promotion programs for individuals with disabilities. *American Journal of Health Promotion, 24*(2), 93–101.

Dunn, W. N. (1994). *Public policy analysis: An introduction.* Englewood Cliffs, NJ: Prentice Hall.

Edberg, M. (2007). *Essentials of health behavior: Social and behavioral theory in public health.* Sudbury, MA: Jones & Bartlett.

Edington, D. W. (2001). Emerging research: A view from one research center. *American Journal of Health Promotion, 15*(5), 341–349.

Edington, D. W., Yen, L., & Braunstein, A. (1999). The reliability and validity of HRAs. In G. C. Hyner, K. W. Peterson, J. W. Travis, J. E. Dewey, J. J. Foerster, & E. M. Framer (Eds.), *SPM handbook of health assessment tools* (pp. 135–141). Pittsburgh, PA: Society for Prospective Medicine.

Educational Resource Information (ERIC). (n.d.). *Eric.* Retrieved April 2, 2011, from http://www.eric.ed.gov/

Edwards, R. W., Jumper-Thurman, P., Plested, B. A., Oetting, E. R., & Swanson, L. (2000). Community readiness: Research to practice. *Journal of Community Psychology, 28*(3), 291–307.

El-Askari, G., & Walton, S. (2005). Local government and resident collaboration to improve health: A case study in capacity building and cultural humility. In M. Minkler (Ed.). *Community organizing and community building for health* (2nd ed., pp. 254–271). New Brunswick, NJ: Rutgers University Press.

Elliott, S. (Ed.). (1998). *Health and productivity management: Consortium benchmarking study, best-practice report.* Houston, TX: American Productivity and Quality Center.

Emont, S. L., & Cummings, K. M. (1989). Adoption of smoking policies by automobile dealerships. *Public Health Reports, 104*(5), 509–514.

Eng, E., & Blanchard, L. (1990–91). Action-oriented community diagnosis: A health education tool. *International Quarterly of Community Health Education, 11*(2), 96–97.

Erfurt, J. C., Foote, A., Heirich, M. A., & Gregg, W. (1990). Improving participation in worksite wellness: Comparing health education classes, a menu approach, and follow-up counseling. *American Journal of Health Promotion, 4*(4), 270–278.

Erickson, W., Lee, C., & von Schrader, S. (2010, March). *Disability statistics from the 2008 American Community Survey (ACS).* Ithaca, NY: Cornell University Rehabilitation Research and Training Center on Disability Demographics and Statistics (StatsRRTC). Retrieved Jun 22, 2011, from http://www.disabilitystatistics.org

Estrada, C., Martin-Hryniewicz, M., Peek, B. T., Collins, C., & Byrd, J. C. (2004). Literacy and numeracy skills and anticoagulation control. *American Journal of Medical Science, 328,* 88–93.

European Centre for Health Policy (ECHP). (1999). *Health impact assessment: Main concepts and suggested approach.* Gothenburg consensus paper. Brussels, Belgium: Author.

Fallon, L. F., & Zgodzinski, E. J. (2012). *Essentials of public health management* (3rd ed.). Sudbury, MA: Jones & Bartlett Learning.

Federal Assistance Division (2011). *The catalog of federal domestic assistance.* Retrieved June 5, 2011, from http://www.cfda.gov

Ferrence, R. (1996). Using diffusion theory in health promotion: The case of tobacco. *Canadian Journal of Public Health,* (Suppl. 2), 24–27.

Fertman, C. I., Spiller, K. A., & Mickalide, A. D. (2010). Developing and increasing program funding. In C. I. Fertman & D. Allenworth (Eds.), *Health promotion programs: From theory to practice* (pp. 233–255). San Francisco: Jossey-Bass.

Fink, A., & Kosecoff, J. (1978). *An evaluation primer.* Washington, DC: Capitol Publications.

Fishbein, M. (Ed.) (1967). *Readings in attitudes theory measurement.* New York, NY: John Wiley & Sons.

Fishbein, M., & Ajzen, I. (1975). *Belief, attitude, intention and behavior: An introduction to theory and research.* Reading, MA: Addison-Wesley.

Fisher, J. D., & Fisher, W. A. (1992). Changing AIDS risk behavior. *Psychological Bulletin, 111,* 455–474.

Fisher, J. D., Fisher, W. A., & Shuper, P. A. (2009). The informational-motivation-behavioral skills model of HIV preventive behavior. In R. J. DiClemente, R. A. Crosby, & M. C. Kegler (Eds.), *Emerging theories in health promotion practice and research* (2nd ed., pp. 21–63). San Francisco: Jossey-Bass.

Fitzpatrick, J. L., Sanders, J. R., & Worthen, B. R. (2004). *Program evaluation: Alternative approaches and practical guidelines* (3rd ed.). Boston, MA: Pearson.

Flint's Youth Violence Prevention Center (FYVPC). (2006). *Photovoice.* Flint, MI: Author. Retrieved April 2, 2011, from http://www.sph.umich.edu/yvpc/projects/photovoice/

Flores, L. M., Davis, R., & Culross, P. (2007). Community health: a critical approach to addressing chronic diseases. *Preventing Chronic Diseases,* 4(4). Retrieved May 12, 2011, from http://www.cdc.pcd/issues/2007/oct/07_0080.htm

Floyd, D. L., Prentice-Dunn, S., & Rogers, R. W. (2000). A meta-analysis of research on protection motivation theory. *Journal of Applied Social Psychology, 30,* 407–429.

Forthofer, M. S., & Bryant, C. A. (2000). Using audience-segmentation techniques to tailor health behavior change strategies. *American Journal of Health Behavior,* 24(1), 36–43.

Fox, S., & Jones, S. (2009). *The social life health information.* Pew Internet & American Life Project. Retrieved March 30, 2011, from http://www.pewinternet.org/Experts/~/link.aspx?_id=62F4D7EFB49C4F9FA384FDC9D3A4B49B&_z=z

Frankish, C. J., Lovato, C. Y., & Shannon, W. J. (1998). Models, theories, and principles of health promotion with multicultural populations. In R. M. Huff & M. V. Kline (Eds.), *Promoting health in multicultural populations* (pp. 41–72). Thousand Oaks, CA: Sage.

French, S. A., Jeffery, R. W., & Oliphant, J. A. (1994). Facility access and self-reward as methods to promote physical activity among healthy sedentary adults. *American Journal of Health Promotion, 8*(4), 257–259, 262.

Friis, R. H., & Sellers, T. A. (2009). *Epidemiology for public health practice.* Sudbury, MA: Jones & Bartlett.

Fry, R. B., & Prentice-Dunn, S. (2006). Effects of a psychosocial intervention on breast self-examination attitudes and behaviors. *Health Education Research, 21,* 287–295.

Gagne, R. (1985). *The conditions of learning* (4th ed.). New York, NY: Holt, Rinehart, Winston.

Galer-Unti, R. A., Tappe, M. K., & Lachenmayr, S. (2004). Advocacy 101: Getting started in health education advocacy. *Health Promotion Practice,* 5(3), 280–288.

Gambatese, J. A. (2008). Research issues in prevention through design. *Journal of Safety Research, 39,* 153–158.

Gambescia, S. F., Cottrell, R. R., Capwell, E., Auld, M. E., Conley, K. M., Lysoby, L., Goldsmith, M., & Smith, B. (2009). Marketing health educators to employers: Survey findings, interpretations, and considerations for the profession. *Health Promotion Practice, 10*(4), 495–504.

General Services Administration (GSA). (2011). *Catalog of Federal Domestic Assistance.* Retrieved June 2, 2011, from https://www.cfda.gov

George, D., & Mallery, P. (2003). *SPSS for Windows step by step: A simple guide and reference.* Boston: Allyn & Bacon.

Getha-Taylor, H. (2008). Identifying collaborative competencies. *Review of Public Personnel Administration, 28*(2), 103–119.

Gilbert, G. G., Sawyer, R. G., & McNeill, E. B. (2011). *Health education: Creating strategies for school and community health* (3rd ed.). Sudbury, MA: Jones & Bartlett.

Gilmore, G. D. (2012). *Needs and capacity assessment strategies for health education and health promotion* (4th ed.). Burlington, MA: Jones & Bartlett Learning.

Gilmore, G. D., & Campbell, M. D. (2005). *Needs and capacity assessment strategies for health education and health promotion* (3rd ed.). Sudbury, MA: Jones & Bartlett.

Gilmore, G. D., Olsen, L. K., Taub, A., & Connell, D. (2005). Overview of the national health educator competencies update project, 1998–2004. *Health Education & Behavior, 32*(6), 725–737.

Gittell, R., & Vidal, A. (1998). *Community organizing: Building social capital as a development strategy.* Thousand Oaks, CA: Sage.

Gittelsohn, J., Dyckman, W., Tan, M. L., Boggs, M. K., Frick, K. D., Alfred, J., Winch, P. J., Haberle, H., & Palafox, N. A. (2006). Development and implementation of a food store-based intervention to improve diet in the Republic of the Marshall Islands. *Health Promotion Practice, 7*(4), 396–405.

Glanz, K., & Bishop, D. B. (2010). The role of behavioral science theory in the development and implementation of public health interventions. *Annual Review of Public Health, 31,* 399–418.

Glanz, K., & Rimer, B. K. (1995). *Theory at a glance: A guide for health promotion practice* (NIH Pub. No. 95–3896). Washington, DC: National Cancer Institute.

Glanz, K., Rimer, B. K., & Viswanath, K. (Eds.). (2008a). *Health behavior and health education: Theory, research, and practice* (4th ed.). San Francisco: Jossey-Bass.

Glanz, K., Rimer, B. K., & Viswanath, K. (2008b). Theory, research, and practice in health behavior and health education. In K. Glanz, B. K. Rimer, & K. Viswanath (Eds.), *Health behavior and health education: Theory, research, and practice* (4th ed., pp. 23–40). San Francisco: Jossey-Bass.

Glasgow, R. E. (2002). Evaluation of theory-based interventions: The RE-AIM model. In K. Glanz, B. K. Rimer, & F. M. Lewis (Eds.), *Health behavior and health education: Theory research, and practice* (3rd ed., pp. 530–544). San Francisco, CA: Jossey-Bass.

Glasgow, R. E., Vogt, T. M., & Boles, S. M. (1999). Evaluating the public health impact of health promotion interventions: The RE-AIM framework. *American Journal of Public Health, 89*(9), 1322–1327.

Goetzel, R. Z., & Ozminkowski, R. J. (2008). The health and cost benefits of worksite health-promotion programs. *Annual Review of Public Health, 29,* 303–323.

Golaszewski, T. (2001). Shining lights: Studies that have most influenced the understanding of health promotion's financial impact. *American Journal of Health Promotion, 15*(5), 332–340.

Golaszewski, T., Allen, J., & Edington, D. (2008). Working together to create supportive environments in worksite health promotion. *The Art of Health Promotion, 22*(14), 1–11.

Golbeck, A. L., Ahlers-Schmidt, C. R., Paschal, A. M., & Dismuke, S. E., (2005). A definition and operational framework for health numeracy. *American Journal of Preventive Medicine, 29,* 375–376.

Goldman, K. D. (1998). Promoting new ideas on the job: Practical theory-based strategies. *The Health Educator, 30*(1), 49–52.

Goldman, K. D., & Schmalz, K. J. (2006). Logic models: The picture worth ten thousand words. *Health Promotion Practice, 7*(1), 8–12.

Goldsmith, M. (2006). Ethics in health education: Issues, concerns, and future directions. *The Health Education Monograph Series, 23*(1), 33–37.

Goldstein, M. G., DePue, J., Kazura, A., & Niaura, R. (1998). Models for provider-patient interaction: Applications to health behavior change. In S. A. Shumaker, E. B. Schron, J. K. Ockene, & W. L. McBee (Eds.), *The handbook of health behavior change* (2nd ed., pp. 85–113). New York: Springer.

Goldstein, S. M. (1997). Community coalitions: A self-assessment tool. *American Journal of Health Promotion, 11*(6), 430–435.

Gomez-Mejia, L. R., & Balkin, D. B. (2012). *Management: People, performance, change.* Boston: Prentice Hall.

Goodhard, F. W., Hsu, J., Baek, J. H., Coleman, A., Maresca, F., & Miller, M. (2006). A view through a different lens: Photovoice as a tool for student advocacy. *Journal of American College Health, 55,* 53–56.

Goodlad, J. I., & Su, Z. (1992). Organization and the curriculum. In P. W. Jackson (Ed.). *Handbook of research in the curriculum* (pp. 327–344). New York, NY: Macmillan.

Goodman, R. M., McLeroy, K. R., Steckler, A. B., & Hoyle, R. H. (1993). Development of level of institutionalization scales for health promotion programs. *Health Education Quarterly, 20*(2), 161–178.

Goodman, R. M., Speers, M. A., McLeroy, K., Fawcett, S., Kegler, M., Parker, E., Smith, S. R., Sterling, T. D., & Wallerstein, N. (1998). Identifying and defining the dimensions of community capacity to provide a basis for measurement. *Health Education and Behavior, 25*(3), 258–278.

Goodman, R. M., & Steckler, A. (1989). A model for the institutionalization of health promotion programs. *Family and Community Health, 11*(4), 63–78.

Goodson, P. (2010). *Theory in health promotion research and practice: Thinking outside the box.* Sudbury, MA: Jones & Bartlett.

Granat, J. P. (1994). *Persuasive advertising for entrepreneurs and small business owners: How to create more effective sales messages.* Binghamton, NY: Haworth Press.

Granello, D. H., & Wheaton, J. E. (2003). *Using web-based surveys to conduct counseling research.* (ERIC Document # ED481144). Retrieved May 30, 2011, from http://www.eric.ed.gov/

Green, L. W. (1989, March). *The health promotion program of the Henry J. Kaiser Family Foundation.* Paper presented at a public lecture at Mankato State University, Mankato, MN.

Green, L. W. (1999). Health education's contributions to public health in the twentieth century: A glimpse through health promotion's rear-view mirror. In J. E. Fielding, L.B. Lave, & B. Starfield (Eds.), *Annual review of public health* (pp. 67–88). Palo Alto, CA: Annual Reviews.

Green, L. W., & Fielding J. E. (2011). The U.S. healthy people initiative: Its genesis and its sustainability. *Annual Review of Public Health, 32,* 451–470.

Green, L. W., Glanz, K., Hochbaum, G. M., Kok, G., Kreuter, M. W., Lewis, F. M., Lorig, K., Morisky, D., Rimer, B. K., & Rosenstock, I. M. (1994). Can we build on, or must we replace, the theories and models of health education? *Health Education Research, 9*(3), 397–404.

Green, L. W., & Kreuter, M. W. (1999). *Health promotion planning: An educational and ecological approach* (3rd ed.). Mountain View, CA: Mayfield.

Green, L. W., & Kreuter, M. W. (2005). *Health program planning: An educational and ecological approach* (4th ed.). Boston, MA: McGraw-Hill.

Green, L. W., & Lewis, F. M. (1986). *Measurement and evaluation in health education and health promotion.* Palo Alto, CA: Mayfield.

Grier, S., & Bryant, C. A. (2005). Social marketing in public health. *Annual Review of Public Health, 26,* 313–339.

Grudzien, L. (2009). *New interim final GINA regulations affect wellness programs.* Retrieved May 15, 2011, from http://larrygrudzien.com/benefits_attorney/new-interim-final-gina-regulations-affect-wellness-programs/

Grunbaum, J. A., Gingiss, P., Orpinas, P., Batey, L. S., & Parcel, G. S (1995). A comprehensive approach to school health program needs assessment. *Journal of School Health, 65*(2), 54–59.

Gurley, L. (2007, April). *Assessing progress on the nation's health promotion agenda: Healthy People 2010.* Presentation at a public lecture at Ball State University, Muncie, IN.

Guyer, M. (1999). Grants: Finding a funding source. *Grant Source* (pp. 1–3). Columbus, OH: Office of the Auditor, State of Ohio.

Haider, M., & Kreps, G. L. (2004). Forty years of diffusion of innovations: Utility and value in public health. *Journal of Health Communication, 9,* 3–11

Hall, C. L. (1943). *Principles of behavior.* New York: Appleton-Century-Crofts.

Hallfors, D., & Godette, D. (2002). Will the principles of effectiveness improve prevention practice? Early findings from a diffusion study. *Health Education Research, 4,* 461–470.

Hancock, T., & Minkler, M. (2005). Community health assessment or healthy community assessment: Whose community? Whose health? Whose assessment? In M. Minkler (Ed.).

Community organizing and community building for health (2nd ed., pp. 138–157). New Brunswick, NJ: Rutgers University Press.

Hanlon, J. J. (1954). The design of public health programs for underdeveloped countries. *Public Health Reports, 69,* 1028–1032.

Harris, J. H. (2001). Selecting the right vendor for your health promotion program. *Absolute Advantage, 1*(4), 4–5.

Harris, J. H., & McKenzie, J. F. (2004). Checklist for selecting health promotion vendors. Retrieved June 8, 2011, from http:// www.welcoa.org/ freesources/pdf/index.php?category=8

Harris, J. H., McKenzie, J. F., & Zuti, W. B. (1986). How to select the right vendor for your company's health promotion program. *Fitness in Business, 1*(October), pp. 53–56.

Harris, M. J. (2010). *Evaluating public and community health programs.* San Francisco: Jossey-Bass.

Hartman, J. M., Forsen, J. W., Wallace, M. S., & Neely, J. G. (2002). Tutorials in clinical research: Part IV—Recognizing and controlling bias. *Laryngosscope, 112,* 23–31.

Haveman, R. H. (2010). Principles to guide the development of population health incentives. *Preventing chronic disease, 7*(5), 1–5. Retrieved May 15, 2011, from http://www.cdc.gov/pcd/ issues/2010/sep/10_0044.htm.

Hayden, J. (2009). *Introduction to health behavior theory.* Sudbury, MA: Jones & Bartlett.

Heaney, C. A., & Israel, B. A. (2008). Social networks and social support. In K. Glanz, B. K. Rimer, & K. Viswanath (Eds.), *Health behavior and health education: Theory, research, and practice* (4th ed., pp. 189–210). San Francisco: Jossey-Bass.

Helitzer, D., Willging, C., Hathorn, G., & Benally, J. (2009). Using logic models in a community-based agricultural injury prevention project. *Public Health Reports, 124*(Suppl. 1), 63–73.

Hergenrather, K. C., Rhodes, S. D., & Bardhoshi, G. (2009). Photovoice as community-based participatory research: A qualitative review. *American Journal of Health Behavior, 33*(6), 686–698.

Hertoz, J. K., Finnegan, J. R., Rooney, B., Viswanath, K., & Potter, J. (1993). Self-efficacy as a target population segmentation strategy in a diet and cancer risk reduction campaign. *Health Communication, 5*(1), 21–40.

Hezel Associates. (2007). *Marketing the health education profession: Knowledge, attitudes, and hiring practices of employers.* Retrieved March 16, 2011 from http://www.cnheo.org/

Hinkle, D. E., Oliver, J. D., & Hinkle, C. A. (1985). How large should the sample be? Part II—The one-sample case for survey research. *Educational and Psychological Measurement, 45*(2), 271–280.

Hitt, M. A., Black, J. S., & Porter, L. W. (2012). *Management* (3rd ed.). Boston: Prentice Hall.

Hopkins, K. D., Stanley, J. C., & Hopkins, B. R. (1990). *Educational and psychological measurement and evaluation* (7th ed.). Englewood Cliffs, NJ: Prentice Hall.

Horne, W. M. (1975). Effects of a physical activity program on middle-aged, sedentary corporation executives. *American Industrial Hygiene Journal,* (March), 241–245.

Hunnicutt, D. (2001). *A dynamic incentive campaign . . . Step-by-step: Walking your way to wellness.* Retrieved May 17, 2007, from http://www. welcoa .org/freeresources/pdf/stepbystep_ic.pdf

Hunnicutt, D. (2007a). The power of planning.*Absolute Advantage, 6*(7), 5–11. Retrieved March 19, 2011, from http://www .welcoa.org/freeresources/index.php? category=8

Hunnicutt, D. (2007b). The 10 secrets of a successful worksite wellness teams. *Absolute Advantage, 6*(3), 6–13. Retrieved March 30, 2007, from http://www.welcoa.org/freeresources/pdf/ 10_secrets.pdf

Hunnicutt, D. (2008a). *Guilty until proven innocent.*WELCOA's *Absolute Advantage, 7*(7), 10–19. Retrieved April 2, 2011, from http:// www.welcoa.org/freeresources/index.php? category=8

Hunnicutt, D. (2008b). *The benefits of conducting a personal health assessment.* WELCOA's *Absolute Advantage, 7*(7), 2–9.Retrieved April 2, 2011, from http://www.welcoa.org/freeresources/ index.php?category=8

Hunnicutt, D. (2009). *Creating a culture of wellness: A WELCOA quick-inventory.* Retrieved May 12, 2011, from http://www.welcoa.org/ freeresources/index.php?category=8

Hunnicutt, D., & Jahn, M. (2011). *Making the case for worksite wellness programs.* Retrieved

March 23, 2011, from http://www.welcoa.org/freeresources/index.php?category=8

Hunnicutt, D., & Leffelman, B. (2006). WELCOA's 7 benchmarks of success. *Absolute Advantage, 6*(1), 2–29. Retrieved March 19, 2011, from http://www.welcoa.org/freeresources/index.php?category=8

Hurlburt, R. T. (2003). *Comprehending behavioral statistics* (3rd ed.). Belmont, CA: Wadsworth/Thomson Learning.

Institute of Medicine (IOM). (2001). *Health and behavior: The interplay of biological, behavioral, and societal influences.* Washington, DC: National Academy Press.

Israel, B. A., Checkoway, B., Schulz, A., & Zimmerman, M. (1994). Health education and community empowerment: Conceptualizing and measuring perceptions of individual, organizational, and community control. *Health Education Quarterly, 21*(2), 149–170.

Issel, L. M. (2009). *Health program planning and evaluation: A practical, systematic approach for community health* (2nd ed.). Sudbury, MA: Jones & Bartlett.

Jacobsen, D., Eggen, P., & Kauchak, D. (1989). *Methods for teaching: A skills approach* (3rd ed.). Columbus, OH: Merrill.

Janz, N. K., & Becker, M. H. (1984). The health belief model: A decade later. *Health Education Quarterly, 11*(1), 1–47.

Janz, N. K., Champion, V. L., & Strecher, V. J. (2002). The health belief model. In K. Glanz, B. K. Rimer, & F. M. Lewis (Eds.), *Health behavior and health education: Theory, research, and practice* (3rd ed., pp. 45–66). San Francisco, CA: Jossey-Bass.

John, R., Kerby, D. S., & Landers, P. S. (2004). A market segmentation approach to nutrition education among low-income individuals. *Social Marketing Quarterly, 10*, 3–4, 24–38.

Johnson, G., Scholes, K., & Sexty, R. W. (1989). *Exploring strategic management.* Scarborough, Ontario: Prentice Hall.

Johnson, J. A., & Breckon, D. J. (2007). *Managing health education and health promotion programs: Leadership skills for the 21st century* (2nd ed.). Sudbury, MA: Jones & Bartlett.

Joint Committee on Terminology. (2001). Report of the 2000 Joint Committee on Health Education and Promotion Terminology. *American Journal of Health Education, 32*(2), 89–103.

Joint Committee on Terminology. (2012). Report of the 2011 Joint Committee on Health Education and Promotion Terminology. *American Journal of Health Education 43*(2).

Kawachi, I., Kennedy, B. P., Lochner, K., & Prothrow-Stith, D. (1997). Social capital, income, equality, and mortality. *American Journal of Public Health, 87*(9), 1491–1497.

Kegler, M. C., & Swan, D. W. (2011). An initial attempt at operationalizing and testing the community coalition action theory. *Health Education & Behavior, 38*(3), 261–270.

Kendall, R. (1984). Rewarding safety excellence. *Occupational Hazards,* (March), 45–50.

Kerlinger, F. N. (1986). *Foundations of behavioral research.* (3rd ed.). Austin, TX: Holt, Rinehart, & Winston.

Keyser, B. B., Morrow, M. J., Doyle, K., Ogletree, R., & Parsons, N. P. (1997). *Practicing the application of health education skills and competencies.* Boston, MA: Jones & Bartlett.

King, A. C., Goldberg, J. H., Salmon, J., Owen, N., Dunstan, D., Weber, D., Doyle, C., & Robinson, T. N. (2010). Indentifying subgroups of U.S. adults at risk for prolonged television viewing to inform program development. *American Journal of Preventive Medicine, 38*(1), 17–26.

King, D. E., Mainous, A. G., Carnemolla, M., & Everett, C. J. (2009). Adherence to health lifestyle habits in U.S. adults, 1988–2006. *The American Journal of Medicine, 122*, 528–534.

Kinzie, M. B. (2005). Instructional design strategies for health behavior change. *Patient Education and Counseling, 56*, 3–15.

Kirsch, I. S., Jungeblut, A., Jenkins, L., & Kolstad, A. (1993). *Adult literacy in America: A first look at the findings of the National Adult Literacy Survey* (NCES 93275). Washington, DC: U.S. Department of Education.

Kirschenbaum, J., & Russ, L. (2005). Community mapping and geographic information systems. In M. Minkler (Ed.). *Community organizing and community building for health* (2nd ed., pp. 450–454). New Brunswick, NJ: Rutgers University Press.

Kline, M. V., & Huff, R. M. (1999). Tips for the practitioner. In R. M. Huff & M. V. Kline (Eds.),

Promoting health in multicultural populations (pp. 103–111). Thousand Oaks, CA: Sage.

Klingner, D. E., Nalbandian, J., & Llorens, J. (2010). *Public personnel management: Contexts and strategies* (6th ed.). New York: Longman.

Kotecki, J. E., & Chamness, B. E. (1999). A valid tool for evaluating health-related WWW sites. *Journal of Health Education, 30*(1), 56–59.

Kotler, P., & Clarke, R. N. (1987). *Marketing for health care organizations.* Englewood Cliffs, NJ: Prentice Hall.

Kotler, P., & Keller, K. L. (2007). *A framework for marketing management.* (3rd ed.) Upper Saddle River, NJ: Pearson/Prentice Hall.

Kotler, P., & Lee, N. (2006). *Marketing in the public sector.* Upper Saddle River, NJ: Wharton School Publishing.

Kotler, P., & Lee, N. R., (2008). *Social marketing. Influencing behaviors for good* (3rd ed.). Thousand Oaks, CA: Sage.

Kotler, P., & Zaltman, G. (1971). Social marketing: An approach to planned social change. *Journal of Marketing, 35,* 3–12.

Krahn G. (2003). Changing concepts in health, wellness and disability. In Institute on Disability and Development (Ed.). *Proceedings of Changing Concepts of Health and Disability: State of the Science Conference and Policy Forum 2003.* Portland: Oregon Health and Science University.

Kramer, L., Schwartz, P., Cheadle, A., Borton, J. E., Wright, M., Chase, C., & Lindley, C. (2010). Promoting policy and environmental change using photovoice in the Kaiser Permanente community health initiative. *Health Promotion Practice, 11*(3), 332–339.

Kreps, G. L., Barnes, M. D., Neiger, B. L., & Thackeray, R. (2009). Health communication. In Robert J. Bensley & J. Brookins-Fisher (Eds.) *Community health education methods: A practical guide* (3rd ed., pp. 73–102). Sudbury, MA: Jones & Bartlett.

Kretzmann, J. P., & McKnight, J. L. (1993). Introduction from *Building communities from inside out: A path toward finding and mobilizing a community's assets.* Retrieved May 29, 2011, from http://northwestern.edu/ipr/publications/books/index.html

Kreuter, M. W., & Skinner, C. S. (2000). What's in a name? *Health Education Research, Theory, and Practice, 15*(1), 1–4.

Kreuter, M. W., Farrell, D., Olevitch, L., & Brennan, L. (1999). *Tailoring health messages: Customizing communication with computer technology.* Mahwah, NJ: Erlbaum.

Kutner, M., Greenberg, E., Jin, Y., & Paulsen, C. (2006). *The health literacy of America's adults: Results from the 2003 National Assessment of Adult Literacy* (NCES 2006–483). Washington, DC: National Center for Education Statistics, U.S. Department of Education.

Lalonde, M. (1974). *A new perspective on the health of Canadians: A working document.* Ottawa, ON: Minister of Health.

Lancaster, B., & Kreuter, M. (2002). Planned approach to community health (PATCH). In L. Breslow (Ed.). *Encyclopedia of public health.* Farmington Hills, MI: Gale Cengage. Retrieved August 13, 2011, from http://www.enotes.com/public-health-encyclopedia/planned-approach-community-health-patch

Lando, J., Williams, S. M., Sturgis, S., & Williams, B. (2006). A logic model for the integration of mental health into chronic disease prevention and health promotion. *Preventing Chronic Disease, 3*(2), 1–5. Retrieved June 9, 2011, from http://www.cdc.gov/pcd/issues/2006/apr.toc.htm

Last, J. M. (Ed.). (2007). *A Dictionary of Public Health* (4th ed.). New York, NY: Oxford University Press.

Lefebvre, R. C. (2006). Partnerships for social marketing programs: An example from the National Bone Health Campaign. *Social Marketing Quarterly, 12*(1), 41–54.

Leventhal, H., & Cleary, P. D. (1980). The smoking problem: A review of the research and theory in behavioral risk modification. *Psychological Bulletin, 88*(2), 370–405.

Levine, R. J. (1988). *Ethics and regulations of clinical research.* New Haven, CT: Yale University Press.

Lewin, K. (1935). *A dynamic theory of personality.* New York: McGraw-Hill.

Lewin, K. (1936). *Principles of topological psychology.* New York: McGraw-Hill.

Lewin, K., Dembo, T., Festinger, L., & Sears, P. S. (1944). Level of aspiration. In J. Hunt (Ed.), *Personality and the behavior disorders* (pp. 333–378). New York: Ronald Press.

Li, C., & Bernoff, J. (2008). *Groundswell: Winning in a world transformed by social technologies.* Boston: Harvard Business Press.

Lindenberger, J. H., & Bryant, C. A., (2000). Promoting breastfeeding in the WIC Program: A social marketing case study. *American Journal Health Behavior, 24*(1), 53–60.

Lindsey, L. L. M., Hamner, H. C., Prue, C. E., Flores, A. L., Valencia, D., Correra-Sierra, E., & Kopfman, J. E. (2007). Understanding optimal nutrition among women of childbearing age in the United States and Puerto Rico: Employing formative research to lay the foundation for National Birth Defects Prevention Campaigns. *Journal of Health Communication: International Perspectives, 12*(8), 733–757.

Lovelace, K. A., Bibeau, D. L., Donnell, B. M., Johnson, H. H., Glascoff, M. A., & Tyler, E. (2009). Public health educators participation in teams: Implications for preparation and practice. *Health Promotion Practice, 10*(3), 428–435.

Luquis, R. R., & Pérez, M. A. (2003). Achieving cultural competence: The challenges for health educators. *American Journal of Health Education, 34*(3), 131–138.

Luquis, R., Pérez, M., & Young, K. (2006). Cultural competence development in health education professional preparation programs. *American Journal of Health Education, 37*(4), 233–241.

Luszczynska, A., & Sutton, S. (2005). Attitudes and expectations. In J. Kerr, R. Weitkunat, & M. Moretti (Eds.), *ABC of behavior change: A guide to successful disease prevention and health promotion* (pp. 71–84). Edinburgh: Elsevier.

MacAskill, S., Stead, M., MacKintosh, A. M., & Hastings, G. (2002). "You cannae just take cigarettes away from somebody and no' gie them something back"; Can social marketing help solve the problem of low-income smoking? *Social Marketing Quarterly, 8*(1), 19–34.

Maibach, E.W., Leiserowitz, A., Roser-Renouf, C., & Mertz, C. K. (2011). Identifying like-minded audiences for global warming public engagement campaigns: An audience segmentation analysis and tool development. *PLoS ONE, 6*(3), e17571. Doi:10.1371/journal.pone.0017571

Marcarin, S. (Ed.). (1995). *Cumulative index to nursing & allied health literature: CINAHL.* Volume 40, Part A. Glendale, CA.

Marlatt, G. A. (1982). Relapse prevention: A self-control program for treatment of addictive behaviors. In R. B. Sturat (Ed.), *Adherence, compliance, and generalization in behavioral medicine* (pp. 329–377). New York: Brunner/Mazel.

Marlatt, G. A. (1985). Relapse prevention: Theoretical rationale and overview of the model. In G. A. Marlatt & J. R. Gordon (Eds.), *Relapse prevention* (pp. 3–70). New York: Guilford Press.

Marlatt, G. A., & George, W. H. (1998). Relapse prevention and the maintenance of optimal health. In S. A. Shumaker, E. B. Schron, J. K. Ockene, & W. L. McBee (Eds.), *The handbook of health behavior change* (2nd ed., pp. 33–58). New York: Springer.

Martinez-Cossio, N. (2008). Developing culturally appropriate needs assessment and planning, implementation, and evaluation for health education and health promotion programs. In M. A. Pérez & R. R. Luquis, R. (Eds.), *Cultural competence in health education and health promotion* (pp. 125–145). San Francisco: Jossey-Bass.

Mausner, J. S., & Kramer, S. (1985). *Epidemiology—An introductory text* (2nd ed.). Philadelphia, PA: W. B. Saunders.

McAlister, A. L., Perry, C. L., & Parcel, G. S. (2008). How individual, environments, and health behaviors interact: Social cognitive theory. In K. Glanz, B. K. Rimer, & K. Viswanath (Eds.), *Health behavior and health education: Theory, research, and practice* (4th ed., pp. 169–188). San Francisco: Jossey-Bass.

McCaul, K. D., Bakdash, M. B., Geoboy, M. J., Gerbert, B., et al. (1990). Promoting self-protective health behaviors in dentistry. *Annals of Behavioral Medicine, 12*, 156–160.

McClendon, B. T., & Prentice-Dunn, S. (2001). Reducing skin cancer risk: An intervention based upon protection motivation theory. *Journal of Health Psychology, 6*(3), 321–328.

McDade-Montez, E., Cvengros, J., Christensen, A. (2005). Personality and individual differences. In J. Kerr, R. Weitkunat, & M. Moretti (Eds.), *ABC of behavior change: A guide to successful disease prevention and health promotion* (pp. 57–70). Edinburgh: Elsevier.

McDermott, R. J., & Sarvela, P. D. (1999). *Health education evaluation and measurement: A practitioner's perspective* (2nd ed.). New York: WCB/McGraw-Hill.

McDonald, M., & Wilson, H. (2011). *Marketing Plans* (7th ed.). United Kingdom: Wiley.

McGinnis, J. M. (2010). Observations on incentives to improve population health. *Preventing chronic disease, 7*(5), 1–4. Retrieved May 15, 2011, from http://www.cdc.gov/pcd/issues/2010/sep/10_0078.htm.

McGinnis, J. M., Williams-Russo, P., & Knickman, J.R. (2002). The case for more active policy attention to health promotion. *Health Affairs, 21*(2), 78–93.

McKenzie, J. F. (1986). Cost-benefit and cost-effectiveness as a part of evaluation of health promotion programs. *The Eta Sigma Gamman, 18*(2), 10–16.

McKenzie, J. F. (1988). Twelve steps in developing a schoolsite health education/promotion program for faculty and staff. *The Journal of School Health, 58*(4), 149–153.

McKenzie, J. F., Wood, M. L., Kotecki, J. E., Clark, J. K., & Brey, R. A. (1999). Establishing content validity: Using qualitative and quantitative steps. *American Journal of Health Behavior, 23*(4), 311–318.

McKenzie, J. F., Luebke, J., & Romas, J. A. (1992). Incentives: A means of getting and keeping workers involved in health promotion programs. *Journal of Health Education, 23*(2), 70–73.

McKenzie, J. F., Pinger, R. R., & Kotecki, J. E. (2012). *An introduction to community health* (7th ed.). Sudbury, MA: Jones & Bartlett Learning.

McKleroy, V. S., Galbraith, J. S., Cummings, B., Jones, P., Harshbarger, C., Collins, C., Gelaude, D., Carey, J. W., & ADAPT Team. (2006). Adapting evidence-based behavioral interventions for new settings and target populations. *AIDS Education and Prevention, 19*(Suppl. A), 59–73.

McKnight, J. L., & Kretzmann, J. P. (2005). Mapping community capacity. In M. Minkler (Ed.), *Community organizing and community building for health* (pp. 158–172). New Brunswick, NJ: Rutgers University Press.

McLeroy, K. R., Bibeau, D., Steckler, A., & Glanz, K. (1988). An ecological perspective on health promotion programs. *Health Education Quarterly, 15,* 351–377.

McLeroy, K. R., Steckler, A., Goodman, R., & Burdine, J. N. (1992). Health education research, theory, and practice: Future directions. *Health Education Research, Theory, and Practice, 7*(1), 1–8.

McMath, B. F., & Prentice-Dunn, S. (2005). Protection motivation theory and skin cancer risk: The role of individual differences in responses to persuasive appeals. *Journal of Applied Social Psychology, 35,* 621–643.

Mercer, S. L., Green, L. W., Cargo, M., Potter, M. A., Daniel, M., Olds, R. S., & Reed-Gross, E. (2008). Reliability-tested guidelines for assessing participatory research projects. In M. Minkler & N. Wallerstein (Eds.). *Community-based participatory research for health: From process to outcomes* (pp. 407–418). San Francisco, CA: Jossey-Bass.

Merrill, R. M., Aldana, S. G., Pope, J. E., Anderson, D. R., Coberley, C. R., Vyhlidal, T. P., Howe, G., & Whitmer, R. W. (2011). Evaluation of a best-practice worksite wellness program in a small-employer setting using selected well-being indices. *Journal of Occupational and Environmental Medicine, 54*(4), 448–454.

Meyer, J., & Rainey, J. (1994). Writing health education material for low-literacy populations. *Journal of Health Education, 25*(6), 372–374.

Mikanowicz, C. K., & Altman, N. H. (1995). Developing policies on smoking in the workplace. *Journal of Health Education, 26*(3), 183–185.

Miller, T., & Hendrie, D. (2008). *Substance abuse prevention dollars and cents: A cost-benefit analysis,* DHHS Pub. No. (SMA) 07-4298. Rockville, MD: Center for Substance Abuse Prevention.

Mindell, J. S., Boltong, A., & Forde, I. (2008). A review of health impact assessment frameworks. *Public Health, 122,* 1177–1187.

Minelli, M. J., & Breckon, D. J. (2009). *Community health education: Settings, roles, and skills* (5th ed.). Sudbury, MA: Jones & Bartlett.

Miniño A. M., Xu J. Q., & Kochanek, K. D. (2010). Deaths: Preliminary data for 2008. *National Vital Statistics Reports, 59*(2). Hyattsville, MD: National Center for Health Statistics.

Minkler, M. (Ed.). (2005a). *Community organizing and community building for health* (2nd ed.). New Brunswick, NJ: Rutgers University Press.

Minkler, M. (Ed.). (2005b). Introduction to community organizing and community building. In M. Minkler (Ed.). *Community organizing and community building for health* (2nd ed., pp. 1–21). New Brunswick, NJ: Rutgers University Press.

Minkler, M. (Ed.). (2005c). Community organizing with the elderly poor in San Francisco's Tenderloin district. In M. Minkler (Ed.). *Community organizing and community building for health* (2nd ed., pp. 272–287). New Brunswick, NJ: Rutgers University Press.

Minkler, M., & Wallerstein, N. (2005). Improving health through community organization and community building: A health education perspective. In M. Minkler (Ed.). *Community organizing and community building for health* (2nd ed., pp. 26–50). New Brunswick, NJ: Rutgers University Press.

Minkler, M., Wallerstein, N., & Wilson, N. (2008). Improving health through community organization and community building. In K. Glanz, B. K. Rimer, & K. Viswanath (Eds.), *Health behavior and health education: Theory, research, and practice* (4th ed., pp. 287–312). San Francisco: Jossey-Bass.

Mokdad, A. H., Marks, J. S., Stroup, D. F., & Gerberding, J. L. (2004). Actual causes of death, in the United States, 2000. *Journal of the American Medical Association, 291*(10), 1238–1245.

Mokdad, A. H., Marks, J. S., Stroup, D. F., & Gerberding, J. L. (2005). Correction: Actual causes of death in the United States, 2000. *Journal of the American Medical Association, 293*(3), 293–294.

Monaghan, P. F., Bryant, C. A., Baldwin, J. A., Zhu, Y., Ibrahimou, B., Lind, J. D., Contreras, R. B., Tovar, A., Moreno, T., & McDermott, R. J. (2008). Using community-based prevention marketing to improve farm worker safety. *Social Marketing Quarterly, 14*(4), 71–87.

Mondros, J. B., & Wilson, S. M. (1994). *Organizing for power and empowerment.* New York: Columbia Press.

Montaño, D. E., & Kasprzyk, D. (2008). Theory of reasoned action, theory of planned behavior, and the integrated behavioral model. In K. Glanz, B. K. Rimer, & K. Viswanath (Eds.), *Health behavior and health education: Theory, research, and practice* (4th ed., pp. 67–96). San Francisco: Jossey-Bass.

Morris, L. L., Fitz-Gibbon, C. T., & Freeman, M. E. (1987). *How to communicate evaluation findings.* Newbury Park, CA: Sage.

Murphy, E. (2004). Diffusion of innovations: Family planning in developing countries. *Journal of Health Communication, 9*(S1), 123–129.

National Association of County and City Health Officials (NACCHO). (2001). *Mobilizing for action through planning and partnerships (MAPP).* Washington, DC: Author.

National Association of County Health Officials (NACHO). (1991). *APEX/PH, Assessment protocol for excellence in public health.* Washington, DC: Author.

National Cancer Institute (NCI). (2002 & 2004). *Making health communication programs work* (NIH Pub. No. 04-5145). Retrieved May 6, 2011, from http://www.cancer.gov/cancertopics/cancerlibrary/pinkbook

National Center for Chronic Disease Prevention and Health Promotion (NCCDPHP), Centers for Disease Prevention and Control. (2009). *The Power of Prevention: Chronic disease . . . the public health challenge of the 21st century.* Atlanta: Author.

National Center for Health Statistics (NCHS). (2011). *Health, United States, 2010: With Special Feature on Death and Dying.* Hyattsville, MD: Author.

National Center for Injury Prevention and Control (NCIPC). (2008; revised 2010). *Adding Power to Our Voices: A Framing Guide for Communicating About Injury.* Atlanta: Author. Retrieved March 28, 2011, from: http://www.cdc.gov/injury.

National Commission for Health Education Credentialing, Inc. (NCHEC). (1985). *A framework for the development of competency-based curricula for entry-level health educators.* New York, NY: Author.

National Commission for Health Education Credentialing, Inc. (NCHEC). (1996). *A competency-based framework for professional development of certified health education specialists.* New York: Author.

National Commission for Health Education Credentialing, Inc. (NCHEC). (2011). *Welcome.* Retrieved March 17, 2011, from http://www.nchec.org

National Commission for Health Education Credentialing. (NCHEC), Society for Public Health Education (SOPHE), & American Association for Health Education (AAHE). (2010). *A competency-based framework for health education specialists—2010.* Whitehall, PA: Author.

National Commission for Health Education Credentialing. (NCHEC), Society for Public Health Education (SOPHE), & American Association for Health Education (AAHE). (2006). *A competency-based framework for health educators.* Whitehall, PA: Author.

National Commission for the Protection of Human Subjects of Biomedical and Behavioral Research. (1979). *The Belmont Report: Ethical Principles and Guidelines for the Protection of Human Subject Research.* Retrieved June 9, 2007, from http://www.nihtraining.com/ohsrsite/ guidelines/ belmont.html

National Highway Traffic Safety Administration (NHTSA). (n.d.). *Traffic safety facts.* Retrieved March 28, 2011, from http://www.nhtsa.gov/ Bicycles

National Institutes for Health (NIH). (2004). *Guidelines for the conduct of research involving human subjects at the National Institutes of Health.* (5th ed.). Retrieved June 21, 2011, from http://ohsr.od.nih.gov/guidelines/GrayBooklet 82404.pdf

National Institutes for Health (NIH), Office of Human Subjects Research (2006). *Guidelines for writing informed consent documents.* Retrieved June 21, 2011, from http://ohsr .od.nih.gov/info/sheet6.html

National Library of Medicine (NLM). (2011). *Fact sheet MEDLINE®.* Retrieved April 2, 2011, from http://www.nlm.nih.gov/pubs/factsheets/ medline.html

National Task Force on the Preparation and Practice of Health Educators, Inc. (1985). *A framework for the development of competency-based curricula for entry-level health educators.* New York: Author.

Neiger, B. L., & Thackeray, R. (1998). *Social marketing: Making public health sense.* Paper presented at the annual meeting of the Utah Public Health Association, Provo, UT.

Neiger, B. L., & Thackeray, R. (2002). Application of the SMART Model in two successful social marketing campaigns. *American Journal of Health Education, 33,* 291–293.

Neiger, B. L., Thackeray, R., Barnes, M. D., & McKenzie, J. F. (2003). Positioning social marketing as a planning process for health education. *American Journal of Health Studies, 18*(2/3), 75–80.

Neiger, B. L., Thackeray, R., & Fagen, M. C. (2011). Basic priority rating model 2.0: Current applications for priority setting in health promotion practice. *Health Promotion Practice, 12*(2), 166–171.

Net.MBA (2002–2010). *CPM-critical path method.* Retrieved June 16, 2011, from http://netmba .com/operations/project/cpm/

Newcomer, K. E., & Wirtz, P. W. (2004). Using statistics in evaluation. In J. S. Wholey, H. P. Hatry, & K. E. Newcomer (Eds.), *Handbook of practical program evaluation* (2nd ed., pp. 439–478). San Francisco, CA: Jossey-Bass.

Norwood, S. L. (2000). *Research strategies for advanced practice nurses.* Upper Saddle River, NJ: Prentice Hall.

Novelli, W. D. (1988). Marketing health and social issues: What works? In R. Dunmire (Ed.), *Social marketing: Accepting the challenge in public health.* Atlanta, GA: Centers for Disease Control.

Nutbeam, D., & Harris, E. (1999). *Theory in a nutshell: A guide to health promotion theory.* Sydney, Australia: McGraw-Hill.

Nye, R. D. (1979). *What is B. F. Skinner really saying?* Englewood Cliffs, NJ: Prentice Hall.

Nye, R. D. (1992). *The legacy of B. F. Skinner: Concepts and perspectives, controversies, and misunderstandings.* Pacific Grove, CA: Brooks/ Cole.

Office of Minority Health (OMH). (2004). *National standards on culturally and linguistically appropriate services (CLAS).* Retrieved June 5, 2011, from http://www.omhrc.gov/templates/ browse.aspx?lvl=2&lvlID=15

Oliver, T. R. (2006). The politics of public health policy. *Annual Review of Public Health, 27,* 195–233.

Ornstein, A. C., & Hunkins, F. P. (1998). *Curriculum: Foundations, principals, and issues* (3rd ed.). Boston, MA: Allyn & Bacon.

Painter, J. F., Borba, C. P. C., Hynes, M., Mays, D., & Glanz, K. (2008). The use of theory in health behavior research from 2000 to 2005: A systematic review. *Annals of Behavioral Medicine, 35,* 358–362.

Parcel, G. S. (1983). Theoretical models for application in school health education research. *Health Education, 15*(4), 39–49.

Parcel, G. S. (1995). Diffusion research: The smart choices project. *Health Education Research: Theory and Practice, 10*(3), 279–281.

Parcel, G. S., & Baranowski, T. (1981). Social learning theory and health education. *Health Education, 12*(3), 14–18.

Parkinson, R. S., & Associates. (1982). *Managing health promotion in the workplace: Guidelines for implementation and evaluation.* Palo Alto, CA: Mayfield.

Pasick, R. J., D'Onofrio, C. N., & Otero-Sabogal, R. (1996). Similarities and differences across cultures: Questions to inform a third generation for health promotion research. *Health Education, 23*(Suppl.), S142–S161.

Patton, M. Q. (1988). *How to use qualitative methods in evaluation.* Newbury Park, CA: Sage.

Patton, R. P., Corry, J. M., Gettman, L. R., & Graff, J. S. (1986). *Implementing health/fitness programs.* Champaign, IL: Human Kinetics.

Pavlov, I. (1927). *Conditional reflexes.* Oxford: Oxford University Press.

Pealer, L. N., & Dorman, S. M. (1997). Evaluating health-related web sites. *Journal of School Health, 67*(1), 232–235.

Pellmar, T. C., Brandt, Jr., E. N., & Baird, M. (2002). Health and behavior: The interplay of biological, behavioral, and social influences: Summary of an Institute of Medicine Report. *American Journal of Health Promotion, 16*(4), 206–219.

Pérez, M. A., & Luquis, R. R. (Eds.). (2008). *Cultural competence in health education and health promotion.* San Francisco: Jossey-Bass.

Perlman, J. (1978). Grassroots participation from neighborhood to nation. In S. Langton (Ed.), *Citizen participation in America* (pp. 65–79). Lexington, MA: Lexington Books.

Pescatello, L. S., Murphy, D., Vollono, J., Lynch, E., Bernene, J., & Costanzo, D. (2001). The cardiovascular health impact of an incentive worksite health promotion program. *American Journal of Health Promotion, 16*(1), 16–20.

Petersen, D. J., & Alexander, G. R. (2001). *Needs assessment in public health: A practical guide for students and professionals.* New York, NY: Kluwer Academic/Plenum.

Petty, R. E., Barden, J., & Wheeler, S. C. (2009). The elaboration likelihood model of persuasion: Developing health promotions for sustained behavioral change. In R. J. DiClemente, R. A. Crosby, & M. C. Kegler (Eds.), *Emerging theories in health promotion practice and research* (2nd ed., pp. 185–214). San Francisco: Jossey-Bass.

Petty, R. E., Wheeler, S. C., & Bizer, G. Y. (1999). Is there one persuasion process or more? Lumping versus splitting in attitude change theories. *Psychology Inquiry, 10,* 156–163.

Pickett, G. E., & Hanlon, J. J. (1990). *Public health: Administration and practice* (9th ed.). St. Louis, MO: Mosby-Year Book.

Poland, B., Krupa, G., & McCall, D. (2009). Settings for health promotion: An analytic framework to guide intervention design and implementation. *Health Promotion Practice, 10*(4), 505–516.

Poole, K., Kumpfer, K., & Pett, M. (2001). The impact of an incentive-based worksite health promotion program on modifiable health risk factors. *American Journal of Health Promotion, 16*(1), 21–26.

Prentice-Dunn, S., McMath, B. F., & Cramer, R. J. (2009). Protection motivation theory and stages of change in sun protective behavior. *Journal of Health Psychology, 14,* 297–305.

Prentice-Dunn, S., & Rogers, R. W. (1986). Protection motivation theory and preventive health: Beyond the health belief model. *Health Education Research: Theory and Practice, 1*(3), 153–161.

Prochaska, J. O. (1979). *Systems of psychotherapy: A transtheoretical analysis.* Homewood, IL: Dorsey Press.

Prochaska, J. O., DiClemente, C. C., & Norcross, J. C. (1992). In search of how people change: Applications to addictive behaviors. *American Psychologist, 47*(9), 1102–1114.

Prochaska, J. O., Johnson, S., & Lee, P. (1998). The transtheoretical model of behavior change. In S. A. Shumaker, E. B. Schron, J. K. Ockene, & W. L. McBee (Eds.), *The handbook of health behavior change* (2nd ed., pp. 59–84). New York: Springer.

Prochaska, J. O., Norcross, J. C., Fowler, J. L., Follick, M. J., & Abrams, D. B. (1992). Attendance and outcome in a worksite weight control program: Processes and stages of change as process and predictor variables. *Addictive Behaviors, 17,* 35–45.

Prochaska, J. O, Redding, C. A., & Evers, K. E. (2008). The transtheoretical model and stages of change. In K. Glanz, B. K. Rimer, & K. Viswanath (Eds.), *Health behavior and health* education: Theory, research, and practice (4th ed., pp. 97–121). San Francisco: Jossey-Bass.

Prochaska, J. O., Redding, C. A., Harlow, L. L., Rossi, J. S., & Velicer, W. F. (1994). The transtheoretical model of change and HIV prevention: A review. *Health Education Quarterly, 21*(4), 471–486.

Putman, R. D. (1995). Bowling alone: America's declining social capital. *Journal of Democracy, 6*(1), 65–78.

Ramaprasad, J. (2005). Warning signals, wind speeds and what next: A pilot project for disaster preparedness among residents of central Vietnam's lagoons. *Social Marketing Quarterly, 11*(2), 41–53.

Redding, C. A., Rossi, J. S., Rossi, S. R., Velicer, W. F., & Prochaska, J. O. (1999). Health behavior models. In G. C. Hyner, K. W. Peterson, J. W. Travis, J. E. Dewey, J. J. Foerster, & E. M. Framer (Eds.), *SPM handbook of health assessment tools* (pp. 83–93). Pittsburgh, PA: Society of Prospective Medicine.

Reeves, M. J., & Rafferty, A. P. (2005). Healthy lifestyle characteristics among adults in the United States, 2000. *Archives of Internal Medicine, 165*, 854–857.

Rich, R. F., & Sugrue, N. M. (1989). Health promotion, disease prevention, and public policy. *Wellness Perspectives: Research, Theory and Practice, 6*(1), 27–35.

Riegelman, R. (2010). *Public health 101: Healthy people–health populations.* Sudbury, MA: Jones & Bartlett.

Rimer, B. K., & Glanz, K. (2005). *Theory at a glance: A guide for health promotion practice* (2nd ed.). (NIH Pub. No. 05–3896). Washington, DC: National Cancer Institute.

Riner, M. E., Cunningham, C., & Johnson, A. (2004). Public health education and practice using geographic information system technology. *Public Health Nursing, 21*(1), 57–65.

Robbins, L. C., & Hall, J. H. (1970). *How to practice prospective medicine.* Indianapolis, IN: Methodist Hospital of Indiana.

Robison, J. (1998). To reward? . . . or not to reward?: Questioning the wisdom of using external reinforcement on health promotion programs. *American Journal of Health Promotion, 13*(1), 1–3.

Rogers, E. M. (1962). *Diffusion of innovations.* New York: Free Press of Glencoe.

Rogers, E. M. (1983). *Diffusion of innovations* (3rd ed.). New York: Free Press.

Rogers, E. M. (2002). Diffusion of prevention innovations. *Addictive Behaviors, 6*, 989–993.

Rogers, E. M. (2003). *Diffusion of innovations* (5th ed.). New York, NY: Free Press.

Rogers, R. W. (1975). A protection motivation theory of fear appeals and attitude change. *Journal of Psychology, 91*, 93–114.

Rogers, R. W. (1983). Cognitive and physiological processes in fear-based attitude change: A revised theory of protection motivation. In J. Cacioppo & R. Petty (Eds.), *Social psychophysiology: A sourcebook* (pp. 153–176). New York: Guilford.

Rogers, R. W. (1984). Changing health-related attitudes and behaviors: The role of preventative health psychology. In J. H. Harvey, J. E. Maddux, R. P. McGlynn, & C. D. Stoltenberg (Eds.), *Social perception in clinical and counseling psychology* (vol. 2, pp. 91–112). Lubbock: Texas Tech University Press.

Rogers, R. W., & Prentice-Dunn, S. (1997). Protection motivation theory. In D. Gochman (Ed.), *Handbook of health behavior research. Vol. 1: Determinants of health behavior: Personal and social* (pp.113–132). New York: Plenum.

Romer, D., & Kim, S. (1995). Health interventions for African American and Latino youth: The potential role of mass media. *Health Education Quarterly, 22*(2), 172–189.

Rosenstock, I. M. (1966). Why people use health services. *Milbank Memorial Fund Quarterly, 44*, 94–124.

Rosenstock, I. M., Strecher, V. J., & Becker, M. H. (1988). Social learning theory and the health belief model. *Health Education Quarterly, 15*(2), 175–183.

Ross, H. S., & Mico, P. R. (1980). *Theory and practice in health education.* Palo Alto, CA: Mayfield.

Ross, M. G. (1967). *Community organization: Theory, principles, and practice.* New York: Harper & Row.

Rothman, A. J. (2009). Capitalizing on opportunities to refine health behavior theories. *Health Education & Behavior, 36*(Suppl. 1), 150S–155S.

Rothman, J. (2001). Approaches to community intervention. In J. Rothman, J. L. Erlich, & J. E.

Tropman, (Eds.), *Strategies of Community Intervention* (6th ed., pp. 27–64). Itasca, IL: Peacock.

Rothman, J., & Tropman, J. E. (1987). Models of community organization and macro practice perspectives: Their mixing and phasing. In F. M. Cox, J. L. Erlich, J. Rothman, & J. E. Tropman (Eds.), *Strategies of community organization: Macro practice* (pp. 3–26). Itasca, IL: Peacock.

Rothschild, M. L. (1999). Carrots, sticks, and promises: A conceptual framework for the management of public health and social issue behaviors. *Journal of Marketing, 63*, 24–37.

Rothschild, M. L., Mastin, B., & Miller, T. W. (2006). Reducing alcohol-impaired driving crashes through the use of social marketing. *Accident Analysis and Prevention, 38*(6), 1218–1230.

Rotter, J. B. (1954). *Social learning and clinical psychology.* New York: Prentice Hall.

Ruof, J., Mittendorf, T., Pirk, O., & von der Schulenberg, J. M. (2002). Diffusion of innovations: Treatment of Alzheimer's disease in Germany. *Health Policy, 1*, 59–66.

Ryan, M., Chapman, L. S., & Rink, M. J. (2008). Planning worksite health promotion programs: Models, methods, and design implications. *The Art of Health Promotion, 22*(16), 1–12.

Sallis, J. F., Owen, N., & Fisher, E. B. (2008). Ecological models of health behavior. In K. Glanz, B. K. Rimer, & K. Viswanath (Eds.), *Health behavior and health education: Theory, research, and practice* (4th ed., pp. 465–485). San Francisco: Jossey-Bass.

Saunders, R. P., Evans, M. H., & Joshi, P. (2005). Developing a process-evaluation plan for assessing health promotion program implementation: A how-to guide. *Health Promotion Practice, 6*(2), 134–147.

Schechter, C., Vanchieri, C., & Crofton, C. (1990). Evaluating women's attitudes and perceptions in developing mammography promotion messages. *Public Health Reports, 105*(3), 253–257.

Selig, S., Tropiano, E., & Greene-Moton, E. (2006). Teaching cultural competence to reduce health disparities. *Health Promotion Practice, 7*(3), 247S–255S.

Shea, S., & Basch, C. E. (1990). A review of five major community-based cardiovascular disease prevention programs: Part I, rationale, design

and theoretical framework. *American Journal of Health Promotion, 4*(3), 203–213.

Sherrill, W. W., Crew, L., Mayo, R. M., Mayo, W. F., Rogers, B. L., & Haynes, D. F. (2005). Educational and health services innovation to improve care for rural Hispanic communities in the U.S. *Education for Health, 18*(3), 356–367.

Simkin, L. R., & Gross, A. M. (1994). Assessment of coping with high-risk situations for exercise relapse among healthy women. *Health Psychology, 13*, 274–277.

Simons-Morton, B., McLeroy, K. R., & Wendel, M. L. (2012). *Behavior theory in health promotion practice and research.* Burlington, MA: Jones & Bartlett Learning.

Skinner, B. F. (1953). *Science and human behavior.* New York: Free Press.

Slater, M. D., Kelly, K. J., & Thackeray, R. (2006). Segmentation on a shoestring: Health audience segmentation in limited-budget and local social marketing interventions. *Health Promotion Practice, 7*, 170–173.

Sleet, D. A., & Cole, S. L. (2010). Leadership for change and sustainability. In C. I. Fertman & D. Allenworth (Eds.), *Health promotion programs: From theory to practice* (pp. 291–310). San Francisco: Jossey-Bass.

Snow, L. (2001). *The organization of hope: A workbook for rural asset-based community development.* Evanston, IL: Institute for Policy Research, Northwestern University.

Soet, J. E., & Basch, C. E. (1997). The telephone as a communication medium for health education. *Health Education & Behavior, 24*(6), 759–772.

Solomon, D. D. (1987). Evaluating community programs. In F. M. Cox, J. L. Erlich, J. Rolhman, & J. E. Tropman (Eds.), *Strategies of community organization: Macro practices* (pp. 366–368). Itasca, IL: Peacock.

Sorensen, G., Rigotti, N., Rosen, A., Pinney, J., & Prible, R. (1991). Effects of a worksite nonsmoking policy: Evidence for increased cessation. *American Journal of Public Health, 81*(2), 202–204.

Spencer, L., Adams, T. B., Malone, S., Roy, L., & Yost, E. (2006). Applying the transtheoretical model to exercise: A systematic and comprehensive review of the literature. *Health Promotion Practice, 7*(4), 428–443.

SPM Board of Directors (SPMBoD). (1999). Ethics guidelines for the development and use of health assessments. In G. C. Hyner, K. W. Peterson, J. W. Travis, J. E. Dewey, J.J. Foerster, & E. M. Framer (Eds.), *SPM handbook of health assessment tools* (p. xxiii). Pittsburgh, PA: Society of Prospective Medicine.

Stacy, R. D. (1987). Instrument evaluation guides for survey research in health education and health promotion. *Health Education, 18*(5), 65–67.

State Health Access Data Assistance Center (SHADAC). (2009). *The impact of wireless-only households on state surveys of health insurance coverage* (Issue Brief #15). Minneapolis: University of Minnesota. Retrieved March 30, 2011, from http://www.rwjf.org/pr/product.jsp?id= 40008

Staten, L. K., Birnbaum, A. S., Jobe, J. B., & Elder, J. P. (2006). A typology of middle school girls: Audience segmentation related to physical activity. *Health Education Behavior, 33*(1), 66–80.

Steckler, A., Goodman, R. M., McLeroy, K. R., Davis, S., & Koch, G. (1992). Measuring the diffusion of innovative health promotion programs. *American Journal of Health Promotion, 6*(3), 214–224.

Steckler, A., & Linnan, L. (Eds.). (2002). *Process evaluation for public health interventions and research*. San Francisco, CA: Jossey-Bass.

Steckler, A., McLeroy, K. R., Goodman, R. M., Bird, S. T., & McCormick, L. (1992). Toward integrating qualitative and quantitative methods: An introduction. *Health Education Quarterly, 19*(1), 1–8.

Strecher, V. J., DeVellis, B. M., Becker, M. H., & Rosenstock, I. M. (1986). The role of self-efficacy in achieving health behavior change. *Health Education Quarterly, 13*(1), 73–91.

Strecher, V. J., & Rosenstock, I. M. (1997). The health belief model. In K. Glanz, F. M. Lewis, & B. K. Rimer (Eds.), *Health behavior and health education: Theory, research, and practice* (pp. 41–59). San Francisco: Jossey-Bass.

Stevens, S. S. (1946). On the theory of scales of measurement. *Science, 103*, 677–680.

Stewart-Brown, S. (2006). *What is the evidence on school health promotion in improving health or preventing disease and, specifically, what is the effectiveness of the health promoting schools approach?* Copenhagen: WHO Regional Office for Europe. Retrieved March 26, 2011, from http://www.euro.who.int/docu ment/e88185.pdf

Strycker, L. A., Foster, L. S., Pettigrew, L., Donnelly-Perry, J., Jordan, S., & Glasgow, R. E. (1997). Steering committee enhancements on health promotion program delivery. *American Journal of Health Promotion, 11*(6), 437–440.

Stunkard, A. J., & Braunwell, K. D. (1980). Worksite treatment for obesity. *American Journal of Psychiatry, 137*, 252–253.

Suggs, L. S., & McIntyre, C. (2009). Are we there yet? An examination of online tailored health communication. *Health Education & Behavior, 36*(2), 278–288.

Sullivan, L.M. (2008). *Essentials of biostatistics in public health*. Sudbury, MA: Jones & Bartlett.

Svenkerud, P. J., & Singhal, A. (1998). Enhancing the effectiveness of HIV/AIDS prevention programs targeted to unique population groups in Thailand: Lessons learned from applying concepts of diffusion of innovation and social marketing. *Journal of Health Communication, 3*, 193–216.

Taylor, L., & Quigley, R. (2002). *Health impact assessment: A review of reviews*. London: NHS, Health Development Agency. Retrieved April 15, 2011, from http://www.who.int/hia/en/

Taylor, S. M., Elliott, S., & Riley, B. (1998). Heart health promotion: Predisposition, capacity and implementation in Ontario public health units, 1994–1996. *Canadian Journal of Public Health, 6*, 410–414.

TechTarget. (2007a). *Gantt chart*. Retrieved June 16, 2011, from http://searchsoftwarequality. techtarget.com/definition/Gantt-chart

TechTarget. (2007b). *PERT-chart*. Retrieved June 16, 2011, from http://searchsoftwarequality. techtarget.com/definition/Pertchart

Tervalon, M., & Garcia, J. (1998). Cultural humility versus cultural competence: A critical distinction in defining physician training outcomes in multicultural education. *Journal of Health Care for the Poor and Underserved, 9*(2), 117–125.

Thackeray, R., & Bennion, S. R. (2009). *Social media matters: Expanding your reach and effectiveness in social marketing*. Paper presented at the Social Marketing and Public Health Conference, Tampa, FL.

Thackeray, R., Fulkerson, K. N., & Neiger, B. L. (2012). Defining the product in social marketing: An analysis of published research from 1999–2009. *A Journal of Non-Profit and Public Sector Marketing, 23*(2).

Thackeray, R., & Hunter, M. (2010). Empowering youth: Use of technology in advocacy to affect social change. *Journal of Computer-Medicated Communication, 15,* 575–591.

Thackeray, R., & McCormack Brown, K. (2005). Social marketing's unique contribution to health promotion practice. *Health Promotion Practice, 6*(4), 365–368.

Thackeray, R., & Neiger, B. L. (2009). A multi-directional communication model: Implications for social marketing practice. *Health Promotion Practice, 10,* 2, 171–175.

Thackeray, R., Neiger, B. L., Hanson, C. L., & McKenzie, J. F. (2008). Enhancing promotional strategies within social marketing programs: Use of Web 2.0 social media. *Health Promotion Practice, 9*(4), 338–343.

Thorndike, E. L. (1898). Animal intelligence: An experimental study of the associative processes in animals. *Psychological Monographs, 2*(8).

Timmreck, T. C. (1997). *Health services cyclopedic dictionary* (3rd ed.). Boston, MA: Jones & Bartlett.

Timmreck, T. C. (2003). *Planning, program development, and evaluation* (2nd ed.). Boston, MA: Jones & Bartlett.

Torabi, M. R. (1994). Reliability methods and numbers of items in development of health instruments. *Health Values, 18*(6), 56–59.

Trickett, E. J. (2011). Community-based participatory research as worldview or instrumental strategy: Is it lost in translational research? *American Journal of Public Health, 101*(8), 1353–1355.

Trust for America's Health (TFAH). (2009). *Prevention for a Healthier America: Investments in Disease Prevention Yield Significant Savings, Stronger Communities.* Retrieved March 22, 2011, from http://healthyamericans.org/reports/prevention08/

Tuckman, B. W. (1965). Developmental sequence in small groups. *Psychological Bulletin, 63,* 384–399.

Tuckman, B. W. (2001). Developmental sequence in small groups: Reprint. *Group Facilitation: A Research and Applications Journal, 3* (Spring).

Retrieved June 4, 2011 from http://dennislearningcenter.osu.edu/references/GROUP%20DEV%20ARTICLE.doc.

Tuckman, B. W., & Jensen, M. A. C. (1977). Stages of small group development revisited. *Group and Organizational Studies, 2,* 419–427.

Turnock, B. J. (2009). *Public health: What it is and how it works* (4th ed.). Sudbury, MA: Jones & Bartlett.

U.K. Office of National Statistics, Social Analysis and Reporting Division. (2001). *Social capital: A review of the literature.* Retrieved April 30, 2011 from www.statistics.gov.uk

United Nations. (1955). *Social progress through community development.* New York: Author.

U.S. Census Bureau (USCB). (2010). *Men and women wait longer to marry.* Retrieved May 29, 2011, from http://www.census.gov/newsroom/releases/archives/families_households/cb10-174.html

U.S. Department of Education (USDE), National Center for Education Statistics (NCES). (n.d.). *National assessment of adult literacy.* Retrieved May 7, 2011, from http://nces.ed.gov/naal/

U.S. Department of Health and Human Services. (1980). *Promoting health/preventing disease: Objectives for the nation.* Washington, DC: U.S. Government Printing Office.

U.S. Department of Health and Human Services. (1986b). *The 1990 health objectives for the nation: A midcourse review.* Washington, DC: U.S. Government Printing Office.

U.S. Department of Health and Human Services. (1990a). *Healthy People 2000: National health promotion disease prevention objectives* (DHHS Publication No. [PHS] 90–50212). Washington, DC: U.S. Government Printing Office.

U.S. Department of Health and Human Services (USDHHS). (2000). *Healthy People 2010* (CD-ROM Version). Washington, DC: Author.

U.S. Department of Health and Human Services (USDHHS). (2001). *Youth violence: A report of the Surgeon General.* Washington, DC: Author. Retrieved June 21, 2011, from http://www.surgeongeneral.gov/library/youthviolence/youvioreport.html

U.S. Department of Health and Human Services. (2003). *Prevention makes common "cents."* Retrieved March 24, 2007, from http://aspe.hhs.gov/health/prevention/

U.S. Department of Health and Human Services (USDHHS). (2005). *The surgeon general's call to action to improve the heath and wellness of persons with disabilities.* Washington, DC: Author. Retrieved June 22, 2011, from http://www.surgeongeneral.gov/library/disabilities/calltoaction/index.html

U.S. Department of Health and Human Services. (2007). *HP 2010 midcourse review: Appendix C: Technical appendix.* Retrieved April 21, 2007, from http://www.healthypeople.gov/data/midcourse/default.html

U.S. Department of Health and Human Services (USDHHS). (2010a). *Healthy People 2020.* Retrieved March 16, 2011, from http://www.healthypeople.gov/2020/default.aspx

U.S. Department of Health and Human Services (USDHHS). (2010b). *Immunization and infectious diseases.* Retrieved March 26, 2011, from http://healthypeople.gov/2020/topicsobjectives2020/overview.aspx?topicid=23

U.S. Department of Health and Human Services (USDHHS). (2010c). *National action plan to improve health literacy.* Retrieved May 8, 2011, from http://www.cdc.gov/healthliteracy/introduction.html

U.S. Department of Health and Human Services (USDHHS). (2011a). *Glossary.* Retrieved June 5, 2011, from http://www.grants.gov/help/glossary.jsp#g

U.S. Department of Health and Human Services (USDHHS). (2011b). *Health communication, health literacy, and e-health.* Retrieved May 6, 2011, from http://www.health.gov/communication/Default.asp

U.S. Department of Health and Human Services (USDHHS). (2011c). *MAP-IT: A guide to using Healthy People 2020 in your community.* Retrieved August 13, 2011, from http://www.healthypeople.gov/2020/implementing/default.aspx

U.S. Department of Health and Human Services (USDHHS), Centers for Disease Control and Prevention. (no date). *Planned approach to community health: Guide for local coordinator.* Atlanta: Author.

U.S. Department of Health and Human Services (USDHHS), Office of Civil Rights (OCR). (n.d.). *Health information privacy.* Retrieved April 2, 2011, from http://www.hhs.gov/ocr/privacy

U.S. Department of Health and Human Services, Office of Substance Abuse Prevention (OSAP). (1991). *The fact is . . . you can prepare easy-to-read materials.* Rockville, MD: Author.

U.S. Department of Health, Education, and Welfare (USDHEW), Public Health Service. (1979). *Healthy people: The surgeon general's report on health promotion and disease prevention* (Publication No. 79-55071). Washington, DC: Author.

U.S. Department of Labor (USDL), Bureau of Labor Statistics (BLS). (2010). *21-1091 health educators.* Retrieved March 17, 2011, from http://www.bls.gov/soc/2010/soc211091.htm

U.S. Department of Labor (USDL). (2011). *Employment characteristics of families, summary.* Retrieved May 29, 2011, from http://www.bls.gov/news.release/famee.nr0.htm

U.S. Department of Labor (USDL). (n.d.). *Summary of the major laws of the Department of Labor.* Retrieved June 21, 2011, from http://www.dol.gov/opa/aboutdol/lawsprog.htm

U.S. Department of Transportation (USDT), National Highway Traffic Safety Administration (NHTSA). (2011). *Countermeasures that work: A highway safety countermeasures guide for state highway safety offices* (6th ed.) (DOT HS 811 444). Washington, DC: Author. Retrieved May 10, 2011, from http://www.nhtsa.gov

U.S. Department of Transportation (USDT), National Highway Traffic Safety Administration (NHTSA). (2010). Seat belt use in 2010—Overall results. *Traffic safety facts.* Washington, DC: Author. Retrieved May 10, 2011, from http://www.nhtsa.gov

U.S. Government Printing Office (USGPO). (2011). *Federal Register: About.* Retrieved June 6, 2011, from http://www.gpoaccess.gov/fr/

University of Kansas. (2011a). *Developing a logic model or theory of change.* Retrieved June 14, 2011, from http://ctb.ku.edu/en/tablecontents/sub_examples_1877.aspx

University of Kansas. (2011b). *Writing a grant.* Retrieved July 31, 2011, from http://ctb.ku.edu/en/tablecontents/sub_main_1301.aspx

University of Nevada, Reno, Cooperative Extension (UNCE). (2003). *Community leaders guide.* Retrieved June 4, 2011, from http://www.unce.unr.edu/publications/files/cd/2001/eb0103.pdf

Utah Department of Health (2011). *The truth campaign: Marketing resources. Tobacco Prevention and Control Program.* Retrieved July 12, 2011, from: http://www.tobaccofreeutah.org/truthmediaresources-feb2004.html

Valente, T. W. (2002). *Evaluating health promotion programs.* New York: Oxford University Press.

van Dam, R. M., Li, T., Spiegelman, D., Franco, O. H., & Hu, F. B. (2008). Combined impact of lifestyle factors on mortality: Prospective cohort study of U.S. women. *British Medical Journal, 337,* a1440.

Van Der Wagen, L., & Carlos, B. R. (2005). *Event management: For tourism, cultural, business, and sporting events.* Upper Saddle River, NJ: Pearson Prentice Hall.

Vogele, C. (2005). Education. In J. Kerr, R. Weikunat, & M. Moretti (Eds.), *ABC of behavior change: A guide to successful disease prevention and health promotion* (pp. 271–287). Edinburgh: Elsevier Churchill Livingstone.

Wagner, E. H., & Guild, P. A. (1989). Choosing an evaluation strategy. *American Journal of Health Promotion, 4*(2), 134–139.

Wallerstein, N. (1987). Empowerment education: Freire's ideas applied to youth. *Youth Policy, 9,* 11–15.

Wallston, K. A. (1992). Hocus-pocus, the focus isn't strictly on locus: Rotter's social learning theory modified for health. *Cognitive Therapy and Research, 16,* 183–199.

Wallston, K. A. (1994). Theoretically based strategies for health behavior change. In M. P. O'Donnell & J. S. Harris (Eds.), *Health promotion in the workplace* (2nd ed., pp. 185–203). Albany, NY: Delmar.

Wallston, K. A., Wallston, B. S., & DeVellis, R. (1978). Development of the multidimensional health locus of control (MHLC) scales. *Health Education Monographs, 6,* 160–170.

Walsh, D. C., Rudd, R. E., Moeykens, B. A., & Moloney, T. W. (1993). Social marketing for public health. *Health Affairs, 12,* 104–119.

Walter, C. (2005). Community building practice. In M. Minkler (Ed.), *Community organizing and community building for health* (2nd ed., pp. 66–78). New Brunswick, NJ: Rutgers University Press.

Wandersman, A., Goodman, R. M., & Butterfoss, F. D. (2005). Understanding coalitions and how they operate as organizations. In M. Minkler (Ed.), *Community organizing and community building for health* (2nd ed., pp. 292–313). New Brunswick, NJ: Rutgers University Press.

Wang, C. C., & Burris, M. A. (1994). Empowerment through photovoice: Portraits of participation. *Health Education Quarterly, 21*(2), 171–186.

Wang, C. C., & Burris, M. A. (1997). Photovoice: Concept, methodology, and use for participatory needs assessment. *Health Education and Behavior, 24*(3), 369–387.

Wang, C. C., Morrel-Samuels, S., Hutchinson, P. M., Bell, L., & Pestronk, R. M. (2004). Flint photovoice: Community building among youths, adults, and policymakers. *American Journal of Public Health, 94*(6), 911–913.

Wang, C. C., Yi, W. K., Tao, Z. W., & Carovano, K. (1998). Photovoice as a participatory health promotion strategy. *Health Promotion International, 13*(1), 75–87.

Warren, M. R. (1963). *The community in America.* Chicago, IL: Rand McNally.

Warren, M. R., Thompson, J. P., & Saegert, S. (2001). The role of social capital in combating poverty. In S. Saegert, J. P. Thompson, & M. R. Warren (Eds.), *Social capital and poor communities* (pp. 1–28). New York: Sage Foundation.

Washtenaw County Public Health (WCPH). (2009). *Youth photovoice: Implementation toolkit.* Ann Arbor, MI: Author

Watson, J. B. (1925). *Behaviorism.* New York: Norton.

Wayman, J., Beal, T., Thackeray, R., & McCormack Brown, K. (2007). Competition. Friend or foe? *Health Promotion Practice, 8*(2), 134–139.

Weinreich, N. K. (1999). *Hands-on social marketing: A step-by-step guide.* Thousand Oaks, CA: Sage.

Weinstein, N. D. (1988). The precaution adoption process. *Health Psychology, 7,* 355–386.

Weinstein, N. D., & Rothman, A. J., & Sutton, S. R. (1998). Stage theories of health behavior: Conceptual and methodological issues. *Health Psychology, 17,* 290–299.

Weinstein, N. D., & Sandman, P. M. (1992). A model of the precaution adoption process: Evidence from home radon testing. *Health Psychology, 11,* 170–180.

Weinstein, N. D., & Sandman, P. M. (2002a). The precaution adoption process model. In K. Glanz, B. K. Rimer, & F. M. Lewis (Eds.), *Health behavior and health education: Theory, research, and practice* (3rd ed., pp. 121–143). San Francisco, CA: Jossey-Bass.

Weinstein, N. D., & Sandman, P. M. (2002b). The precaution adoption process model and its application. In R. J. DiClemente, R. A. Crosby, & M. C. Kegler (Eds.), *Emerging theories in health promotion practice and research: Strategies for improving public health* (pp. 16–39). San Francisco, CA: Jossey-Bass.

Weinstein, N. D., Sandman, P. M., & Blalock, S. J. (2008). The precaution adoption process model. In K. Glanz, B. K. Rimer, & K. Viswanath (Eds.), *Health behavior and health education: Theory, research, and practice* (4th ed., pp. 123–147). San Francisco: Jossey-Bass.

Weiss, C. H. (1984). Increasing the likelihood of influencing decisions. In L. Rutman (Ed.), *Evaluation research methods: A basic guide* (2nd ed., pp. 159–190). Beverly Hills, CA: Sage.

White, S., & Dillow, S. (2005). *Key concepts and features of the 2003 National Assessment of Adult Literacy* (NCES 2006-471). Washington, DC: National Center for Education Statistics, U.S. Department of Education.

Wilbur, C. (1983). Live for life—The Johnson & Johnson program. *Preventive Medicine, 12*(5), 672–681.

Williams, J. E., & Flora, J. A. (1995). Health behavior segmentation and campaign planning to reduce cardiovascular disease risk among Hispanics. *Health Education Quarterly, 22*(1), 36–38.

Wilson, M. G. (1990). Factors associated with, issues related to, and suggestions for increasing participation in workplace health promotion programs. *Health Values, 14*(4), 29–36.

Windsor, R., Clark, N., Boyd, N., & Goodman, R. M. (2004). *Evaluation of health promotion, health education, and disease prevention programs* (3rd ed.). Boston, MA: McGraw-Hill.

W. K. Kellogg Foundation (WKKF). (2004). *Logic model development guide.* Battle Creek, MI: Author.

W. K. Kellogg Foundation (WKKF). (2008). *Using logic models to bring together planning, evaluation, and action: Logic model development guide.* Battle Creek, MI: Author. Retrieved March 26, 2011, from http://www.wkkf.org/knowledge-center/publications-and-resources.aspx

World Health Organization (WHO). (2009). *Milestones in health promotion: Statements from global conferences.* Retrieved May 12, 2011, from http://www.who.int/entity/healthpromotion/Milestones_Health_Promotion_05022010.pdf

World Health Organization (WHO). (2011). *Health impact assessment: Why use HIA?* Retrieved April 15, 2011, from http://www.who.int/hia/about/why/en/index.html

Wright, P. A. (Ed.). (1994). *Technical assistance bulletin: A key step in developing prevention materials is to obtain expert and gatekeepers' reviews.* Bethesda, MD: Center for Substance Abuse Prevention (CSAP) Communications Team.

Wurzbach, M. E. (Ed.). (2002). *Community health education and promotion: A guide to program design and evaluation* (2nd ed.). Gaithersburg, MD: Aspen.

Yamane, T. (1973). *Statistics: An introductory analysis* (3rd ed.). New York, NY: Harper & Row.

Zara, S., Briss, P. A., & Harris, K. W. (Eds.). (2005). *Guide to community preventive services: What works to promote health.* New York, NY: Oxford University Press.

Name Index

Subject Index

Text Credits

Chapter 2 **p. 20** "Securing Support from Top Management" by Larry S. Chapman, from *Art of Health Promotion.* Copyright © 1997 by the American Journal of Health Promotion. Reproduced with permission.

Chapter 4 **pp. 99–102** "Basic priority rating model 2.0: Current applications for priority setting in health promotion practice" by Brad L. Neiger, R. Thackeray, and M. C. Fagen from *Health Promotion Practice,* vol. 12, no. 2. Copyright © 2011 by Sage Publications. Reprinted with permission; **pp. 106–107** *Health Impact Assessment: Why Use HIA?* from WHO website, 2011. http://www.who.int/hia/about/why/en/index.html. Copyright © 2011 by World Health Organization. Reprinted with permission.

Chapter 5 **pp. 124–125** *Health Promotion and Education Research Methods: Using the Five-Chapter Thesis/Dissertation Model,* by R. R. Cottrell and J. F. McKenzie. Copyright © 2011 by Jones & Bartlett Learning. Reprinted with permission.

Chapter 7 **p. 163** "Capitalizing on Opportunities to Refine Health Behavior Theories" by Alexander J. Rothman, from *Health Education & Behavior.* Copyright © 2009 by Society for Public Health Education. Reprinted with Permission; **pp. 173, 175–177** "Protection Motivation Theory and Preventive Health: Beyond the Health Belief Model" by Steven Prentice-Dunn and Ronald W. Rogers, from *Health Education Research: Theory And Practice,* 1986, Volume 1(3). Copyright © 1986 by Oxford University Press. Reprinted with permission.

Chapter 8 **p. 220** "Integrating Adult Learning Principles into Training for Public Health Practice" by Rebecca L. Bryan, Matthew W. Kreuter, Ross C. Brownson, from *Health Promotion Practice* 10(4). Copyright © 2009 by Society for Public Health Education. Reprinted with Permission; **pp. 229–232** "Practical Tips for Influencing Public Policy" by E. M. Auld, from *Health Education & Behavior.* Copyright © 1997 by Sage Publications. Reprinted with permission.

Chapter 10 **p. 299** *Collins English Dictionary 10th Edition* © William Collins Sons & Co. Ltd 1979, 1986 © HarperCollins Publishers 1991, 1994 (Third updated edition), 1998, 2000, 2003, 2005, 2006, 2007, 2009.